HEALTH

4

Life

USER MANUAL

Dr. Mike Van Thielen
PhD. Holistic Nutrition

Awesome cartoons, illustrations and cover design by Artist PEREGO © 2013.

Visit www.artofperego.com

For additional copies of the book, contact your local book seller or visit us at:

www.Health4Life.info

The website also contains FREE Downloads, Dr. Mike's VIDEO BLOG, an Interactive APP, and HEALTH FREEDOM Products and gear.

Produced by:

FriesenPress

Suite 300 – 852 Fort Street
Victoria, BC, Canada V8W 1H8

www.friesenpress.com

Distributed to the trade by The Ingram Book Company

Table of Contents

To Justin,

yours in Optimal

Health,

Dr. Mike

Inspired by: :)

Kira & Eryn Van Thielen, my two beautiful daughters.
The principles and practices of **ORTHOPATHY.**
The millions of SICK people around me.

WARNING

Prerequisites to read this book:

BE OPEN MINDED

"It is exceedingly difficult to secure an honest hearing for any criticism of authority. Established beliefs are extremely invulnerable because they are accorded infallibility by the masses who are educated to believe they will be damned for thinking, and because of this, few will tolerate opposition of any nature to anything they have been educated to believe. People who have their thinking done for them are always intolerant."

J.H. Tilden.

Our wisdom lies in our willingness to learn. In other words, keep an open mind and investigate before condemning new and revolutionary thought. This book presents facts to the reader with an open mind. That is to say, the reader with an open mind will arrive at the basic truth just with some clear reasoning and willingness to embrace new thought. A reflective denial and scorn of a natural law only perpetuates misguided beliefs and is counterproductive to good health and wellbeing. Trying to break these laws of human life merely demonstrates the law and only hits back and hurts. We must rise above these ages of wrong thinking and wrong living, embrace the natural laws of human life and the healing power of the living body and in doing so obtain health freedom.

Health Freedom is a term I use throughout the book to indicate and reinforce the fact that we are FREE to do with our health what we want. We can have doctors, insurance companies, the FDA, and big or small pharmaceutical companies control (read: ruin) our health and wellbeing OR we can take control of our own health and regain and maintain optimal health. We can choose to be sick and suffer OR we can choose to be healthy and happy. In this book, I share with the reader my C.L.E.A.N. Living principles (refer to chapter 4; 4.2) and show him/her HOW to obtain HEALTH FREEDOM and live a healthy and happy life.

USE YOUR COMMON SENSE

This book lays it all out in a simple, organized, common-sense format. It allows you to acquire a new understanding of health, a revolutionary new conception of the essential nature of disease, a new attitude towards the body and the laws which govern it, a new outlook on the causes of ill health (or so called disease) and the only way to recover from such a condition.

With some clear thinking, a paradigm shift and a grain of common sense, this book will lead you to health freedom by showing you how to regain control of your health and live a happy life.

BE CAUTIOUS ABOUT RESEARCH

For several reasons, I don't use any references to research in this book.

Research is mostly fraud and biased, and is commonly funded by the companies who will profit from the skewed results.

Even if research is executed within the correct standards set forth and not funded by possible beneficiaries, it's still INVALID. Why?

1. Research NEVER represents a real life situation. For example, research often isolates a single nutrient and studies

this nutrient while fact remains that nutrients NEVER work alone. Nutrients work in synergy with hundreds of other nutrients and are involved in millions of complex chemical reactions per second. (For more info, refer to chapter 14).

2. Research NEVER takes into account the inherent healing power of our body and therefore ALWAYS comes to the wrong conclusions (refer to chapter 3; 3.4). Drugs for example are DEAD matter and cannot act, and only can be acted upon (refer to chapter 17; 17.1).

This book uses FACTS of simple BIOLOGY and PHYSIOLOGY, and incorporates examples of Mother Nature to back up its undisputable TRUTHS.

So if you happen to question some of these truths, simply review any biology, physiology, or natural law book or reference. Use your common sense instead of being misled by so called research based on false schools of thought and wrong hypothesis.

FOREWORD

I wanted to use this page to explain my style of writing: I DON'T HAVE ONE. I'm NOT a writer, and I didn't pay a professional to write my book either. I'm a motivational speaker and I'm passionate about health, wellness and nutrition. In this book I'm just talking to you. So hopefully you won't get stressed by the typos and grammatical mistakes. If you do I recommend you read that little book titled "Don't Sweat the Small Stuff" or have your doctor prescribe you some Prozac or Paxil (I'm serious about the former and despise the latter).

I won't bother you with details, fiction, and myths. I will get straight to the point and use plain and simple language. I am candid and brutally honest. I have only ONE GOAL, and that is, without any ulterior motive, to help you regain your health. I will tell you the unvarnished truth and often there is no delicate way to do it. Just keep an open mind and finish the book... I promise you won't regret it.

This book reveals the good and the bad about the very BEST way to achieve optimal health. I go right for the jugular when it comes to YOU improving your health. I would like you to enjoy your journey to a healthier, happier life!

I talk about SICKNESS, bad doctor's practices, scams and myths and put to rest what many THINK they know but really DON'T. I have been in field of HEALTH for over 2 decades and sought the advice of many HEALTH experts.

By telling it the way it is, you can decide for yourself whether being healthy is a priority for you or not, and whether the Action Plan in this book is the right tool to guide you to optimal health and happiness.

My mission is to help those of you who REALLY AND TRULY want to regain their health and live longer. Too many people like to talk about health, wellness, nutrition and exercise but NEVER take action. If you follow the concepts in this book, I am confident you will improve your health. The ONLY reason you will not improve your health may very well be due to lack of discipline, lack of motivation or refusal to embrace the revolutionary concepts in this book, because these concepts are contrary your current habits and beliefs.

If you are NOT ready yet, DON'T waste your time reading this book. Try to get a refund or give it to someone who may benefit from it. Yes, this book goes right at it...

Now, let's get started and find out how simple it is to REGAIN CONTROL OF YOUR HEALTH and achieve HEALTH FREEDOM.

INTRODUCTION

Let's start with my personal story...

As a youngster growing up in my country of origin, Belgium, I was very competitive minded. In 1st grade we had school competitions (sports) and the top athletes of each class qualified to represent the school in the district competition and then eventually in the national competition. I qualified for every sport... I was on the soccer and basketball team, and I was the fastest runner in my class but I failed to win one sport: swimming. A good friend of mine was a member of the local swim team and he royally beat me on a regular basis. I didn't like it and I decided to join the local swim team. For the next 20 years or so, I was a competitive swimmer with some modest achievements, including some age-group national titles and records.

In my early swimming years I wasn't aware of the importance of nutrition and/or supplements, even though I clearly remember my mother, grandmother and grandfather making sure I ate a good steak before every swim meet. My great grandmother who lived next door even made my brother and I some fresh squeezed lemon juice when we came home on our bicycles from school every day. She thought that we needed some good vitamins prior to our swim workout at the local community pool.

As I grew older and decided to enroll in the Physical Education program and later in the Physical Therapy program at the University of Brussels (V.U.B.), I learned more about the human body, its physiology and biomechanics, and some about nutrition. My interest in optimal physical performance was spiked and I started to self study and investigate this field. For a brief time I even traveled with the Flemish delegation (Flandres is the northern part of Belgium) of the Belgian Olympic Swim Team as the Physical Therapist and Technical Advisor in preparation for the Olympic Games in Atlanta in 1996.

In 1997 I moved to Florida and after working briefly in a hospital setting, I decided this was not my calling. I started to work in a private setting and was introduced to acupuncture and herbal medicine.

After witnessing better results when combining therapy with 'alternative medicine', I went back to school and received my Master of Science in Oriental Medicine and my license as an Acupuncture Physician. I completed Certifications in Homeopathy and Homotoxicology, Acupoint Injection Therapy, Laser Therapy, Biopuncture, Chinese Herbal Medicine, Bio-Identical Hormone Replacement Therapy (BHRT) among others.

Allopathic and Natural Medicine

A few thousand patients later, I wasn't convinced that this alternative medicine was the right approach either. ***Conventional medicine, drugs and surgeries are the devil for sure***, but even my more natural approach seemed to lack long-lasting results.

Approaching my 40's and also concerned about the health and welfare of my two beautiful children, I continued to look into new advances and technologies in the health industry. I attended many conventions and lectures. A light bulb finally went off and I decided to go back to basics, after all I was known among my peers to simplify things. I decided to get my PhD in Holistic Nutrition and expand my knowledge in this field. The program presented by the Natural College of Health was nothing less than outstanding.

I was introduced to some of the greatest names in NATURAL HYGIENE, including Dr. Isaac Jennings, Dr. Trall, Vincent Priessnitz, Sylvester Graham, Theodor Hahn, Schroth Rausse, Felix Oswald, J.H. Tilden, Herbert M. Shelton and others. These men are the true pioneers of Natural Hygiene. My personal bible "HUMAN LIFE – IT'S

PHYLOSOPHY AND LAWS" by Herbert M. Shelton prompted me to write this book. Much of the credit of this book goes to Mr. Shelton and the Natural Hygiene movement.

What I found was a shift in my paradigm. I certainly was a step ahead of what is called allopathic medicine (drugs and surgeries) by offering 'natural treatments' but I was still part of the problem... until now. The problem with all alternative or natural therapeutic approaches (acupuncture, naturopathy, herbal medicine, homeopathy, chiropractic and many more) is that just like allopathic medicine, it is *a cesspool of therapeutic systems and methods trying to cure or to resolve a medical problem*. The 'natural' therapeutic approach is certainly less ruinous to its victims. It kills less, but it doesn't cure more.

The controversy between the various schools of healing has been fought around the question: "what is the proper way to aid nature?" Nobody seems to ever have thought of the primary question: "Does nature require aid?" Dr. Benedict Lust stated once: "Naturopathy is systemized drugless healing". In other words, if one system or method fails, we'll try another one.

Any non-allopathic method, regardless of its true relation to vitality, is called natural and nobody dares to challenge this idea. One of the main purposes of this book is to point out the TRUE natural method, based on the principles and practices of Orthopathy and Natural Hygiene. The terms drugless and natural are not synonyms.

So this book is far from just another wellness or health book. I don't promote single nutrients or advocate natural therapeutic methods or systems. I don't present any magic bullets, elixirs, or cures to any so called diseases. I know the FDA uses the word CURE for the pharmaceutical drugs... preposterous. Nothing cures! Not a drug, not a nutrient, not a food, not a therapy... ONLY the body has the ability to cure itself.

Every living tissue continuously strives for optimal health while dead or inorganic matter such as a drug cannot act and only can be acted upon by the body. When we feel sick and we present with symptoms such as fever, chills, headache, nausea, vomiting or whatever, it is just an internal action of the body in an attempt to expel a virus, bacteria, or other pathogen or toxin and restore optimal health. It is not a disease.

This book

This book will present the reader with a simple, organized, systematic presentation of the **ONLY TRUE natural method to regain control of your health and achieve health freedom and happiness**.

I applaud the people who initiated the so called 'Wellness Revolution' and have partially succeeded in creating some awareness among the people in regards to the flawed foundation of our health care system and the natural alternatives that are available to improve one's health. This may have been the first baby step, but is far from the solution or the real 'cure'. So-called wellness experts and hundreds of other's with knowledge (but not understanding) in health, natural medicine and supplements are part of the problem.

The reader will learn in this book that not just one nutrient can correct or cure a disease, and that health can never be achieved while disregarding the laws of human life. Many so called wellness experts (whether or not they have fancy titles such as M.D. or PhD) are totally uninformed as how to achieve optimal health. Beyond those who are uninformed, there are those who, under the guise of expertise, are intentionally and unintentionally pandering worthless supplements to the public.

So I finally found the answer to living a healthy and happy life. I started practicing it not too long ago and started changing some of my habits. Nobody said it will be easy, but it certainly will be worth it!

I have always been a teacher by nature, I love to talk and share information and I love to motivate and help people. Locally, I do it one person at the time and that's great but my aspirations are much higher (yes, I still have a competitive mind-set and when I'm passionate about something there's no stopping me). That's why I decided to write this book and share a wealth of life-saving information with you. Keep an open mind as I debunk several well-established misconceptions that you believe in right now. Keep reading and with some clear thinking you will discover the truth. If you find the truth, it will change your life. My only goal: change peoples' lives and show them the path to health freedom. If you can't find or see the truth, read with a closed mind, or resist a paradigm-shift, you may burn this book (even though recycling it would be better).

I don't take credit for the ideas and concepts in this book, nor do I pretend it's all coming from my bright, genius mind. It's a synopsis of years of education and experience in this field which has led to the ONLY answer to TRUE Health. What I do take credit for is the simplification of this valuable and life-saving information, the action plan you can follow, and the fact that my goal is to bring this information to every human soul on the planet.

You are about to experience a PARADIGM-SHIFT

In order for most people to find the truth about health, a paradigm-shift needs to occur. What is a paradigm-shift? Some call it the 'Aha' experience when they finally 'see' things from another or opposite perspective. It's as though a light were suddenly turned on inside. Many people experience a fundamental shift in thinking when they face a life-threatening crisis and suddenly see their priorities in a different light, or when they suddenly step into a new role (such as that of a husband or wife, parent or grandparent, manager or leader).

I first learned about the paradigm-shift when reading and studying Steven R. Covey's 'The 7 Habits of Highly Effective People' (still one of my favorites and highly recommended if you didn't read it yet). To further clarify this phenomenon, I'll use a direct example out of this book. The story made an impression on me and has stuck with me since. Here it is:

Mr. Covey was sitting quietly on a subway in New York one morning. Some people were reading a newspaper, some were lost in thought, and some were just resting with their eyes closed. It was calm and peaceful. Then suddenly, a man and his children entered the subway car. The children were so loud and rambunctious that instantly the whole climate changed. The man sat down next to Mr. Covey and closed his eyes, apparently oblivious to the situation. The children were yelling back and forth, throwing things, even grabbing people's papers. It was very disturbing. And yet, the man sitting next to Mr. Covey did nothing about it. It was difficult not to feel irritated. One could not believe that this man could be so insensitive as to let his children run wild like that and do absolutely nothing about it, taking no responsibility at all. It was easy to see everyone on the subway felt irritated. So finally, with what Mr. Covey felt was unusual patience and restraint, he turned to the man and said: "Sir, your children are really disturbing a lot of people. I wonder if you couldn't control them a little more?" The man lifted his gaze as if to come to a consciousness of the situation for the first time and said softly: "Oh, you're right. I guess I should do something about it. We just came from the hospital where their mother died about an hour ago. I don't know what to think, and I guess they don't know how to handle it either".

Can you imagine how you would feel if you were Mr. Covey at that moment? His paradigm shifted. Suddenly he SAW things differently, and because he saw things differently, he THOUGHT differently, he FELT differently, he BEHAVED differently. Mr. Covey's irritation vanished. Mr. Covey didn't have to worry any longer about controlling his attitude or his behavior; his heart was filled with the man's pain. Feelings of sympathy and compassion flowed freely. "Your wife just died? Oh, I'm so sorry! Can you tell me about it? What can I do to help?" Everything changed in an instant.

I hope this example of a paradigm-shift illustrates the importance of keeping an open mind and trying to look at things from the other side, to try to understand the other person's point of view. It takes effort to first listen and then understand that 'other' perspective. This is how one creates a paradigm-shift. In this book, hopefully you will experience a similar paradigm-shift, one that shifts from a flawed health system in which you currently believe to the truth about health and a way to enjoy true health freedom.

A note to physicians and other health care professionals:

Ask yourself and be honest, and allow yourself some time to think this over: are you really helping people with their health problems or are you merely masking the symptoms? Do you really believe that pharmaceuticals and surgeries are the answer to disease or ill health? Do you believe drugs, surgeries, food, supplements, therapy, natural or alternative medicine practices and methods or systems cure disease? Or do you believe that only our bodies have the ability to heal themselves? This is your paradigm. You have been fed through professional school, sales solicitations from drug company representatives, insurance companies, etc. that this current health system works, that pharmaceutical drugs cure, and that current research saves lives. I hope this book causes a major paradigm shift in your thinking and that you end up joining us in the education of your patients in true health and achieving health freedom.

If we cannot practice the healing art with a higher purpose than monetary gain, preying upon the ignorance or blind trust of the people, would it not be better for ourselves and the rest of the world that we choose another job, or, in the alternative, helped reform the health care system as we know it?

What if you would learn **HOW to regain your health** and achieve optimal health by just complying with the laws of human life and following a simple action plan?

What if you could *teach all your patients* how to do the same? What if you could get them off their prescription drugs and show them how to get healthy again?

What if you would be able to *promote health* and finally stop treating disease?

Would you not be a **REAL doctor** then? I bet you would finally feel some real satisfaction in your work. You would be passionate. You would absolutely love it. You would be able to REALLY GIVE to others something that is priceless... health! You would be a true hero. You would be part of a revolution. You would look back at your life and be proud. You made a difference. So, read this book with an open mind, experience the paradigm-shift and join me in the health freedom movement.

If you are not a physician or health care professional, you can do exactly the same. If you love this book and WHEN it changes your life, share it with your family, friends and loved-ones and spread the word.

So who is this book for?

This book is for those who wish to be or stay healthy, be happy and live longer. You already know that you won't stay healthy or become healthy by taking prescription medications, eating toxic, synthetic and processed foods, ignore healthy practices and depend on someone else's advice. And you already figured out that *many* doctors don't help you to get healthy, but rather mask the symptoms of the underlying cause.

How much time do you spend going to the doctor? How much money do your prescription and over-the-counter medicines cost each month? Do you want to die at a young age? Do you want to end-up spending your last years in and out of the hospital, coping with the ramifications of strokes, heart attacks, Alzheimer, diabetes or cancer? Do you want to spend your savings on hospital and medical bills? Do you want your loved-ones or children to commit their lives to help you because you are unable to take care of yourself? OR, do you want to live your dreams and stay healthy, enjoy your retirement, travel, and see your grand-kids grow up? Frankly, *the choice is yours!*

Don't blame others, or the government, or the drug companies, or the marketing scams of major companies luring you into buying stuff that's just BAD for you. Blame yourself and get over it right now! There's nothing you can do about the past, you can't predict the future BUT YOU CAN **CONTROL THE PRESENT**, and the present is a GIFT.

So, Correct the Situation: TAKE ACTION, **TAKE RESPONSIBILITY**. ONLY YOU CAN CHANGE YOUR HEALTH, YOUR ROAD MAP and YOUR FUTURE (and also influence the health of your kids and loved-ones). You just have to break some habits, acquire new habits and COMMIT. This book shows you HOW! I will be your COACH...BUT ultimately YOU have to EXECUTE.

You also know that many health or wellness programs out there are usually just some quick-fix, one-size-fits-all approaches to supposedly improve your health while selling you their supplements. These programs may have seemingly short-term benefits but lack lasting results and true longevity, and contribute to the exacerbation of ill health.

HOW am I going to optimize my health and get back on track, you ask? It's easier than you think. Don't enroll in a program and waste your hard earned money. Don't walk into a health food store and just start buying any supplement that someone else recommended or your doctor or a celebrity wellness expert told you to buy. Don't ask anyone without true knowledge in health (I mean health, not disease... even though they are the same), and don't ask anyone with any secondary interests or gains. Just READ this book and TAKE ACTION!

The approach in this book is logic, pure and simply COMMON SENSE, but YOU need to take responsibility and follow the Health 4 Life ACTION PLAN. Anybody can do it, and EVERYONE feels the benefits... almost IMMEDIATELY!

This book has the answers you have been looking for. It tells you HOW to take control of your health, enjoy life, and live longer with no major financial investment (you already bought this book) and no special knowledge required...just an open mind and some common sense!

A Short Note before you get started

Some passages and parts of this book are repetitive. This is done purposefully to assure that every reader gets the full knowledge and understanding necessary to succeed in changing his or her life for the better. Sometimes, explaining the same thing in more than one way allows for the reader to REALLY get it. Repetition of important information also promotes retention of the information.

I also wanted to prepare and warn you about the first 3 chapters. The first 3 chapters are pretty BOLD, straight-forward, and sometimes interpreted as 'negative'. This is because I expose what I see as the flaws of our current medical system. Even more importantly I make you aware of the health condition you are in right now. It's not pretty. However it's the only way to wake you up and create awareness. It's also the only way to create a paradigm-shift which is crucial for you to succeed in regaining control of your health.

Luckily, from Chapter 4 on, reading will be more pleasant. Content is positive and energetic. I'm confident you will encounter many 'a-ha' experiences which will change your life. Some stuff will boggle your mind and your first reaction may be: "NO WAY". I just ask you to keep an open mind, to think about it and be honest... so you can and will find the truth.

NOW is the time to undo years of mistreatment to your body and mind. I will show you HOW to DO this.

No matter what your current level of health may be, I have a PLAN for you. This plan WORKS, guaranteed. This is a NEW START, a new beginning. This is your YEAR ZERO. Year Zero is the year at which you start to make the RIGHT CHOICES in life. Year Zero starts TODAY by reading this book and implementing the ACTION PLAN (chapter 18).

My ACTION PLAN shows you the path to HEALTH FREEDOM (chapter 3) by simply incorporating my C.L.E.A.N. LIVING principles (chapter 4; 4.2):

Control emotions and feelings.
Listen to the warning signs of your body, avoid overstimulation and overindulgences.
Enough rest, sleep and sunshine.
Active lifestyle.
Natural and clean air, water and food.

HOW IS THIS BOOK DIFFERENT?

This book is different from other health and wellness books for several reasons:

NOT JUST ANOTHER HEALTH & WELLNESS BOOK

This book is not just another health or wellness book with emphasis on a therapeutic model or system, or a new supplement, or a fad diet or whatever new secret. This book is unique in that is goes far beyond therapeutic methods or systems that focus on 'curing' a disease. This book uses the principles of Natural Hygiene and teaches the laws of human life. This book will show the reader what health REALLY is and exposes the flawed foundation of the current 'health' system. With an open mind, some common sense and clear thinking, the reader will find the truth about health and disease, and ultimately will become his or her own 'doctor'.

THE R3 WELLNESS MODEL

My revolutionary wellness model 'R3' (Restore, Resolve, Rejuvenate) provides the consumer and health care provider unprecedented access to success and is the cornerstone for anyone to regain *CONTROL* over their health and live a longer, happier life. So how is this R3 wellness model different? Because access to success lies in restoring normal body functions prior to trying to resolving medical issues or health problems.

Let me explain. Regardless the type of health care practitioner one chooses to get help from, the vast majority of health care practitioners will try to resolve your problem. A medical doctor may prescribe medication, a chiropractor may prescribe manipulations and adjustments, an acupuncturist may perform acupuncture and prescribe Chinese herbal medicine, a naturopath may recommend a diet or certain nutritional supplements, etc. Unfortunately, their approach is premature. Let me use the following analogy. Take a wounded soldier on the battle field and give that soldier a powerful weapon to defeat the enemy. What is that wounded soldier going to do with that powerful weapon on the battle field? Wouldn't it make much more sense to drag that wounded soldier off the battle field, heal that soldier and only then give him or her that powerful weapon to defeat the enemy? I thought so! The same holds true for a person with a medical problem. Almost every health care practitioner tries to resolve that medical problem by prescribing a treatment or intervention. This is a low-success rate approach!

So when it comes to regaining control of your health or fighting a disease or medical condition, one has to balance and normalize bodily functions first prior to trying to resolve that medical condition or disease. The soldier needs to be strong and healthy prior to fighting the enemy. Dr. Mike's R3 wellness model shows you how to *RESTORE your health prior to trying to RESOLVE any medical issue or disease.* This approach guarantees great results, all the time.

KEYS TO SUCCESS

I seek to not only SIMPLIFY health and wellness practices for you, but DRIVE you and MOTIVATE you towards your own health freedom. I have helped people worldwide and I want to equip you as well with a simple, practical, organized and affordable action plan to guarantee success in regaining and obtaining optimal health.

My core goal is providing not only education, knowledge and awareness but also a simple *ACTION PLAN.* Most people equate knowledge with power, but that's not accurate. According to Napoleon Hill (Think & Grow Rich), knowledge is only potential power. Knowledge must be organized and must be applied to a definite purpose; it must be molded into a practical action plan in order to obtain the riches. There are plenty of wellness 'experts' and wellness coaches out there, even conventional doctors (MD's) that specialize in health and wellness. They all educate the consumer and sell their products. However, the consumer reading the articles, watching T.V. or you-tube videos and listening to podcasts is unable to reap the health benefits from that newly acquired knowledge. Why? The consumer is unable to put the new knowledge into practice. A practical organized action plan is missing with ultimately NO RESULTS.

No pun intended when I talk about so-called wellness experts. They are certainly a major driving force in the wellness revolution and great educators reaching a broad audience. But if we have to take their advice, we will end-up with 6612 supplements. Get my point? There is no ACTION PLAN, no starting point, no evaluation or interim evaluation, progress markers, objective tests etc. It's an overload of information causing confusion and possible harm. This book provides a simple, step-by-step ACTION PLAN, unlike any other, that has proven to be highly effective.

Another key element is *MOTIVATION*. Many consumers read about health and wellness, 'good' foods and 'bad' foods, risk factors to health etc. but no action is ever taken. My mission is to MOTIVATE people FIRST, and THEN provide them with a simple ACTION PLAN. How do we motivate? We educate the consumer through a simple, understandable, fun, interactive (this book, seminars and webinars), and most of all PASSIONATE learning experience. We are the 'ANTHONY ROBBINS' of health. We present the reader with easy to understand vocabulary, using analogies and examples to assure the reader UNDERSTANDS the what, why and how. We present FACTS about YOUR HEALTH and the road of destruction you are on right now. We create *awareness* about your current 'health' situation and the scary statistics that you are part of. We get the reader excited and motivated, we promote compliance, and we show them how to record their progress and results.

This book presents you with the <u>KNOWLEDGE</u> and <u>SKILLS</u> you need to REGAIN CONTROL OF YOUR HEALTH. Unfortunately that's not enough to succeed. You need the <u>WILLINGNESS</u> to take action to succeed, something ONLY YOU can bring to the table. That's why we present you with the HARD FACTS and truths about your current health practices, paint a picture of your miserable future if you continue those devastating health practices, and present you with an easy solution. You will need to fight to stop some of your bad habits and implement new healthy habits.

According to Stephen R. Covey, *habits* are exactly that: an intersection of knowledge, skill and desire or willingness. Knowledge is the theoretical paradigm, the WHAT TO DO and the WHY. Skill is the HOW TO DO. And desire or willingness is the motivation, the WANT TO DO. In order to make something a habit in our lives, we have to have all three. It's sometimes a painful process. It's a change that has to be motivated by a higher purpose, by the willingness to subordinate what you think you want now for what you want later. But this process produces happiness, "the object and design of our existence". Happiness can be defined, in part at least, as the fruit of the desire and ability to sacrifice what we want now for what we want eventually.

There you have it! That's why this book and our approach to REGAIN CONTROL OF YOUR HEALTH is different and SUCCESSFUL.

DISCLAIMER

The ideas, suggestions and action plan in this book are not intended as a substitute for the medical advice of a trained professional. Actually they are, but my lawyer advised me that a legal disclaimer is intended to protect me from lawsuits by those who will claim that they relied on my book to the exclusion of conventional medicine.

So let me clarify that this book is intended for you to regain control of your health, and obtain and maintain optimal health. I suggest you retake that control and ask your physician to help you in your quest to optimal health. Your physician should be delighted to help you, by carefully monitoring vitals and progress, and helping you to get off ALL the harmful drugs.

If there is doubt about the truth due to lack of common sense, failure to keep an open mind, or failure to think clearly, please consult your physician or rely on some research and tests conducted by pharmaceutical companies. I'm sure there is a drug out there that can temporarily mask your symptoms while wreaking more havoc in your body and promoting life threatening so called disease. This drug only requires a simple swallow every day, hardly any effort at all compared to respecting the laws of human life and living healthier and happier.

Possible **ADVERSE REACTIONS** that may be caused by implementing the Action Plan in this book:

Energy, joy, happiness, deep sleep, strength, freedom of pain, alertness, good memory, great vision, good appetite, increased flexibility, absence of disease, absence of depression, absence of suicidal thoughts, great libido and sex drive, vital complexion, healthy looking skin, desire to throw your drugs in the garbage, desire to enjoy life, feelings of empowerment, feelings of self-esteem and control of life, thoughts of helping others, uncontrollable need to throw away walking aids and useless supplements, desire for optimal health, crazy thoughts of becoming your doctor's doctor, clear mind, controlled emotions, mental vitality, optimal body composition, feeling of fulfillment, absence of worry, absence of stress, more money in your pocket which was not spent on medical bills and drugs but on vacations and fun, and many more not listed here.

Chapter 1 – Nutritional Suicide, Homicide and Genocide

1.1 Health is the Rule, Disease the Exception

Let's start with clarifying some terminology:

Life is the state of being alive. It's a condition in which humans, animals and plants exist with capacity for exercising their functions. **Perfect life** is that condition in which those functions are exercised perfectly. **Death** is the cessation of life. Between these two extremes of perfect life, on one hand, and death on the other, are found all those various degrees of health and disease which exist today. From this point of view, both health and disease are states or conditions of being or life.

Health consists of the correct condition and action of all the vital powers and properties of the living body. This condition requires the proper development and optimal function of all the organs and tissues of the body and a close adherence to the laws of life. Health is the normal, natural state of all organic existence; it is spontaneous and the result of the normal operation of the organs and functions of the living body. Living matter cannot be otherwise than healthy if the conditions of health are present (you will learn what these conditions are later in this book). Life always strives toward perfection. We can conclude that it's much easier to be in a good state of health than to have poor health.

The human body is one unit. No part of the body can be affected independent of other parts. Each organ has its particular function to perform, yet no organ can perform its function independently of the others, and no organ can sustain itself by its own function alone. The digestive system digests food for the whole body, the lungs supply oxygen and eliminate carbon dioxide for the entire body, the kidneys and the skin excrete toxins and waste products from the whole body, the heart and vascular system carry blood and oxygen throughout the entire body and so on. This clearly illustrates the dependence of each organ upon the whole system and the whole system upon each organ, and shows that the function of not one single organ can be impaired without affecting the whole system as a consequence. Furthermore, as long as life continues each tissue and organ, whether in a state of health or disease, is at its post, ready and disposed to perform its particular function to the full extent of its ability.

Today's 'specialists' in medicine treat each part of the body as though it were independent from the rest of the body. Organs (tonsils, gallbladder etc.) are removed surgically by the millions contributing to the increased liability of disease and the weakened constitution of our species... stupidity at best!

Health thus depends not only on the perfection of the organism but also upon the conditions under which life exists. Just like animals, human beings require air, water, food, light, and freedom from violence along with rest, exercise and cleanliness (hygiene). Under these natural conditions, health is potential in life and is as inevitable as the rise and fall of the tides. Living matter cannot be other than healthy if the conditions of health are present. However, it lies in man's power to place himself under conditions other than those of health and therefore impair his health.

Health is a state of physical, mental, emotional and spiritual well-being. PERFECT Health is a perfect balance of physical, mental, emotional and spiritual well-being resulting in a disease-free *body, mind & soul*, with all bodily systems functioning in balance and harmony.

Perfect health expresses itself:

1. *Physically* as an optimal body composition (ratio of body fat,

lean muscle mass, water balance etc.) with a strong muscu-loskeletal system, plenty of energy reserve (no unexplained fatigue) and a healthy appearance (skin, complexion).

2. *Mentally* as a focused, organized, alert, problem-solving, positive thinking, and proactive human being FREE of con-fusion, loss of memory, lack of attention.

3. *Emotionally* as a healthy balance between one's emotions such a joy, fear, grief, anger, worry; expressed appropriately and under control.

4. *Spiritually* as peace with a 'higher being' or belief system; and using that belief system to guide one's values and prin-ciples.

When body, mind (mental & emotional aspects), and soul (spiritual aspect) are balanced, perfect health is achieved. Therefore, the current 'health system' should be renamed 'disease system' because our entire 'health system' is based on disease. It's about treating or masking symp-toms, ignoring the underlying cause, prescribing drugs and prescribing more drugs to mask the side-effects of the other drugs. It's about keeping us all alive as long as possible so more drugs can be sold. Sounds hor-rible, but think about it...is it true? Your common sense and observation will tell you...just step out-of-the-box for a minute!

Our modern **health standard** is ridiculously low and represents a false picture of health. A true health standard would be the highest possible degree of healthy action in a perfect organism; anything short of this is impaired health (disease). Today people are sick and far from perfect health, and those whom we call healthy are nothing more than less sick than the average person... yes, that includes you and me! All you have to do is open your eyes and look at wild animals in nature, or compare us with primitive men or cavemen.

Look at thousands of wild fish or eagles, or antelopes, or lions or goril-las, or whatever, and find that they are all sound and healthy. These wild animals in nature are beautifully and symmetrically developed and present a uniform type, totally free of all the disease known to man. Have you ever heard or seen a wild lion, gorilla or eagle with diabetes, a-fib, pneumonia, cancer, Alzheimer, COPD? Have you ever seen a fat one? Not only do these wild animals not suffer from any diseases, they don't exhibit any deformities.

Now let's look at us... deformities and defects are everywhere, and beauty, strength, and symmetry are absent in both sexes. We are rapidly becoming a race of bald heads, false teeth, glass eyes, prosthetic legs, obesity, pimples, blotches, fatigue, weakness, fear, worry, restlessness, insomnia, war, crime, irritability, addiction, sickness and so on. These observations along with the presence of hospitals, doctor's offices, drug stores, prisons, coffee shops, whore houses, health magazines, asylums and sanitariums are all evidence and prove that man's health standard borders on death. We rely on cosmetic products, make-up, hair dressers, beauty salons etc. to make us 'beautiful' and hide our real appearance. Both sexes seem to be content with imitation. Even so called beautiful women are like masterpieces in oil (they look good from far but far from good), and the average middle-aged man has problems with getting an erection. Cavemen and Indians (before white man changed their way of living) lived long, exhibited well developed muscles, a power-ful bony framework, great strength, vigorous health, sound and strong teeth (without the aid of a tooth brush or tooth paste), and didn't know of any disease.

Mankind today has degenerated far below this natural health standard. As long as the average man is able to get out of bed in the morning, and is able to eat three meals per day (which is two too many) with the aid of various condiments (sauces, dressings) to whip up his appetite, and with the use of coffee, soda, tobacco, alcohol and other stimulants gets himself through the work day, he is considered healthy. His friends are satisfied with his 'healthy' appearance. If however, he should get sick and suddenly die, they exclaim "how sudden! He was a picture of

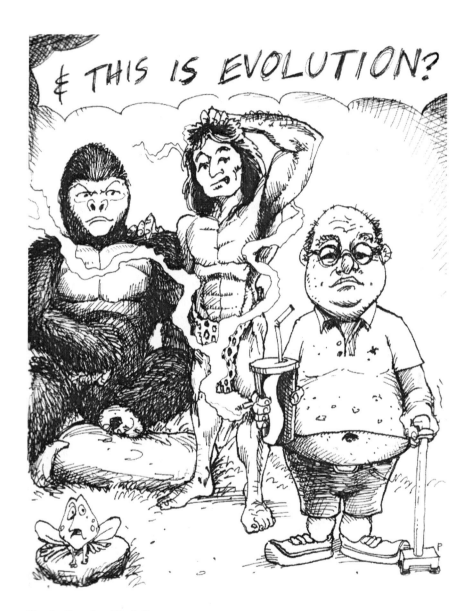

Illustration 1 – Evolution

perfect health." A picture, indeed! How low the standard! Even those among us that are considered healthy or consider themselves healthy today because they are not suffering and don't take any prescription drugs, will suffer tomorrow.

Today's normal standards for body weight, blood pressure, heart rate, urine acidity, cholesterol, hormone levels etc. are all mere averages of what a bunch of abnormal and overstimulated men and women represent. *Normality cannot be found by averaging up abnormality*, rather it should approach the ideal or optimal.

Some would argue that 'we must be healthier because we live longer today than ever before'. Let's look at the facts. The average person does not live longer than before, to the contrary, many more people die young (40's, 50's, 60's). Agreed that some people live to be a hundred... but not many. Most of us are kept alive with drugs, surgeries, CPR and technologies... and given another chance (or more than one), but death is near unless one changes his or her lifestyle and obeys the laws of human life. We should all live to be at least 120 years! This is just going by the animal standard. Animals live on average, from five to seven times the length of time they require to reach complete physical maturity. Oh, I forgot to mention, this is 120 years disease-free!

The human being, masterpiece of creation, subject to disease while both plant and animal kingdoms present beauty and perfection in their tendency towards normal. Sad that such low standards are held up and defended by the so called brightest minds of the dominant schools of medicine.

If you dare, stand in front of a big mirror, take your clothes off and ask yourself whether or not your body looks the way it should, based on the perfect creation and compared to wild animals? Are you overweight? Are you symmetrical? Are you abundant of strength and flexibility? Do you exhibit smooth, healthy skin? Do you have a vital complexion? Are you full of energy? Does your body reflect its full potential? If not, should you be ashamed of how you have treated this perfect gift so far, and shouldn't you start doing something about it right now? At least you are because you are reading this book! Keep at it! You must understand that your body always strives for perfection and strives for perfect health. It's your mistreatment of your body that causes less than perfect health.

You can now understand that:

HEALTH IS THE RULE, DISEASE THE EXCEPTION.

1.2 Disease is the Cure

Disease is indeed the exception. It has been a misconception also. We have been taught since youth that disease is the enemy and that this enemy needs to be conquered through drugs and surgery. Failing body parts are removed, organs and systems are poisoned and cells are destroyed by the toxic chemicals we call pharmaceuticals. Our health impairs further and more drugs are prescribed and swallowed to suppress the additional symptoms of imbalance in the body and to counteract the toxic side-effects of the initial drugs. This is a vicious, detrimental cycle that has taken over and we enter our 'golden' years crippled and sick. The misconception here is that disease is an outward manifestation of an inward imbalance, a demon harassing us. Disease is NOT an attack from the external environment (outside), it's merely a state of health. So called germs and pathogens are ALWAYS around but we only get sick when our internal environment is weak or compromised. That's why certain people (weak ones) get the flu during cold season, and the stronger ones don't. It obviously has nothing to do with the presence of germs or viruses or pathogens. It's a weak constitution that welcomes them. More clarification will be found in chapter 2.

Answer the following questions:

If our body creates a fever to speed up metabolism to deal with and correct an internal imbalance, is it prudent to ingest a drug or non-food toxin to suppress that fever? Is it prudent to immerse in cold water to reach homeostasis (balance, eg. a normal temperature in this case)?

If our body creates swelling and inflammation to initiate the healing process (increase circulation, remove waste, repair tissue etc.) around the ankle joint after spraining it for example, is it prudent to apply ice and counteract the body's attempt to heal?

Is osteoporosis a disease crying for drugs or the end-result of the body robbing the bones of alkaline minerals to buffer acids ingested from years of improper diet, all in an attempt to keep us alive and maintain our blood pH at 7.2-7.35?

Do we suffer from aspirin or Prozac or Coumadin deficiency? Do we suffer from acupuncture or chiropractic deficiency?

The answer to all questions is a definite 'NO'. The origin or cause of disease is NOT an enemy from the outside but an internal act of physiology by the body in an attempt to stay alive or in perfect health. Why would we interfere with that? No matter what the interference, it's always wrong!

We can conclude that:

DISEASE IS THE CURE.

Nutrition is the process of nourishing or being nourished, especially the process by which a living organism assimilates food and uses it for growth and for replacement of tissues. It is whatever we consume to keep our organism (body, mind, spirit) in perfect health.

In perfect health, our body receives the right nutrients from the food we consume. This food is digested, assimilated and converted to vital energy. This energy is used to carry out all metabolic processes and functions necessary to maintain health and stay alive. The vital energy is used to build, repair and renew cells, tissues and organs.

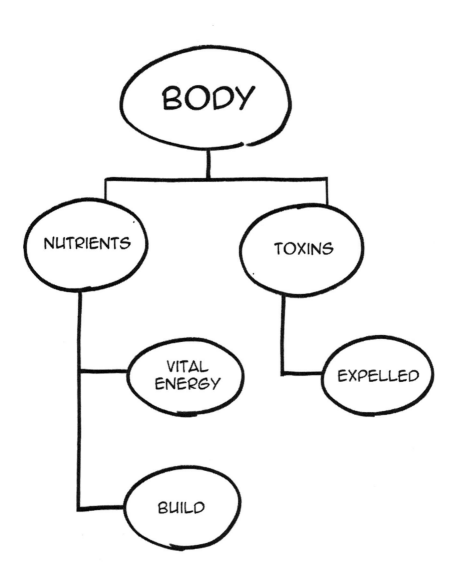

Illustration 2 – Perfect Health Model

The body is constantly exposed to toxins from the external environment and toxins from our food. In perfect health the body uses vital energy to quickly remove these toxins, impurities, and wastes from the body.

Now that we learned about life, health, death, disease and nutrition... let's move on and take a closer look at nutritional suicide, homicide and genocide.

1.3 Nutritional Suicide

The vast majority of us are committing **nutritional suicide**. Unlike shooting a bullet straight through your brain, nutritional suicide is a very slow, self-inflicted and self-destructing process. Both result in early death but the latter with a lot more suffering along the way.

Most of the time this process of nutritional suicide is unintentional, but that's not an excuse. It's time to be responsible for your own body. It's time to be educated about the unbelievable creation that is YOU. And it's time you start respecting that creation and treat it like it should be treated... anything else would be very ungrateful.

Your toaster, your hair dryer, your washing machine, your DVD player, your car, they all come with a user manual or at least an instruction guide on how to properly use and maintain your equipment. *Did you ever get a user manual for your body upon birth?* I didn't. But we all should have received one! This book can be that user manual (or use the extended version by Herbert M. Shelton 'Human Life – Its philosophy and laws). And every parent should teach their child this user manual, including how to respect the rules and laws of human life and provide the necessary conditions for your body to stay in perfect health.

The Standard American Diet: S.A.D.

The world population has grown out of proportion and there is not enough food from nature (whole foods) available to feed every mouth. Industrialization and commercialization have caused the mass-production of synthetic and processed foods, containing harmful preservatives, antibiotics, colorings and toxins which are foreign to the body and cause plenty of diseases. These include but are certainly not limited to allergies, immune-diseases, degenerative disease, cancers and more (I'll explain later how that works).

At the same time, these synthetic, processed foods do NOT contain any nutritional value. In other words, our body does NOT get the nutrients it needs to function properly and replace itself AND is continuously forced to use useful nutrients like vitamins, minerals and enzymes to neutralize the harmful toxins we ingest.

We have become slaves of the industrialization and commercialization of our food and drinks, and we have become slaves of civilization and the high demands of society and our jobs. We live in a state of emergency.

The Dalai Lama, when asked what surprised him most about human-ity, answered "Man. Because he sacrifices his health in order to make money. Then he sacrifices money to recuperate his health. And then he is so anxious about the future that he does not enjoy the present: the result being that he does not live in the present or the future; he lives as if he is never going to die, and then he dies having never really lived."

Although our genetics didn't change (much), many more diseases developed and even our children have to cope with more and more conditions such as diabetes, obesity, allergies, ADD/ADHD, etc. Why is that? Because of our current lifestyles we ignore the laws of human life and disrespect the needs of our body. We have no time for a healthy meal, we abuse our body with drugs, alcohol and other stimulants, we consume man-made foods not recognized by our body, we overindulge, we stress, we are emotionally unstable and the list goes on and on…

Let's have a look at our current eating practices and some trends:

We hardly eat any fruits and vegetables compared to the man-made junk. Although an increase in the consumption of fruit and vegetables is noted… WOW, you may think…but hold on: 18% of all vegetables consumed are French fries! Yes, French fries are potatoes.

A decrease in consumption of foods high in fat is also noted because people wrongly assume that fat makes you fat. BUT there has also been an increase in the consumption of foods with added fat such as fried foods and butter.

Cheese consumption increased by 250% due to the increase in pizza and cheeseburger consumption.

According to a UNC-study, the calorie content of food has increased also. For example, the calorie content in soft drinks increased by 49, fries by 68, salty snacks by 93, hamburgers by 97, and Mexican food by 133.

Visits to restaurants increased by 200%, resulting in higher fat and sugar consumption.

All processed and canned foods contain numerous toxins (preservatives, antibiotics, colorings etc.) and gross failure of the FDA to execute its only job (protect public health) results in thousands of products on our shelves, unfit and detrimental to the human body. These foods and products continue to get worse and worse with the introduction of more deadly ingredients.

Look at the gigantic increase in 'diet' products for example which replace regular sugar for carcinogenic or cancer causing, synthetic, cheaper sugar substitutes. Furthermore, the consumer is misled by the marketing scams of the manufacturers who can get away with labeling anything but the truth (what ingredients are in their product) and promote their products incorrectly as 'natural' or 'diet' or 'low fat' or 'no cholesterol' etc.

Besides the direct consumption of all these un-natural foods and drinks, and all their toxins, humans are further exposed to other forms of body pollution. In life, lack of knowledge comes at a very high price (and is for sure the number 1 cause of death; it's not heart disease…trust me). It can easily cost us our most precious commodity, our health! We live in a highly toxic world where our water is undrinkable, our food is poisoned with thousands of chemicals, and our air is polluted. On top of that we already established that our food is also virtually devoid from any nutrients. As people, we try to compensate for this lack of nutrients by eating much larger quantities; and to make things worse, only few of us exercise regularly and are able to cope with the stresses of life.

Since the start of the Industrial Revolution, thousands of new chemicals have been introduced to our environment. These cell-damaging and deadly toxins are invisible and insidious. Like a remorseless killer, they break down all body systems at the cellular level. This process is slow (day by day) and undetectable, UNTIL disease finally signals its presence. The first sign may be a harmless rash OR a deadly cancer.

Some scary statistics…

1. There are currently well over 10,000 different chemicals used in food processing and preservation. The average American is exposed to 50,000 chemical agents in his lifetime and only a small fraction of these have been studied for their effects on humans.

2. Almost 1.5 billion pounds of pesticides are sprayed on wheat and vegetable crops in the U.S. each year…that's more than 5 pounds per person! According to experts, only 2% of these pesticides actually serve to protect the crops while 98% is absorbed by air, water and the food itself. There are currently well over 1,500 different organophosphate pesticides used in over 50,000 products in North America alone. These pesticides were developed in Nazi Germany in the 1930's and their chemical agents were used during WWII. Currently, they are classified as weapons of mass destruction and are banned in most nations (another great job by the FDA who's really looking out for us).

3. There are also another 24.6 million pounds of antibiotics utilized in factory farming per year. A sampling of the average grocery store milk showed the presence of over 80 different antibiotic residues (more about milk later).

4. The average American consumes 150 pounds of sugar and 566 cans of soft drinks (soda or 'liquid candy fortified with carcinogens and biological warfare chemicals')... each year. What if I also told you that on average, each year, we consume 150 slices of pizza, 120 pastries or desserts, 120 orders of French fries, 190 candy bars and 45 large bags of potato chips. Looking at these astonishing numbers it is no surprise that every other American is chronically ill!

5. Oh, I almost forgot! Our pharmaceutical drugs (the ones that are supposed to 'cure' us) also contain a fair amount of these harmful and toxic chemicals (additives as well as environmental pollutants).

Besides all these toxic exposures, we use shampoos, conditioners, hair coloring products, hair spray, gels, body lotions, tooth pastes, cosmetic products of all kinds (toners, moisturizers, bleaching agents, tanning agents etc.), sunscreen, deodorant, nail polish, eyeliner, make-up etc. which all contain more than one harmful, toxic chemical that may easily penetrate our largest organ, the skin. Once absorbed by the skin, these toxins end up in our bloodstream and are spread throughout the body wreaking havoc at every level. They affect every organ and cell and cause our body to yet again operate in a state of emergency, trying to expel or neutralize these toxins, requiring useful nutrients and lots of energy. Eventually, our cells and tissues are literally 'swimming' in contamination.

This constant circulation of toxins taxes the immune system which must continually strive to destroy these toxins. Eventually the body's own cleansing and detoxification system becomes overburdened.

I hope you agree that it is impossible to avoid the constant onslaught of toxic waste from every possible angle...unless you move away from civilization back into nature (that would be ideal but we need to be realistic also). Just be aware of this daily, toxic onslaught and try to MINIMIZE this onslaught by educating yourself and being aware of these SILENT KILLERS. Avoid these toxic exposures as much as possible while simultaneously putting a healthy detoxification practice into place to regularly and effectively rid your body of these toxins.

Whether you like it or not, whether you are sick already or not, whether you wrongly assume you are healthy right now just because you are not yet diagnosed with a degenerative disease and you are not taking any prescription drugs yet, you are definitely committing nutritional suicide. You are just waiting for that day to come, the day that will change your life suddenly, unexpected… the day they diagnose you with a disease which has been developing for years, but only now expresses itself with unpleasant symptoms because your body has been fighting and neutralizing it for years and years.

Your body has given you many warning signals but you completely ignored them. Now you will pay the price for the abuse you inflicted on your body, for making it work in a state of emergency, all the time trying to break-down, dissolve, neutralize, excrete and store man-made, unnatural substances and toxins forced into your body by YOU. YOU are responsible and being irresponsible comes with a price tag: your health and your life. But it's never too late to turn things around, after all, your body forgives and continues to strive for perfect health (it cannot do anything else).

We do have THE POWER to improve our health and well-being, and we have to do it one step at the time. Optimal nutrition is a key factor; how well these nutrients are absorbed by our body is another key factor; and how well and regularly we eliminate waste products and harmful toxins from our body, is yet another vital key along with respecting the laws of human life.

So wake up people! I know you are addicted to food and I know we all prefer to take the path of least resistance, but the price is simply too high! Agreed? Then stop committing nutritional suicide!

1.4 Nutritional Homicide

Now that you are aware you are committing nutritional suicide, you can understand that you also may be committing nutritional homicide. Luckily for you this kind of homicide is not recognized as an actual act of violence in the justice system and therefore goes unpunished.

But that doesn't mean you aren't committing the crime... because that's exactly what it is. You are poisoning human life and promoting disease and death. I know that most of you are doing it unintentionally and unwittingly, but not anymore. You know now, which means you need to act now. If not, how can live with the fact you are killing everyone you feed and raise in your family, your children and your loved-one?

Not only are you feeding them these poisons and slowly killing them and setting them up for a life of sickness, disease, and prescription drugs... but you fail to raise them and educate them about their physical body, their creation, and how to respect that creation, how to live by the laws of human life, how to maintain that creation and how to have it function in perfect health, which all leads to the purpose of life... happiness.

Besides your children and loved-ones, maybe as part of your job or volunteer work you feed children in a school, patients in a medical setting, people in a restaurant, the homeless, travelers on a cruise, etc. Yes, you are an accomplice in their homicide also.

And what about your pet? Unfortunately, these domestic animals are subject to their master and unlike us they do not have any control of their health. They can only consume what they are given. Most pets consume man-made foods (I don't know of any pets that don't) and therefore end up with the same diseases as their human counterpart: arthritis, diabetes, cancer etc. The treatment is similar to the treatment of human so called diseases (drugs, surgeries etc.) and interferes with the healing capabilities of the body. Can we consider this animal abuse? You decide.

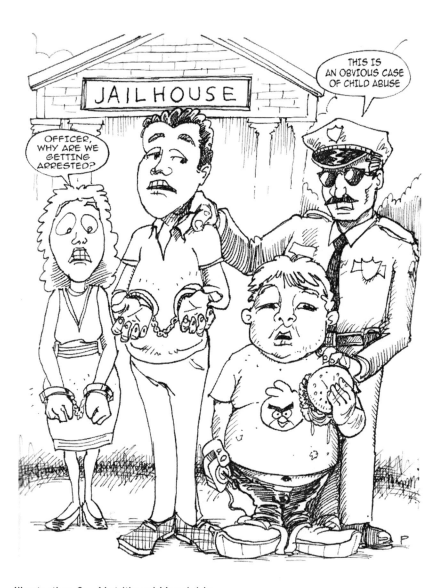

Illustration 3 – Nutritional Homicide

1.5 Nutritional Genocide

Can this get any worse? Sure! What if you are working for the FDA or you're part of the FDA, or what if you are a drug representative or have anything to do at all with pharmaceutical companies, or what if you are part of a company (whether a multi-level network marketing company or not) that sells nutritional supplements that don't work (the vast majority – more later in this book), or what if you are a lobbyist or part of the government approving all this toxic waste to enter our bodies, or what if you are a doctor or other health care professional and prescribe drugs or useless treatments, or what if you sell or market shampoos, conditioners, hair colorings, deodorants, skin care products etc., what if you are a distributor or work for a company that distributes any of these products, what if.... Then you are guilty of genocide in the first or second degree...

I know it sounds over the top at first, but with what you know now... it is the truth and nothing but the truth. I know that these statements are frowned upon, but they are nothing but facts and hopefully cause a shift in your paradigm.

It's time to stop helping these industries achieve their money-hungry goals accomplished at the expense of us, the people. Whether they are operating or not, it's still in your control whether you consume and use all these toxic, un-natural, detrimental products or not; and it's also up to you if you want to continue to be part of this genocide.

The human race has lowered its standards of health, and more and more disease is present today... more and more babies born with defects and disabilities, a mutation from a perfect healthy body as seen in cavemen to a very poor copy of that today. Luckily, all of this is reversible by simply following your instruction manual and following the laws of human life. Save yourself, save your children and loved-ones, save your friends and family, save others.

So there you have it. That's where we are today, and tomorrow doesn't look any better if we continue this non-sense and allow the authorities to benefit financially from poisoning us on purpose.

1.6 Key Points

Our body is the perfect creation and will always strive for perfect health, therefore health is the rule and disease is the exception.

Health depends on the perfection of the organism and the conditions under which life exists. Humans require air, water, food, and light, freedom from violence, rest, exercise and hygiene.

Disease is nothing more than an internal act of physiology by our body in an attempt to stay alive, or to regain perfect health. Disease itself is the cure. Degenerative diseases and cancers are caused by the continuous neglect of the human body and the laws of human life.

Our modern health standard is ridiculously low and what we consider healthy today is far from perfect health. Current health standards and 'normality' are merely averages of what a bunch of abnormal, overstimulated men and women represent. Our health standard should at least approach ideal or optimal.

Due to civilization, industrialization, and commercialization we are consuming nutrient-depleted, man-made foods and drinks and using man-made products (drugs, cleaning detergents, soaps, cosmetic products, toothpaste etc.), all of them loaded with toxins, colorings, preservatives, antibiotics, pesticides etc. Furthermore, we are exposed to a multitude of environmental toxins including dirty air and dirty water. The constant onslaught of these toxins taxes our body and results in an overburdened system, prone to chronic disease and cancer.

You are committing nutritional suicide. Help yourself and do something about it.

You may be committing nutritional homicide. Help your children and loved-ones and do something about it.

You may be committing nutritional genocide. Help thousands of other people and do something about it.

It's time to take responsibility for your behavior now that you are finally aware of it. Keep reading and discover the truth. Put the Action Plan in motion and save yourself, your loved-ones and everyone else. You and only you can do this! You can't count on the government, the FDA, the advice of your doctor or Dr. Oz.

Chapter 2 – Aging Theories & Disease

In this chapter, I'm going into more detail with regard to the HOW and WHY of certain key concepts. It may be confusing at times to some of you, but no worries. You have two options when things get a little confusing:

1. Read the paragraph again and dissect the message; repeat until you understand.

2. Ignore and keep on reading. You may get an understanding when more info is presented later in this book.

Here we go...

Several theories have tried to answer the age old question: why do we age and eventually die? What can we do to extend the boundaries of our own existence?

Advances in genetics and molecular biology uncovered some of the answers, and it's important to therefore expand on the Free Radical Theory in this chapter.

Besides this Free Radical Theory, several other aging theories exist, most of them being what we call *'structural damage' theories*. These theories are based on the concept that the molecular components of the cell begin to malfunction and break down over time. When many cells malfunction, eventually tissues and organs are affected and degenerative disease takes form.

The 'Wear and Tear' theory (1982) stipulates that because of the daily use and abuse our body literally wears out and that aging occurs when this wear and tear exceeds the body's ability to repair.

The 'Waste Accumulation' theory proposes that our cells accumulate more and more waste products as part of our normal metabolic processes. The build-up of this toxic waste compromises function as we age.

The 'Errors and Repair' theory engages the concept that aging is caused by damage to our DNA (genetic structure) due to faulty repairs. Accumulation of these faulty repairs leads to errors in protein manufacturing, therefore accelerating aging.

There are several other structural damage theories, but I assume you are getting the idea. Besides these structural damage theories we also have *'Programmed Obsolescence' theories* which stipulate that aging and death are the inevitable consequences of the workings of an internal biological clock. This clock is programmed at conception and decides when cells can no longer function and reproduce at a rate sufficient to maintain health.

2.1 Free Radicals & Antioxidants

The Free Radical Theory was first proposed in 1954 by Dr. Denham Harman. Today, the majority of degenerative disease is believed to involve free radical activity. Of course, as we will discuss later, degenerative diseases are not really separate entities but rather different forms of expression of chronically impaired health.

What are Free Radicals?

Don't get stressed over this stuff if it's not clear... just keep on reading.

Most of us have heard of 'free radicals' before, but what are they?

As you probably remember from your old high school days, atoms consist of a nucleus, neutrons, protons and electrons. The number of protons (positively charged particles) in the atom's nucleus determines the number of electrons (negatively charged particles) surrounding the atom. Electrons are involved in chemical reactions and are the substance that bonds atoms together to form molecules. Normally, bonds don't split in a way that leaves a molecule with an odd, unpaired electron. But when weak bonds split, free radicals are formed. Free radicals are very unstable and react quickly with other compounds, trying to capture the needed electron to gain stability. Generally, free radicals attack the nearest stable molecule, 'stealing' its electron. When the 'attacked' molecule loses its electron, it becomes oxidized and therefore a free radical itself, beginning **a chain reaction**. Once the process is started, it can *cascade*, disrupting the living cell, resulting in impaired health (if not counteracted by potent, natural antioxidants).

In short, *free radicals* are atoms, molecules and molecular fragments with unpaired electrons making them *very reactive and unstable*. Therefore, free radicals can cause substantial *damage to the structure of the molecules in the cell*, impairing their function.

Where do Free Radicals come from?

Some free radicals arise normally during *metabolism*. Sometimes the body's *immune system* cells purposefully create them to neutralize viruses and bacteria. However, *environmental* factors such as industrial wastes, chemical residues, radiation, metals, cigarette smoke, pesticides and herbicides, and any material that is foreign to the body (called xenobiotic) can also spawn free radicals. Even certain *foods* such as processed and preserved meats and beverages (alcohol, coffee) are loaded with potent free radical generators. The most critical free radicals include hydrogen, hydrogen peroxide, hypochlorous acid, superoxide ion and singlet oxygen.

How does the Body deal with these Free Radicals?

Normally, the body can handle these highly reactive free radicals with endogenous (from within the body) and dietary (food intake) anti-oxidants. Antioxidants neutralize free radicals, stopping them dead in their tracks before they can cause structural damage to the cell. But if antioxidants are unavailable, or if the free-radical production becomes excessive, damage can occur.

The first line of defense against free radicals consists of three protective enzyme systems, which convert those free radicals into harmless substances such as water and oxygen. It is believed that with age, this enzyme system fails due to an impaired ability to make important functional proteins.

The second line of defense comes from the antioxidants we consume. Antioxidants neutralize free radicals by donating one of their own electrons, ending the electron-'stealing' reaction. The antioxidant nutrients themselves don't become free radicals by donating an electron because they are stable in either form. They act as scavengers, helping to prevent cell and tissue damage that could lead to cellular damage and disease. In this process, the antioxidant itself is altered chemically.

Antioxidants

Some of the many potent *dietary antioxidants* include vitamins (A, C, E, B1, B3, B5, B6 & B12), minerals (selenium, zinc, copper, manganese), mangosteen, beta-carotene, CoQ10, grape seeds, pomegranate, aloe vera, various berries, cloves, turmeric, cinnamon, cacao, bioflavonoids and hundreds of other plant-nutrients. Simply put, they come from Mother Nature's fruit and vegetables, plants and herbs!

Some of the *endogenous antioxidants* (produced within the body itself) include many of the body's natural enzymes, coenzymes, and sulfur containing molecules such as glutathione and n-acetyl-cysteine.

Some antioxidants, after they have neutralized a free radical and are altered chemically, are regenerated by the presence of other antioxidants. This is a good reason to consume a multitude of various antioxidants (a variety of fruits and vegetables plus a supplement containing a wide spectrum of antioxidants). Furthermore, various antioxidants also work in different areas of the cell. We can conclude that *antioxidants thus work together as a team* and therefore eating a monotone diet or supplementing with one single or few nutrients/antioxidants would be insufficient to control the free radicals in our body.

Balance is required

Not everything about free radicals is bad news though. Free radicals play a central role in *respiration* and a number of other biological processes. They are crucial in the *body's immune response* also, destroying bacteria and other pathogens. Free radicals even assist in initiating the *inflammatory response*. So while we can't live without free radicals, we can't live with too many of them either. The key is balance! The body requires an optimal nutritional state, moderate exercise, adequate rest, and a clean environment. We must make sure that we have sufficient antioxidant stores in our cells while simultaneously avoiding the exposure to free radicals from our environment and our diet. When the balance is impaired and an excess of free radicals causes damage to the cell, the process of degenerative disease and accelerated aging starts. Our cells oxidize and our body slowly rusts away.

2.2 Chronic Inflammation – The Silent Killer

By definition, inflammation is a normal action by the body as part of its defense against pathogens or injury. The symptoms of *acute inflammation* are redness, heat, swelling, and pain (for example a sprained ankle). The symptoms of *chronic, systemic* (involving the whole system) or *silent* inflammation are entirely different and if un-checked turn into degenerative disease. Silent inflammation causes the body to turn on itself and the immune defense system attacks the organs and tissues. In response to this systemic attack from within, the body produces even more inflammation and free radicals resulting in a perpetuating cycle. Spreading like wild fire, this systemic inflammation damages cells, tissues, organs, and arteries. It compromises the immune system while stimulating cancer growth. It's the first step toward *degenerative disease*.

Studies show conclusively that systemic inflammation is involved in allergies, Alzheimer's, anemia, ankylosing spondylitis, aortic valve stenosis, arthritis, cancer, Crohn's disease, congestive heart failure, diabetes, fibromyalgia, fibrosis, hypertension, heart attack, Huntington's disease, irritable bowel syndrome, kidney disease, lupus, metabolic syndrome, MS, osteoporosis, Parkinson's disease, psoriasis, stroke etc. Of course... as we will learn in more depth later, all degenerative diseases are just various expressions of the same condition: chronic impaired health.

To pick an example, cardiovascular disease, is finally regarded as an inflammatory process much like rheumatoid arthritis and no longer a result of high cholesterol or cholesterol blockage, which always has been a myth to say the least (more in chapter 15). Paul Ridker, a Harvard cardiologist, identified several principal clinical markers for systemic inflammation (C-reactive protein or CRP, fibrinogen, homocysteine etc.) and showed a highly significant correlation between the levels of these markers and cardiovascular disease: the higher the level of the marker (a signaling molecule that initiates inflammation), the greater the risk for cardiovascular disease. Several studies show that cholesterol most likely does not pose any danger itself.

Systemic or chronic inflammation is also the underlying cause of excess body fat and the inability to lose weight, regardless the efforts taken with popular diets and weight loss programs.

So instead of dealing with the ramifications of any of the above degenerative diseases or getting involved with allopathic medicine (drugs and surgery) and receiving radical treatments, wouldn't it be wiser to just take preventative measures to reduce and control this systemic inflammation today?

So what causes this systemic inflammation?

To understand the dynamics, one has to know about <u>Eicosanoids</u> (what a tongue twister). These eicosanoids are a large group of fat-like substances derived from essential fatty acids through our diet. They play the central role in <u>regulating the levels of inflammation in our body</u>. Some of these eicosanoids are inflammatory and yet others are anti-inflammatory. In a healthy body there is a dynamic balance between these opposing eicosanoids.

The *inflammatory* ones (prostaglandins which cause pain and leukotrienes which cause swelling) are certainly necessary in the body's efforts against acute trauma and infection but their excess initiates degenerative disease. It pays to know that these inflammatory ones are manufactured from arachidonic acid (AA) which is found in animal-based products such as red meats and shellfish. AA is also manufactured within the body from an *omega-6* essential fatty acid (linoleic acid). Rich sources of linoleic acid are borage oil, primrose oil and black current seed oil. This pathway which manufactures the inflammatory eicosanoids is controlled by an enzyme: COX-2. Vitamin E (in the form of gamma tocopherol only) and curcumin (found in the Indian spice turmeric, which is also a great pain reliever) both block the activity of COX-2. Oh, and yes this is a much better approach than swallowing poisonous Celebrex pills that also attempt to block COX-2 but with lots of adverse reactions (the body tries to expel poisonous substances).

The *anti-inflammatory* eicosanoids are manufactured from eicosapentaenoic acid (EPA will do) which is derived from alpha-linoleic acid (ALA will do). ALA is an essential omega-3 fatty acid. Rich sources of omega-3 fatty acids are fatty cold water fish (salmon and sardines) and canola, flax seeds and pumpkin seeds. Another essential *omega-3* fatty acid is DHA which converts into EPA. So, both EPA and DHA manufacture these anti-inflammatory eicosanoids but they also block the formation of AA. In other words, they kill two birds with one stone: they produce not only anti-inflammatory eicosanoids but they also block the production of the inflammatory eicosanoids.

Optimal health is achieved when the inflammatory and anti-inflammatory eicosanoids are in balance. Disease is promoted when these eico-sanoids are out of balance because a cascade of systemic (silent) inflammation arises.

Interesting to note is that high insulin levels increase oxidative stress and promote the conversion of AA, therefore increasing inflammatory eicosanoids. As you already know, high insulin levels are the result of a chronic sugar overload, a state of insulin resistance or the hormonal effects of excess fat.

As inflammation rises, so does cortisol, an anti-stress hormone that will try and reduce the inflammation. But it places a heavy burden on all the organs by increasing blood pressure, elevating blood-sugar levels and suppressing the immune-system.

Both the systemic inflammation and elevated levels of cortisol are responsible for degenerative diseases.

But no worries! *All we have to do is balance the production of inflamma-tory and anti-inflammatory eicosanoids, right? Yes.*

How to achieve Balance?

The current problem is that the S.A.D. (Standard American Diet) is loaded with omega-6 fatty acids (which promote inflammation) and lacks omega-3 fatty acids (which reduce inflammation).

So we must simultaneously:

1. Reduce the dietary intake of AA (which produces omega-6 fatty acids) present in animal products (red meats and shellfish) and foods high in saturated fats,

2. Reduce the dietary intake of linoleic acid present in borage oil, primrose oil and black current seed oil,

3. Increase the dietary intake of fatty cold water fish (salmon and sardines) and canola, flax seeds and pumpkin seeds,

raw nuts and grains,

4. Consider supplementing with a high-quality cold-pressed fish oil or krill supplement (omega-3, not omega-6, or at least the right balance),

5. Increase the dietary intake of vitamin E (gamma tocopherol), and consider turmeric (curry blends) and anti-inflammatory foods.

Some of the most potent anti-inflammatory foods are:

Cruciferous vegetables (broccoli, Brussel sprouts, kale and cauliflower), Kelp (Kombu, wakame and arame are good sources), certain fruits (blueberries, strawberries, citrus fruits, papaya, cherries), ginger, garlic, onions, green tea, extra virgin olive oil, sweet potatoes and others.

Some more foods that promote inflammation and need to be removed or reduced:

Sugar is everywhere. Try and limit processed foods, desserts and snacks with excess sugar, and opt for fruits low in sugar.

Dairy is one of the worst foods men can consume (refer to chapter 15). Milk is a common allergen that can trigger inflammation, stomach problems, skin rashes, hives and even breathing difficulties.

Trans-fats increase bad cholesterol, promote inflammation, obesity and resistance to insulin. They are found in fried foods, fast foods, commercially baked goods, such as peanut butter and items prepared with partially hydrogenated oil, margarine and vegetable oil.

Common Cooking Oils: Safflower, soy, sunflower, corn, and cottonseed promote inflammation and are made with cheap ingredients.

Regular consumption of alcohol causes irritation and inflammation to numerous organs.

Refined products have no fiber and have a high glycemic index. They are everywhere: white rice, white flour, white bread, pasta, pastries etc. Try to replace them with minimally processed grains.

Artificial food additives: Aspartame and MSG are two common food additives that can trigger inflammatory responses. Omit them completely from the diet.

More about meats:

The meat of animals which are fed with grains like soy and corn is highly inflammatory. These animals also gain excess fat and are injected with hormones and antibiotics.

Always opt for organic, free-range meats which have been fed natural diets. Red meat contains a molecule that humans don't naturally produce called Neu5GC. Once you ingest this compound, your body develops antibodies which may trigger constant inflammatory responses.

The Link

Inflammation is now thought to be the initiating factor in up to 98% of all disease. Please note that there is a critical link between oxidative stress and inflammation: oxidative stress promotes inflammation as inflammation promotes oxidative stress.

With the knowledge and understanding you acquired so far in this chapter you can clearly see that the onslaught of free radicals and the systemic inflammation in our body are detrimental to our health and need to be dealt with, not when degenerative disease and cancer pop their ugly head but NOW when it's not too late to reverse the situation.

The Solution

Looking at the solution to combat free radicals and oxidation (antioxidants) and the solution to combat systemic inflammation (vegetables, fruits, natural substances), we can already see yet again that the dietary creations from Mother Nature are the solution, while man-made poisons are the cause. Just by putting our body in the necessary conditions for optimal health (clean water, clean air, clean food, rest etc.) we can regain and maintain optimal health. Don't be one of the millions whose health is squandered by the current medical system that only deals with symptoms and never addresses the cause.

2.3 What is Toxemia?

Toxemia is defined as toxins in the blood.

Metabolism is defined as the normal functions and processes of the body to maintain health and life.

In a healthy body, cells are constantly being built (anabolism) and destroyed (catabolism) as part of normal metabolism. The destroyed tissue is toxic matter and in a healthy body this toxic matter is eliminated from the blood and body.

However, when the body's energy to fulfill this crucial job of elimination is dissipated to attend to emergencies, the toxins retain in the blood. This is called toxemia.

The accumulation of these toxins continues until the energy is restored by removing the cause (the emergency).

What we call disease is just nature's effort to eliminate toxin from the blood and body (e.g. vomiting, diarrhea, fever, rash). All so called diseases are crises of toxemia.

Emergencies or Bad Habits

So what are these emergencies or bad habits that take the body's energy away from doing its job in eliminating these toxins? These emergencies include physical as well as mental/emotional ones:

1. Improper diet, overeating, eating several meals per day,

eating when not hungry, etc.

2. Too much excitement, too much entertainment, too much stimulation.

3. Too much light and noise.

4. Overwork.

5. Lack of rest and sleep.

6. Competition (school, work, sports).

7. Drugs and surgeries.

8. Vaccines and serums.

9. Use of stimulants such as coffee, tobacco, drugs, energy drinks etc.

10. Stress of any kind.

11. Self-pity, irritability, fear, anxiety, worry, grief, anger, shock.

12. Self-indulgence, egotism, selfishness, ambition and disappointment, envy, dishonesty.

13. Any excess emotion (e.g. jealousy).

All of these 'state of emergencies' or 'bad habits' put an unnecessary burden on the body. The body has to use vital energy to deal with and attend to these emergencies by constantly eliminating these 'extra' toxins from the body. If the bad habit or emergency is not removed, the body is forced to keep operating in overdrive and eventually toxins build up (called toxemia).

When more toxins build-up than the body is able to eliminate, disease processes are started in an attempt to purge these 'extra' toxins from the body. This expresses itself in *acute symptoms* (fever, chills, rash, diarrhea, vomiting etc.).

This disease process can be stopped at any time by simply removing the cause (which is the bad habit). However, conventional medicine has no clue to what the cause of such so called disease is and interferes with the body's effort to eliminate toxins. The prescription of drugs to reduce the fever or stop diarrhea or vomiting only halts the healing process.

If the bad habit continues, the disease process becomes more and more intense and continues. Why? The body has no other choice but to continue to try and eliminate these toxins in order to preserve health and life. At this stage symptoms may include pneumonia, bronchitis, gastritis, stomach ulcer etc. The stomach ulcer may be surgically removed and the pneumonia or bronchitis may be treated with antibiotics, but as long as the cause (bad habit) remains, the disease process continues to evolve, resulting in degenerative disease, cancer and death.

2.4 Acute Disease and Symptoms

We already established that disease is merely a state of impaired health and that the symptoms are just an expression of that impaired health in an effort to regain optimal health. But I know some of you are not convinced yet so I'm going to clarify this further and use some simple examples.

Germs

Every new school of 'science' arises with new theories, new dogmas, and new doctrines but with the same arrogance and bigotry as the previous schools. Often these new things are nothing but teachings by the schools, asserted to be scientifically proven when in actuality they only have been accepted by self-constituted authority.

So is the germ-theory yet another unsubstantiated, false 'scientific' theory in which the 'scientist' spends countless time finding specific germs for each disease. If only the 'scientist' would realize that unity of disease exists, in other words that all disease originates from a common cause. This common cause is certainly not the attack of a germ.

What are germs?

Germs are bacteria. Bacteriologists usually divide germs in two classes: saprophytic and parasitic. Saprophytic germs (98% of all germs) live off dead organic matter while parasitic germs (2% of all germs) survive off a living host.

What do they do?

Saprophytic germs are scavengers, breaking down and transforming dead matter into usable forms for the nourishment of growing vegetation. Plants and animals wouldn't survive long without the presence of these germs. Therefore humans depend on germ life.

An example is a healthy, beautiful deer that has never been sick (wild animals don't know what sickness is). The deer gets shot by a hunter. All the functions of life cease. If left alone, the corps starts smelling foul after just a few hours and after a few more hours we have a mass of putrid flesh, swarming with bacteria (germs). The germs are multiplying rapidly and are destroying the body of the deer. A few days later, the germs have turned all flesh into inorganic matter; they consumed it and returned it to its primitive elements (dust). Question: why did the germs not do this while the deer was alive? Germs don't attack living, healthy flesh.

Parasitic germs always live off a living host and are said to produce disease. It's stated that these parasitic germs differ from the saprophytic germs in that they can produce toxins. The fact is that both groups of germs are harmless and identical but that non-toxic germs can only become toxic in a toxic environment (yes, read that sentence again). Germs are powerless against the healthy body.

Germs cannot cause disease

It's not the so called germs or pathogens in our external environment that make us ill. They are ALWAYS there: in the air, in the water, in our food, in our drinks… they have always been there, they are there now and they will always be there.

We cannot escape them and attempting to destroy them is folly. We cannot avoid germs. We can only prevent their invasion by being in great health.

We are constantly exposed to them and yet we are not always feeling sick, right?

It's *the condition of our internal environment* that dictates whether or not that pathogen will wreak havoc and sickness or not. When our body is in a state of good health, the pathogen is neutralized as fast as it enters the body or even prior to entering the body (tonsils acting as guards, sneezing etc.). When our health is compromised due to our poor life-style choices, bad food and drink choices, our daily stress or an imbalance of emotions, our internal environment is compromised.

So, the war with the pathogen is then fought on the inside, not the outside! To illustrate this even further (yes, it's really important to grasp this truth) I'm going to use an analogy used by Michael Murray. Let's use New York City as the setting and let's imagine that the garbage collectors didn't come and collect the piles of garbage in front of each apartment for weeks. Then rats would be running all over the streets enjoying the garbage festival, wouldn't they? Now, killing the rats wouldn't do much to solve the problem, would it? They would keep on coming from everywhere until the garbage was taken away, right? The rats are always in New York City; what would draw them out on the streets would be piles and piles of garbage. Let's translate that to our bodies: the germs or pathogens are always there in our external environment and what draws them out and welcomes them are a pile of toxins in our body (weak internal environment).

Think about this… what if someone states something like "6 kids out of my son's class all got this flu that's going around". What does that mean? Does it mean that germs are biased? Or does it mean that germs have the ability to be selective or take part in racial profiling? Or maybe it just means that 6 kids have a compromised internal environment at the time of exposure, and the other 7 kids (let's say there are 13 kids in the class) are in a state of good health at that same time of exposure. Again, it's not the external environment that causes symptoms and disease, but a compromised or weak internal environment. It's also in these situations that people use the term 'contagious' while all that seems to be contagious these days is poor health, not the so called germs.

Many studies also confirm this simple truth about germs. One of the more recent studies conducted a comparison of two controlled groups of children of the same age. One group of children grew up on farms exposed to all kinds of germs typically associated with farm animals. At the same time, the second controlled group of children lived in a city environment, and they were protected (as much as one can of course) from germs by their parents. The children who grew up on the farms had significantly less incidence of disease.

Paranoia

Something that cracks me up every time I see it is the germ paranoia of people. I see them use antiseptic and antibacterial soaps, gels, sprays and wipes and get this toxic junk smeared over their hands and what not, even wiping off the shopping carts in the supermarket or the door handle before they touch it. OMG. Did you know that we survived germs for thousands of years without antiseptic and antibacterial soaps, gels, sprays and wipes? Of course, we are more susceptible to them today because YOUR INTERNAL ENVIRONMENT is COMPROMISED. Enough said.

The only reason one could justify the use of these poisons on your skin is to protect the weak, for example if one is working with sick patients. Still, the sick and weak patient will not be protected from the billions of germs he or she is exposed to daily (for example, according to germ theorists, only through the nose alone over 14,000 germs pass on average every hour) regardless the hand washing and antibacterial soap use.

<u>Germs Conclusion</u>

It's simple, clear and common sense that germs do not cause disease. They may play a factor in disease but only when they enter a compromised body.

The medical profession is hard pressed for a means to save the flawed germ theory. They first professed that germs cause disease, but since the presence of germs does not cause disease, they have to have an 'unknown cause' which causes the germs to cause disease. This solves their dilemma. Strange I think, a science based on the 'unknown'.

Would the promotion and cultivation of a healthy body not be far more sensible in the defense against these germs or pathogens as opposed to the ridiculous efforts to immunize everyone with vaccines and serums? Their toxicity further compromises the health of the already sick person, and more germs will enter the body wreaking havoc.

What SYMPTOMS really are

I'll start with an example which I will use to clarify what symptoms really are:

Bad eating causes acid fermentation which irritates the mucous membrane of the stomach. In a healthy body, the toxins entering the stomach are expelled through acts of indigestion such as vomiting.

Prolonged <u>irritation</u> however will cause <u>inflammation</u> and prolonged inflammation then causes <u>ulceration</u> of the stomach, resulting in thickening and hardening of the mucous membrane of the stomach ending up in stomach <u>cancer</u> at last. This last step occurs because of degeneration of the stomach due to lack of oxygen and nutrients which causes toxins and septic waste to enter the bloodstream.

Along the course of this disease process various symptoms show up.

In the early stages we see attacks of indigestion and gastritis: stomach sickness, nausea and vomiting. Nervous people may present with nervous symptoms such as headaches and insomnia while some women may exhibit symptoms of painful menstruation etc.

As the disease becomes more chronic, some may present with anemia, infection or ulceration (intestinal or gastric) while others may present with bleeding (from ulcer), food retention (toxic build-up expelled by vomiting every few days caused by partial closing of the pylorus) and so on. Cancer may be next.

When we look at this example we can conclude several things. First and most importantly, *we can stop this disease process at any time by taking away the cause: bad eating habits.* Science can study pathology (organic change) till doomsday without shedding any light on the cause. Physicians should know that these early stages of disease are purely functional and that no interference is necessary. When the irritation stops, normal functioning is resumed. However, when irritation continues, the pathology evolves.

So let me ask you: will drugs to stop vomiting or anti-inflammatories help in the early stages? Will surgically removing a stomach ulcer be beneficial? Of course not, it's a waste of time. It's a pure symptomatic treatment, most likely aggravating and worsening the pathology by interfering with the body's healing process.

Second: the stomach pain, indigestion, poor appetite, headache, nausea, vomiting, gastritis, heavy menstrual cramps, anemia, stomach ulcers, intestinal ulcers, internal bleeding, cancer etc. are ALL JUST SYMPTOMS. They are ALL *expressions and attempts of our body to expel the toxins.* If the cause and irritation is not taken away, the symptoms and pathology evolve. These symptoms are not a disease (for example: a stomach ulcer is NOT a disease, it's a symptom) and studying these symptoms is a waste of time, and treating them also.

The same holds true for every other pathology or disease process in our body. The common cold or a 'running nose' for example will at first cause irritation and then inflammation (periodic and functional). If the irritation is not stopped, the inflammation will become more intense and continuous, eventually causing thickening and hardening of the mucous membrane and an organic change of the organ. Chronic, degenerative disease or cancer is the end-stage.

What is Acute Disease?

Now that we are clear on what symptoms REALLY are, let's define acute disease. You already know! Acute disease is nothing more than *a curative process* in which the body defends against pathogens and toxins, expelling them from our body.

The living system acts on food (from nature) to build, replenish and renew tissues and organs. This is called digestion and assimilation. The living system also acts on drugs, poisons, impurities, dead matter, infections and everything else not useful or usable in our organic body by resisting, expelling, and purifying processes such as running a fever, having chills, coughing, sneezing, sweating, fainting, vomiting, getting a rash, having diarrhea etc. (symptoms). It's simply a vigorous effort of the body to remove useless and harmful matter and restore balance and optimal health.

In short, acute disease is really not a disease. The symptoms of the body – wrongly labeled acute disease - are a functional and vital part of the body's attempt to eliminate toxins and obtain perfect health.

2.5 Degenerative Diseases Explained

Well, if you paid attention, you can answer already what degenerative diseases really are, how they are caused, and how we can 'cure' them.

Toxemia is the cause of any so called disease and if unchecked and continued, the disease state progresses and ends as a chronic degenerative disease, cancer and death. We can extrapolate that theory to our free radical theory and the systemic inflammation. A build-up of free radicals (unchecked by potent antioxidants) or an ongoing systemic

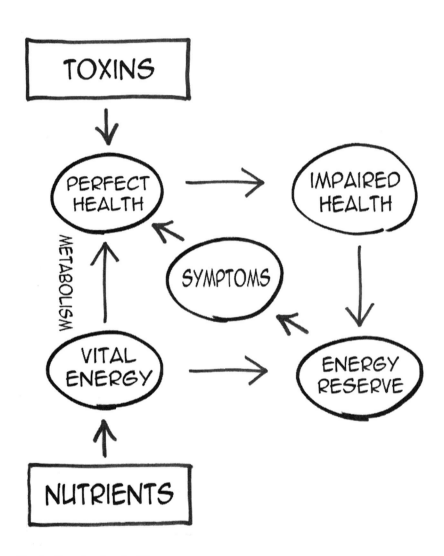

Illustration 4 – Acute Disease

inflammation (due to an imbalance of inflammatory and anti-inflammatory eicosanoids) both result in a build-up of poisons or toxins in our blood, tissues, organs and body.

In any acute 'disease', the symptoms (fever, cold, vomiting, diarrhea, poor appetite, headache, pain, swelling, indigestion, nausea etc.) are only an attempt of the body to eliminate toxins from the body. If not interfered with (drugs, foods) and if the cause (not the symptoms) or bad habit is removed, optimal health will return very soon (as soon as the poisons are expelled). When the bad habit or cause continues, the disease will only progress as the body is unable to eliminate the toxins produced by normal metabolism because its energy is used to check the toxins from the emergency (bad habit). The cold becomes pneumonia and the stomach pain becomes a stomach ulcer and eventually stomach cancer.

No matter what the degenerative disease, they are all an expression of the same cause: toxic accumulation. They all develop over a lifetime and are the product of our dietary and lifestyle choices. They are our life sentence.

Years in the Making

We have taken our health for granted and assume that this perfect creation that was given to us can be abused over and over again. Trust me, our body can take a lot, if not we wouldn't make the age of 2.

Every living cell strives for perfect health, all the time. It can't do otherwise. Today in our modern society, we are 'too busy', everything gets in the way of eating healthy, rest and sleep, exercise, and cleansing.

Today, over 80% of Americans suffer from chronic disease. Unfortunately, most people accept the onset of these chronic, degenerative diseases such as arthritis and diabetes as an inevitable result of the aging process while the truth is that all of these can be prevented. Yes, even cancer! Now that you know that cancer is just the result of toxemia, you not only can prevent cancer but also stop it in its tracks.

These degenerative diseases however pass under our radar. They don't happen overnight and they take decades to develop. All that time your body has been trying to stop this ongoing process but you have been stealing its energy to deal with your bad habits and emergencies and you failed to remove these bad habits or causes of toxemia.

Then suddenly, after 10, 20 or 30 years symptoms appear and the doctor diagnoses you with a degenerative disease. Immediately, the doctor comes out with his or hers heavy artillery (drugs, surgery, radiation etc.) but cutting, burning, and poisoning won't reverse the disease state. Only removing the cause and placing your body in the right conditions for perfect health can.

What about cancer?

Just as any other degenerative disease, cancer is the end-stage of toxemia (unchecked toxic build-up, free radicals galore, systemic inflammation), in which the blue-print of our molecules (DNA) has been damaged.

Since President Nixon (1971) declared the 'War on Cancer' and despite the billions of dollars poured into this campaign and the flawed research on cancer over the years, survival rates have not significantly improved. Of course not!

First of all, there is no cure. The cure only exists in taking away the cause of cancer, which is toxemia. Regardless of this oversight by conventional medicine, the profiteering by a multibillion dollar industry influencing and manipulating our politics and research cannot be ignored. Even if there was a magic bullet or cure for cancer (which there is not and never will be), it would not be in the financial interest of the drug manufacturers, oncologists, hospitals, nursing homes, medical equipment manufacturers (PET scans), etc. to find it.

Ignorance and stupidity are the terms to describe the research on cancer (and any other so called disease). One can study pathology to infinity but will never find the cause, and suppressing symptoms will not cure the disease. Critics have called the 'War on Cancer' a 'medical

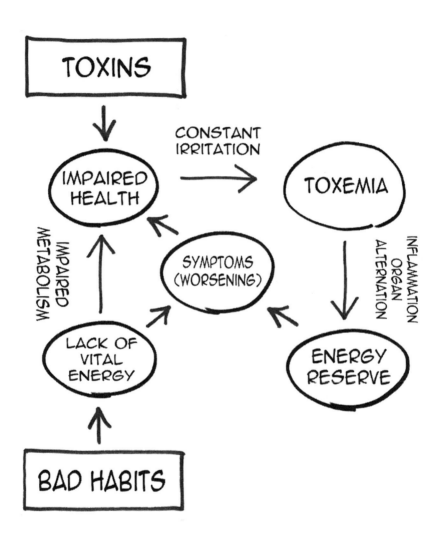

Illustration 5 – Degenerative Disease

Vietnam'. Linus Pauling (Nobel laureate) stated: "Everyone should know that the war on cancer is largely a fraud". We have been and still are desperately looking for a magic bullet, an elixir, a miracle drug while ignoring the underlying cause.

Just as with degenerative diseases, cancer is the result of long-standing deficiencies in the body's physiological and nutritional status. Just as with degenerative diseases, cancer can be prevented and resolved by removing the REAL cause (not symptoms) and placing the diseased body in the right conditions for healing (rest, clean air, clean water, clean food).

2.6 Key Points

As part of normal metabolism, a healthy body continuously removes toxic matter.

Our poor lifestyle choices, poor food choices, daily stresses and indulgences, and unbalanced emotions rob energy from our body so it can no longer carry out its task of removing toxic matter effectively.

If toxins build up (*toxemia*), degenerative disease is initiated and will continue to progress unless the cause is removed. The cause is one or more poor lifestyle choices.

Free radicals are necessary for certain bodily functions, but when in excess and unchecked will cause a cascade of damage to all living cells and tissues in the body.

Free radicals can be neutralized prior to causing cell damage by potent, natural antioxidants. *Antioxidants* work as a team and therefore a variety of vegetables and fruits containing these antioxidants must be consumed.

Inflammation in our body is controlled by fatty substances called eicosanoids. A balance of inflammatory and anti-inflammatory eicosanoids maintains health, while an excess of inflammatory eicosanoids causes chronic inflammation, also labeled systemic or 'silent' inflammation. Systemic inflammation attacks the body's own tissues and organs and this attack causes even more inflammation along with more free radicals, resulting in a perpetuating cycle. Degenerative disease and cancer is the result.

Symptoms are just an expression of the body in a state of impaired health in an effort to remove toxins and useless matter from to body and restore optimal health. Symptoms are not diseases and do not need any medicine nor any form of treatment.

Acute disease is merely a *curative process* of the body that doesn't require any interference, while *degenerative disease* is the unchecked build-up of toxins resulting in more intense and continuous symptoms. Degenerative disease doesn't require any interference either; drugs and treatment only robs more energy and worsens the disease state.

Only when the cause of disease (lifestyle habit) is removed, the body can heal when placed in the right conditions.

Chapter 3 – Health Freedom

In this chapter you will discover the truth about WHAT really HEALS and WHAT really KILLS, and WHO is responsible for your health.

Over the last few decades more and more people have finally been questioning the medical monopoly and its lack of results, along with its killing list. Medical errors and overtreatment are the 3rd leading cause of death in the U.S. Over 100,000 people per year, in the U.S. alone, die because of these errors or wrong interventions.

During the Vietnam War (1955-1975) 47,424 Americans gave their life. WWI caused 53,402 American casualties and WWII 291,557 over a 4 year period (1941-1945), which averages 72,890 deaths per year. On 9/11 almost 3,000 people lost their lives. Keep in mind that these wars are single events, while the 100,000 Americans that die because of medical errors and overtreatment is continuous, YEAR AFTER YEAR!

The problem is that most of these mistakes are attributed to not only human error, but also lack of communication between different disciplines, equipment failure, diagnostic error resulting in wrong treatment, misinterpretation of results etc. Even though efforts are made to reduce these mistakes, this approach is obsolete. The arrogance and short-sightedness of the medical profession is beyond belief. Constantly making efforts to try and fix details while forgetting about the big picture. The big picture is HEALTH. The CAUSE of so called disease is bad habits and poor lifestyle choices.

If the medical profession would educate the people in HEALTH, and address the one and only cause of all disease, and STOP chasing symptoms like a crazy madman shooting in the dark, we even wouldn't have a term 'medical errors' and we would have 100,000 less deaths per year. Yes, it's that simple. No interventions that interfere with the healing process of the body, no poisons to interfere with this healing process, no drugs, no surgeries.

Conventional medicine has ONLY ONE place in our society: TRAUMA. Yes, that's it. If one gets into a car accident or suffers a life-threatening trauma (fall, gun-shot wound etc.), emergency medicine can save a life.

All other conventional medicine activity should be stopped in its tracks! Really, is this guy serious you may ask? Of course! Did you not just read that the medical profession kills over 100,000 Americans each and every year? Only the acute trauma patients benefit from this system. I know 'other' emergencies end-up at the ER also, but these are merely crises of toxemia, end-stages of degenerative disease, death around the corner... and even if this person is so-called 'saved' in the ER, we all know it's just a matter of time. A little time was bought. The person wasn't saved; saving that person would mean to address the cause of his or her disease and place the body in the conditions needed to recover from that disease.

Every trip to the doctor, a specialist, or 'alternative' health care professional results in one or another way of trying to resolve a medical problem or disease. A treatment, a drug, a nutrient, a new method, surgery... they all interfere with the body's intrinsic power to heal. This artificial approach and attempt to try and circumvent the laws of life is very costly while simply following the laws of life would be much cheaper and easier. However, the artificial approach does allow the medical professional to exploit the suffering of millions of people whose health is destroyed by drugs and mutilating surgeries.

Health care professionals are nothing but a product of their environment, their education. This education in the medical schools is not based on science (sure, science of the 'unknown cause') but merely on thought (schools of thought), dogmas and false hypothesis. The emphasis is on pathology, disease and symptoms and the drugs that mask these symptoms until worse symptoms pop up. It's preoccupied with useless details while ignoring the cause of all disease and while ignoring the fact that there is only one cause of all disease. This faulty education in the schools of medicine has caused these thoughts to crystalize into habits. The eradication of these habits is very difficult. Only a paradigm-shift can cause such an event.

3.1 Your Doctor: Foe or Fab?

Let's not call your doctor a foe, but let's not call him or her fab either. Let's call your doctor a product of his or her environment. Your doctor or health care professional may have great knowledge in pathology, symptomatology, and pharmacology (drugs) but unfortunately has NO understanding of them. Your doctor doesn't know WHAT disease or pathology REALLY is, what SYMPTOMS really are, what ACUTE disease really is and WHY degenerative disease rears its ugly head. Your doctor has no clue as to what the cause of disease is. He or she wrongly assumes that diabetes is the cause of the numbness in your feet while both are just symptoms; he or she wrongly assumes that Parkinson's is the cause of gait abnormality and tremors while Parkinson's itself is a symptom complex. Your doctor just doesn't understand.

We don't need more knowledge, we need more understanding.

Your doctor is the product of a faulty medical system based on faulty thoughts, science that's not science at all, and a relentless arrogance to stick with its dogmas and doctrines in a relentless attempt to keep its head above the water. But the end is near.

The people are awakening. The information is out. The system is crashing. And (if willing) the doctors can open their eyes and start being part of the HEALTH FREEDOM movement, educating people on health and the laws of human life.

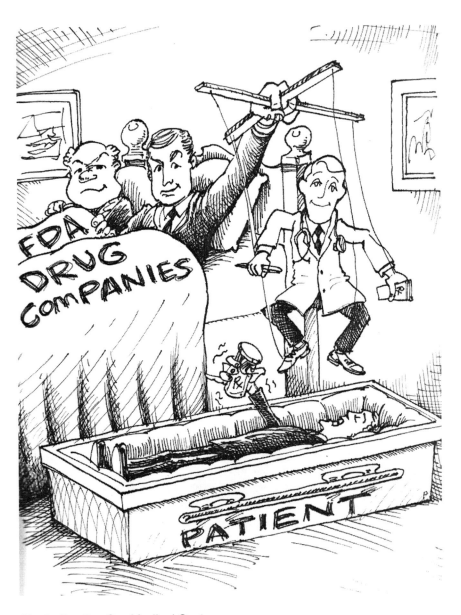

Illustration 6 – Our Medical System

It's not your doctor's fault: he or she has been corrupted by the medical profession. This profession is the most powerful and organized in the world and has captured the schools, government, army and navy, and all commercial and industrial organizations. It dictates what can and cannot be taught in school, and the press is biased and close-minded and wouldn't hesitate a second to lie in the interest of medicine. Your doctor's education is based on thoughts that sadly are wrong and your doctor was pulled into the current faulty medical system. These doctors are like a puppet on a string, influenced and bossed around by their medical associations, insurance companies and pharmaceutical companies. If you are a doctor reading this, don't get all bent out of shape and realize this truth, rise above it and start really helping and healing your patients.

In my modest opinion, about 40% of doctors and health care professionals still really care about their patients. Some of them actually really believe that they are helping their patients, while others realize that their intervention is not the solution but they don't know what else to do. The other 60% couldn't care less anymore: they don't listen to the patient, they have lost their bedside manner and lack empathy. They are part of a system that prescribes drugs and cuts open body parts. They are stuck in a material world, milking the system for the financial gain so the bills can be paid. Sad but true.

3.2 Drugs & Surgeries

I know I repeat myself, but repetition makes the mind remember, and if repeated enough a habit is created. In this case, a good habit, a RIGHT habit.

<u>What are drugs?</u>

Pharmaceutical drugs are synthetic, man-made poisons manufactured in a laboratory. The purpose of their existence is so that certain people monetarily benefit from the suffering of millions of people. While the solutions to suffering and so called disease are present in Mother

Nature, these natural forms of healing plants, herbs and foods cannot be patented. In other words, a drug company could not make any substantial profits from suggesting and selling a natural remedy.

So what they do is find the food, plant or herb in Mother Nature with the healing properties for a certain so called disease, then identify the so called active nutrient containing those healing properties, and then try and synthetically copy that nutrient in a laboratory.

As much as they try, each of those drugs comes with a wash list of side-effects, while its natural counterpart is (most of the time) safe and doesn't cause any side-effect. Why is that? A food, or herb or plant contains thousands of nutrients, all of them working in synergy.

Isolating a single nutrient is not only pure non-sense but changes the dynamics and inhibits or totally abolishes its benefits. That's what happens with many supplements also. But the drug companies have to take it a step further. Once they isolate that single, active nutrient they now have to make a fake copy of it in the laboratory, and then patent the drug so cash can be made.

Dead matter cannot ACT

Drugs and pills are just dead, poisonous matter. No living properties. Did you know that only life things can act? Did you know that dead stuff can't do anything? I'm just being facetious. You don't have to 'know' this, it's common sense. Some dead poison cannot act, drugs cannot DO anything. It's our body, our living system, which acts upon the dead matter or the drug in this case. Our body reacts to the intake of these poisons by trying to expel them and purify the body.

That's also why each drug has a wash-list of side effects. I know you laugh when you see these T.V. commercials for drugs, right? For example a drug for depression that may cause suicidal thoughts? LMAO.

These so called side effects are all different attempts of the body to expel the toxic drug. They may differ from person to person. Each person's state of health is different and the conditions at the time of ingesting the drug may be different. So some people may experience vomiting and nausea and dizziness while other may experience headaches, heavy menstrual cramps, fatigue etc. People already in a severely compromised state of health may just die.

Can you also see now how absurd it is to perform an autopsy to determine the cause of death? Dead matter doesn't act, it's dead. Sure, one may find cancer in the dead body, but that's NOT the cause of death.

The cancer is the end-stage of a long-term degeneration of a tissue or organ, merely the last symptom. Maybe, one finds out that a heart attack was the cause of death after autopsy? Again, the heart attack was the last symptom, certainly not the cause of death. The cause started decades ago - poor lifestyle choices - ignored all along.

<u>Surgery</u>

Unless performed after a trauma such as a fall or car accident, surgeries never save lives. They only speed up life so death approaches sooner. In the best case, they buy a little time.

Cutting out an ulcer or a tumor is just cutting out a symptom while ignoring the cause. By cutting out a tumor or ulcer or abscess or cyst or whatever, the cause is not taken away and the disease process just continues and worsens, most likely aggravated by the surgical intervention.

Wouldn't it be much easier to halt the disease in its tracks by removing the cause? The body will heal itself, ALWAYS and CONSTANT as long as we are alive, when we put it in the RIGHT conditions for healing.

Removing entire organs, really? Debilitating and mutilating a human life for the sake of a few thousand dollars. We already established that the body functions as a unit and that each organ depends on the whole body and that the whole body depends on each and every organ and the vital functions it carries out.

How dare they take out a gallbladder? The surgeon suggests 'explorative surgery' to see if the gallbladder is 'diseased' and even when found in good shape they take it out anyway because "the gallbladder is useless". Truth be told, they remove the gallbladder because otherwise the surgeon wouldn't be able to charge for the surgery.

In the case of the gallbladder, surgery is usually recommended to the patient when there's inflammation of the gallbladder (cholecystitis). This inflammation is due to a build-up of bile caused by gallstones blocking the tube leading to the gallbladder. So why are there gallstones? Guess! Yes, poor food and drink choices cause the aggregation of chemicals (calcium and/or cholesterol) to form a 'stone' inside the gallbladder.

Gallstones can be reversed. However, they didn't appear overnight and they won't go away overnight either. And eventually passing them will be quite painful. So, both surgeon and patient opt for the easy way out. Over 500,000 gallbladders are removed in the U.S. each year.

But since when is an organ useless? Each organ carries out vital functions. Let's discuss that gallbladder for example.

The functions of the gallbladder:

1. Store bile for the liver (the liver produces bile, excess bile is stored in gallbladder).

2. Concentrate bile (make it usable and highly effective).

3. Deliver bile to the small intestine and stomach when needed for digestion. Bile breaks down fats to its usable forms and neutralizes stomach acids.

4. Bile acts as an antioxidant and helps remove toxins from the body.

So what happens when the gallbladder gets surgically removed?

1. There is no longer a storage place for the bile so the liver dumps the bile directly into the small intestine. The small intestine receives too much bile and gets irritated which

may result in IBS (Irritable Bowel Syndrome).

2. The quality of bile is impaired and therefore the digestion of dietary fats, including essential fatty acids is impaired. People without a gallbladder miss out on all essential fatty acids (omega-3). As we learned in chapter 2, an imbalance of omega-6 (inflammatory) and omega-3 (anti-inflammatory) fatty acids will cause systemic inflammation, excess cortisol and toxic build-up. Classic signs of omega-3 (EPA) deficiency are impaired function of the nervous system, learning difficulties, irritability, heart disease, impaired blood sugar control etc...ending in degenerative disease and maybe cancer.

3. Possible chronic diarrhea due to excess bile in the large intestine.

4. Digestive problems and pain.

Does the surgeon educate the patient on the long-term consequences? Of course not! That may scare the patient. It's downright CRIMINAL and EVIL.

I could give a similar example for the unnecessary removal of the tonsils, and any other supposedly non-important organ but bottom line is that the body works as a unit. If an organ is removed, the body is forced into physiological compensation.

Examples are increased sight in one eye after the other eye is destroyed, the increase in size of the remaining lobes of a lung after a lobe has been removed, an increase in the size of one kidney after surgical removal of the other one.

We see this all the time: first there is an increase in the size of the cells of the remaining tissue or organ (hypertrophy) to do the extra work, and if that isn't sufficient there will be an increase in the number of its cells (hyperplasia). However, there is a limit to the body's compensation powers and when this limit is reached serious damage is done.

Surgeries are most often unnecessary and performed because of ignorance and greed. One of our local hospitals (Halifax Hospital) is currently under investigation because of allegations that several of their neurosurgeons performed unnecessary spinal procedures (spinal fusions, etc.) solely for profit without medical necessity. Initial estimates are that these surgeons fraudulently charged Medicare, Medicaid and other insurances between $750 million and $1 billion. We are just talking about a small 900-bed, local hospital. What do you think that means on a national scale? I picked on a local hospital because they were just in the local news, however nearly EVERY hospital and surgeon commits these crimes.

3.3 Diagnostic Tests

Allopathic or conventional medicine is focused on diagnosing. However, once diagnosed and given a name, allopathic medicine doesn't have the solution or cure anyway. What's the point in diagnosing then? You decide.

Diagnostic tests include X-rays, MRI's, CAT-scans, EMG, EEG, EKG, mammograms, blood work among many others. I could write a whole separate book on these but it wouldn't get us any closer to being healthy.

The bottom line is that conventional medicine is trying to NAME a SYMPTOM and that doesn't help at all in correcting the cause of disease and achieving optimal health. If someone is diagnosed with MS (Multiple Sclerosis) then the MS is exclaimed to be the cause of all other symptoms, while MS is merely a symptom-complex itself. The cause lies in poor lifestyle choices and so the cure lies in removing those poor lifestyle choices.

Caution! Whatever is seen on pictures (a bulging disc, torn ligament, tumor, ulcer, plaque etc.) is surely there but is NOT necessarily the reason or cause of the pain or discomfort, or symptom. Too often the link is made between what's seen on a test and the complaint of the patient, resulting in a wrong assessment or diagnosis, resulting in the wrong treatment. Regardless, any treatment would be wrong anyway.

Many of these diagnostic tests are not even reliable, yet they are performed by the thousands because insurance pays for them. For example, the *EMG/NCV* test, a test doctors like to use when patients report pain, usually in conjunction with muscle weakness and/or neuro-logical symptoms.

This EMG/NCV test is an Electromyography and nerve conduction velocity test. They are actually two tests performed simultaneously. The first tests for proper muscle response to a signal sent in its direc-tion, while the second determines if any abnormal responses are due to nerve damage. These tests were developed and used during WWII to determine motor deficit in wounded soldiers. The test is effective in assessing the alpha-motor muscle fibers and gamma-motor muscle fibers. However, 95% of patients reporting pain today come without a motor deficit. The pain originates from the smaller Alpha-delta pain fibers and the C-type pain fibers. This means that only 5% of patients presenting with pain are true candidates for this test.

Furthermore, the test is not always as conclusive as some medical pro-fessionals would like us to believe. Ten to fifteen percent of the NCV tests performed come back with a false positive result, and for some of the diseases which are tested for with EMG, it has been reported that 30-40% of the negative results were false negatives. The reason for this is because the patient must also have accompanying muscle weak-ness for the EMG test to be effective. So, even if there is actual nerve damage, without muscle weakness, it cannot be determined.

Even though this type of test is mostly worthless, it doesn't necessarily worsen the disease or impair health further unlike the many RADIATION tests. To take a picture of your body or body-part, X-rays, all kinds of scans, mammograms etc. use ionizing radiation. The wavelength of this radiation is very-short and powerful, so powerful it splits the nucleus of atoms in your body. In short, this radiation destroys living cells.

Another example is *mammograms*. Not only is a mammogram ineffec-tive in that it has never been proven to save lives, it actually does quite the opposite. False positive diagnoses are very common – as high as 89 percent – leading many women to be unnecessarily and harmfully treated by mastectomy, more radiation, or chemotherapy.

Health hazards of mammography have been well established. John Gofman, M.D., Ph.D. – a nuclear physicist and a medical doctor, and one of the leading experts in the world on the dangers of radiation – presents compelling evidence in his book *'Radiation from Medical Procedures in the Pathogenesis of Cancer and Ischemic Heart Disease'* that over 50 percent of the death-rate from cancer is in fact induced by x-rays.

Now consider the fact that the routine practice of taking four films of each breast annually results in approximately 1 rad (radiation absorbed dose) exposure, which is about *1,000 times greater than that from a chest x-ray.*

Even the American Cancer Society lists high-dose radiation to the chest as a medium to high risk factor for developing cancer.

What's even more important is that there are many other risk factors for breast cancer that can be assessed without mammograms. And to make things worse, there is actually a test available that uses no mechanical pressure or ionizing radiation, and can detect signs of breast cancer as much as 10 years earlier than either mammography or a physical exam: **thermography**. But the medical profession looks the other way, as expected (because insurance companies don't pay for this test).

We can discuss all other diagnostic tests available to impair your health, promote cancer and misdiagnose you, but I'm sure you get the point. Please don't just come to any hasty decisions when it comes to having one of these tests done. You can no longer blindly follow the advice of your doctor for two reasons: (1) your doctor does not understand health and disease and is merely a puppet on a string, just doing what every other doctor does and what he or she has been fed in medical school; and (2) many of them are eager to make the easy extra cash.

3.4 Only Your Body Can Heal Itself

I'm quite sure you understand that our body is immensely complex and ingenious, but can you really grasp the complexity of our CREATION? We can build a rocket and put a man on the moon and we can build and control a nuclear plant (not always though) but we are far from understanding the human body.

<u>Complexity of our Body</u>

Our body has an estimated 100-200 trillion cells (impossible to grasp this number which is larger than the amount of stars in the entire milky galaxy). Each single cell performs an estimated few million chemical reactions per second. So if we want to know the estimated number of chemical reactions occurring in our body at any given second during our entire life, we need to multiply 100 trillion with a few million. Next time someone asks you if you are busy, answer: "extremely".

Every time a blood cell in the lungs takes on an oxygen molecule, that's a chemical reaction. Every time a cell in the pancreas produces an insulin molecule, multiple chemical reactions are involved. Every time a nerve cell in our eye or brain fires, a cascade of ions travel through the nerve cell, which is essentially thousands of chemical reactions, which cascade out to thousands of other nerve cells, and so on.

Each and every cell in our body has 100,000 receptors on its outer membrane. The RNA or messenger of each cell 'tells' these receptors constantly what the cell needs to carry out its functions effectively, and repair, rebuild and renew itself. The receptors then 'stick out their neck' and scan the environment (extracellular fluid) for the nutrients the cell asked for.

If due to our S.A.D. (Standard American Diet) these nutrients are not available, then our cells are forced to use less potent, often incompatible, replacement parts. It's like using a copy instead of an original, and when the process continues and copies are made of copies we end up with malfunctioning of the tissues and organs, cell mutation (cancer) and degenerative disease. So all we have to do from this point of view is

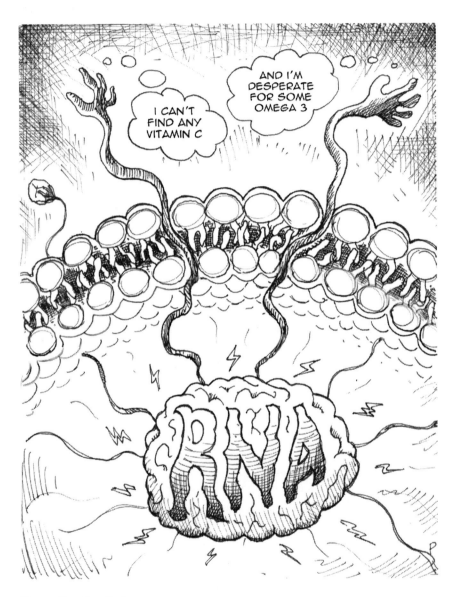

Illustration 7 – Cell

provide our body with all the essential nutrients, all the time.

As you can understand the complexity of this human body, do you really believe we are meant to interfere with this CREATION? DO you believe we are supposed to ingest man-made foods and poisons and drugs to intoxicate that great gift? Do you think we are supposed to remove limbs and organs to the benefit of our body? Of course not!

Do we need to understand the complexity of all functions and processes of the body?

The answer is: NO. And even if we wanted to, we simply cannot and will never be able to comprehend the complexity and magnitude of the workings of our body.

All we need to do is realize that the body knows what it's doing. The body and every living cell in it, always (from birth to death) strive for perfect health. All we need to do is LISTEN to our body and put our body in the RIGHT CONDITIONS in times of impaired health AND in times of perfect health.

One of these right conditions is clean food of course. We must make sure our body receives all the nutrients necessary to do its job.

The Powers

The following are some of the most vital powers our body possesses. These powers prove that our body cures itself, as does all living matter.

POWER of REPAIR

Each and every cell, tissue and organ *repairs* and renews itself constantly, by its own intrinsic power. No evidence is needed as both physiologists and lay-men know. As a result of the daily operations wear and tear of the tissues occurs and our body constantly repairs these tissues. If this power wouldn't exist, we wouldn't make the age of 2 weeks.

POWER of REGENERATION

Not only does our body repair tissues, it also *regenerates* destroyed tissues. All parts of the body have been shown to grow and re-grow under the right conditions. Examples are wounds, abrasions, cuts, broken bones etc. Even when parts of other species are used (grafting) successful growth of new tissue is observed.

POWER of REPRODUCTION

This power is more easily observed in the lower organism where animals and plants reproduce lost parts. Examples are worms, salamanders and lizards, craw-fish etc. who all successfully reproduce lost parts, in full and completely. Moreover, these new parts are new, young and more vital than the lost, older parts. In the lower animals we even see that when cutting up a worm in several pieces, each piece reproduces a perfect individual. In the human body we can see this power when broken bones heal.

POWER of REJECTION

This is the power of our body to eliminate and excrete all waste. This waste includes the useless waste generated within the body as a result of normal metabolism, and the toxins ingested through food, air, and water. All organs and orifices of the body react against inorganic, dead matter and they all are self-cleansing. The chief organs here are the skin, lungs, kidneys, liver and lymphatic glands, bowels, and mucus membranes.

When health is impaired due to toxemia (toxin build-up), the body employs more aggressive actions to expel these toxins. These actions are wrongly called 'disease' while they are merely abnormal efforts of organic house cleaning. We could say that the body has its own detoxification program in place. When this program or process of detoxification is overburdened (chronic toxemia), the body is forced to make further adaptations in an effort to stay alive. Examples are hypertrophy (increase in size or enlargement) of certain glands and/or organs to meet the extra demands for detoxification, or the presence of cysts and abscesses (the body envelops and deposits harmful substances).

POWER of ADAPTATION

Our body quickly adapts itself and accommodates itself to the ever changing conditions, from within the body and from the external environment. On a summer day the body will cool itself by sweating, and to meet physical activity demands the body will increase heart rate, blood flow etc. It's a normal process of adaptation.

Another example of adaptation is seen after drinking your first beer or smoking your first cigarette, which is followed by an aggressive effort of the body to expel this new toxin (violent vomiting, nausea etc.). When the ingestion of these toxins becomes frequent and habitual, the body seems to react less violent and eventually doesn't react anymore. This is a self-protective adaptation. The body gave plenty of warning signs and the individual keeps ignoring them. The intoxication will be dealt with differently as the violent vomiting requires too much energy. Toxemia will be the result.

Even during a state of impaired health or so called disease, the body alters its functions to meet the existing conditions. The body will reduce certain functions to conserve energy while increasing other functions in the body which are meant to actively meet and overcome the foes of life. A simple example is that one of a fever in which the temperature of the body rises while the appetite decreases. The rise in temperature is necessary to repair the damages. The increased heat production requires increased oxidation, which calls for more oxygen and faster circulation. Both respiration and heart action increase. Even though these two are regarded 'symptoms of acute disease' they each serve a purpose to an end. While this heat production requires more energy, the body needs to save or conserve some energy in other places. The body doesn't want to spend any energy on digestion while combatting the pathogen, so a symptom of 'poor appetite' urges the body NOT to consume anything.

POWER of HIEARCHY

Our creation has placed the most vital organs in the least exposed and protected places of the body. These places are also the most accessible. The brain is carefully wrapped in two membranes. In between these 2 covers, fluid serves as a shock absorber and all of this is encased with hard bone. The heart and lungs are protected by the ribcage and sternum, yet easily accessible, and so on.

When short or deprived of nutrients, the body will continue to nourish the most vital organs while consuming fat first and then other tissues in the reverse order of importance. Yet another great example of the preservation of life at all times.

During a fast, the diseased tissue is first broken down and absorbed. Diseased tissue includes exudates, effusions, deposits, infiltrations and growths, even tumors. All this matter was deposited in the adipose tissue which is simply tissue that connects more important tissues and parts of the body. Now you can see why our body removes this fat tissue first… because it contains the dead matter and deposits that were stored there at times of impaired health. The power of self-repair needs no outside assistance, just the normal conditions of animal and plant life.

We can conclude that with all the powers our body possesses for repair, regeneration, renewal, removal, development etc. it does not need any help from us. No therapeutics, no medicine of any kind, no intervention of any kind. The cure is simply the healing or repair process of our body. As we know not to intervene we also know we must place our body in the right conditions to heal. These right conditions are hygienic conditions.

3.5 Time to Take Control

Yes, it's time to take CONTROL of our HEALTH. As you can understand now, we don't need any help from any health care professional. They would only intervene. It's my hope however that every health care professional reads this book and studies this subject and the natural laws of human life so that he or she can educate the people on health and disease and the one and only cure.

Since ONLY your body can heal, it's ONLY YOU that can make sure it does heal by respecting the laws of human life. YOU are in TOTAL CONTROL and this total control is a GREAT POWER. And as stated in the Spiderman movie: 'WITH GREAT POWER COMES GREAT RESPONSIBILITY'. Upon birth you were given this creation and it's your responsibility to cherish it, nourish it, love it, enjoy it, maintain it, optimize it.

Human versus Animal

What separates us from the animals? The best answer is: AWARENESS and the FREEDOM TO CHOOSE our RESPONSE.

Animals have an instinct and they respond to any stimuli with that instinct. That instinct is set by Mother Nature; it's always the best solution in that particular situation. The purpose of that instinct is survival (of the individual and of the species) and the continuous quest for perfect health.

Humans are more complex. Humans are not only able to respond (response-ability) but they can choose their response, while animals can't. Human beings are therefore responsible for their own lives. Our habits and behavior are a function of our decisions, not our conditions. We can make the right choices or we can make the wrong choices. Unfortunately, we all have become slaves of these wrong choices.

The choices we make are based upon our values, habits, independent will, self-awareness, imagination, and conditioning. When it comes to our health and eating practices we have been conditioned wrongly.

This explains why animals in the wild are so perfect and healthy and don't know of any disease. Their instincts make them do the right things. Humans have the possibility or choice to make other decisions and therefore do wrong things, detrimental to the individual and to the species.

So even though this freedom to choose our response has caused us harm as a human species, it also allows us to make the necessary corrections and adjustments, and regain control of our health and our lives.

With the knowledge and understanding you acquire in this book, you can consciously make that better choice the next time there's a stimulus.

Now you can see why you need that paradigm-shift and why it was necessary to shed light on the flaws of our current healthcare system and our poor eating habits and lifestyle choices, and how they affect our health and our life. The first few chapters were negative in nature, but there was no other way to expose the truth. The following chapters will be more pleasant and positive as we learn how to regain control of our health and as we experience more 'a-ha' moments.

You may assume it's going to be difficult to turn around your health, but I guarantee it's going to be worth it. Simply follow the Action Plan and you will be ABSOLUTELY AMAZED on how you will feel and look. You probably never felt ALIVE recently and have to jog your memory for those days when you were a kid and full of energy. Those days are coming back if you just DO WHAT NEEDS TO BE DONE.

3.6 Key Points

Our current healthcare system causes over 100,000 direct deaths per year in the U.S. alone. Doctors simply don't understand health and disease.

The medical profession is based on dogmas, doctrines and thoughts which is not science. Science and truth can only be found in the laws of Mother Nature.

Drugs and surgeries are evil acts in an attempt to remove or mask symptoms and receive monetary gains at the expense of human suffering; so are most diagnostic tests.

The complexity of our body and the powers it possesses will always be incomprehensible to the human brain. There is no need to even try. Just know that ONLY THE BODY CAN HEAL and that we are RESPONSIBLE for putting that body in the RIGHT CONDITIONS for perfect health.

Humans, unlike animals, have the freedom to choose their response. This freedom has cost humanity a huge price: its health and happiness. Fortunately, we can utilize this awareness and choose to regain CONTROL of our health.

CHOOSE HEALTH FREEDOM.

Chapter 4 – Laws of Human Life

Finally! We are going to learn HOW to regain control of your health and obtain optimal health and happiness. The previous chapters were an awakening, but necessary to expose the truth about the current medical system and about the abuse you inflict on your own body.

Now that you are aware, let's do something about it! Remember that we can choose our response and that ONLY YOU are in charge and in TOTAL CONTROL of your HEALTH because ONLY the BODY can heal itself.

Now, it's going to be exciting, fun and mind-opening. Let's get started with the natural laws of human life.

The laws of life have been adopted and simplified from "Human Life – Its Philosophy and Laws" by Herbert M. Shelton.

We have talked about these laws up to this point and I'm sure you have been wondering what these laws are. They are as true and solid as the law of gravity, and when we respect and comply with them perfect health is achieved.

These natural laws are formulas which describe uniformities or regularities of nature. These uniformities are not coincidences but intrinsically necessary conditions.

We do not have to know the essential nature of life in order to intelligently obey its laws. An electrician for example must not know what the nature of electricity is in order to provide us with power, light and heat. No matter what the electrician's hypothesis or ideas in regards to the nature and essence of electricity are, he or she must obey and observe by its laws. These laws are fixed and ideas or theories about them don't change them.

Animals in the wild cannot do anything but respect and live by these natural laws because their instinct guides them to do so. That's why these wild animals are in such perfect health.

Humans have the ability to choose their response and make their own decisions. Unfortunately, this uniqueness has cost humans lots of harm and suffering by making the wrong decisions and ignoring the natural laws of human life.

4.1 The Laws

LAW of SELF-PRESERVATION

From the smallest microscopic single cell to the most complex living organism, every particle of living matter is under the control of a vital force or life energy and is endowed with the instinct of self-preservation. All living matter will do whatever it takes, in a very well organized matter, to preserve life and its species or race.

LAW of ACTION

Living organisms possess the power of action. They can move themselves and other matter as well. The action of this living organism under various conditions when subjected to various stimuli does NOT represent the action of these conditions or stimuli upon the living organism, but rather the RESPONSE of the living organism to the conditions or stimuli. This response, or power, or action is from within. We already established that dead matter cannot act and is lifeless. Lifeless matter cannot move itself, it can only be moved, it is passive.

This action is directly proportional to the amount of power. If the power is high, the response is high and if the power is low the response or action is low.

This law is best illustrated with drugs, laxatives (Epson salt) for example. One assumes that these drugs 'act on the bowels'. The question is: which one acted and which one is acted upon? The bowel acts, the salts are acted upon. The salts cannot give power to the bowels as they do not possess power.

You may ask why does the bowel act so fast after ingestion of these salts? Self-preservation is the answer. These salts or any other chemical drug for that matter are destructive to the cells, fluids and tissues of the body, impairing their functions and health. They act as irritants and their irritation is in direct proportion with their destructiveness. The bowels act upon them to purge or eliminate them from the body as fast as possible. This action is VITAL action.

LAW of POWER

The vital action requires power. This power comes from within and not from without. The salts mentioned earlier will not produce any movement in a dead person, nor will other drugs. Even the body of a very diseased person near dead won't respond to medicines because the power is absent.

Vital force or power is the cause of the action. The presence of the drug is just the stimulus for the action. Any condition, or drug, or treatment will just be the stimulus and may be acted upon by the living organism.

Also note that the living organism will NEVER tolerate the presence of dead matter and therefore will always try to expel and eliminate that dead matter.

The action of a living organism is in proportion to the need of action and the amount of power available to complete the action.

In the case of stimulants (alcohol, coffee, energy drinks, certain drugs etc.), power or strength is felt only in its expenditure. The stimulant possesses no power and only occasions the expenditure of power possessed by our body. The stimulant does not add power. Therefore, one 'crashes' after using the stimulant. First one feels stronger while he is growing weaker and then one feels weaker when he or she is actually growing stronger through the recuperation of power. In other words, a period of apparent vigor or stimulation is followed by a period of fatigue or depression. These two effects are normal with the use of power and further discussed in the law of dual effect.

LAW of DISTRIBUTION

The body delicately controls and distributes the vital power to all cells and tissues as long as there is enough power available. When the body is short of power, the body wisely appropriates and discriminates this power where most needed. It always does the best it can with the power at its disposal. However, with a shortage of power, functions are impaired and not carried out optimally or effectively.

LAW of DUAL EFFECT

We already saw an example of this law when discussing the action of stimulants or tonics. These drugs (including coffee, tobacco, energy drinks etc.) only take away the strength they appear to give. The initial and brief effect of these tonics is the vital resistance of the body to expel the tonic or toxin, and the energy felt is nothing but the expenditure of vital energy of the body. The secondary effect of the tonics (fatigue, weakness etc.) is due to exhaustion of the vital powers and destructive effects upon the tissues of the body. A tonic medicine first strengthens and then debilitates. This illustrates the law of dual effect.

If the habitual user of any drug stops its use for a few days, the user will experience the secondary effects in their fullness. If he or she returns to use the drug, the symptoms disappear. The 'disease' is cured by its cause: coffee cures headaches and tobacco steadies the nerves. I'm just being sarcastic of course. The only cure is to take the cause away, and let the body rid the toxins (yes, it may be a violent process).

You can see once again that medicine has it wrong. The nomenclature of medicine is wrong: tonics are a-tonics and stimulants are really depressants, opium and anti-spasmodics are spasmodics etc. Why? Medicines should be named according to their lasting effects, not their temporarily effects.

Work and exercise consume vital energy and thus result in an appearance of increased vigor. This is their first effect (energy expenditure). The second effect is fatigue, tiredness and decreased vigor (energy recuperation).

Sleep and rest produce weakness and laxity as their first effect (recuperation) and increased vigor and alertness as a secondary effect (lasting result). One must be 'weak' (read: rest and sleep) in order to be strong.

In short, the law of dual effect makes sure that energy is recuperated after it has been spent.

LAW of LIMITATION

This law assures that when vital powers are used up so much that life is threatened, the organism will stop any further unnecessary expenditure.

A good example is prescription medicines. When a patient takes the medicine on a daily basis and the body has to use vital power on a daily basis to deal with and try to expel this medicine, energy will soon run very low. The body then will stop reacting to this bad habit of the ingestion of medicine.

This is why doctors have to increase the dosage of that medicine after a while. This may happen a few times. When the dosage can no longer be increased and the patient doesn't respond to this medicine anymore, the doctor usually opts to try another medicine and the whole process starts over again. Sounds familiar? I thought so. The same is true with other stimulants, bad foods and drinks, bad habits, overindulgence, excess emotions etc. This law simply says: "enough is enough" when needed to preserve life.

LAW of SPECIAL ECONOMY

The body builds up a reserve of vital energy whenever it can. All excess vital energy, above current energy expenditures, is stored to be used in future times of special need. This vital energy reserve is the best guarantee against disease. All emergencies (use of stimulants – better called irritants or depressants – and consumption of un-natural foods and drinks, overindulgences, unbalanced emotions, overwork and over-stimulation or excitement etc.) use the body's reserve energy and power to overcome them. Sleep, rest, nutrient rich food, clean air and clean water build up this energy reserve. When we spend more energy than is available, toxemia happens and disease starts and progresses, unless the cause is removed.

Natural examples include growth and development. These processes take place is 'spurts'. Periods of rapid growth alternate with periods of slow growth. During periods of rapid growth the body needs lots of energy to complete its tasks of development while during periods of slow growth the body is accumulating energy and power in preparation for the period of rapid growth. So a period of work does require a period of rest.

LAW of VITAL ACCOMMODATION

We can use the example of tobacco again to illustrate this law. The first smoke usually causes a very powerful reaction: headache, nausea, vomiting, weakness, poor appetite etc. The poisonous character of tobacco alarms the body which responds with this powerful reaction to expel the poison. This is a warning sign of the body. A pretty clear sign, no? But many choose to ignore that warning sign and light up another cigarette.

With repetitive use of tobacco, the organism responds less and less powerfully and eventually doesn't respond at all. The body adapts itself as much as possible to the habitual use of this toxin. No energetic effort is made to expel the toxin anymore. In this case, the body will harden and thicken the mucous membranes and the (at first) sensitive linings of the mouth, throat, stomach, intestines and bowels to guard against the constant irritation to which the body is now ignorantly subjected. The same process would take place with the habitual use of any other irritant such as alcohol, coffee, tea, spices and condiments (salt, pepper, mustard, ketchup, all dressings etc.), mouthwashes, man-made foods and drinks, and so on.

If the body cannot overcome such habitual poisoning, it must learn to endure it in order to survive or perish. But keeping the body accustomed to the action of irritants and poisons is a very expensive business, resulting in toxemia.

Other examples of this law of accommodation are the adaptations made when one lives in a cold versus a warm climate, or the cushions that are formed on the feet of people who walk bare foot or the calluses on the hands of a manual laborer.

All of these bad habits are of no immediate danger to life but when continued will cause several crises as the body has to accommodate itself. If a habit doesn't cause immediate danger, that doesn't mean it's not destructive. Drinking a cup of coffee produces an immediate feeling of well-being while drinking a glass of orange juice doesn't. However, when we look at the secondary effects (long-term effects) we can clearly conclude that coffee is injurious while orange juice is beneficial.

LAW of SELECTIVE ELIMINATION

We are already familiar with this law. The body has the ability to be selective in which substances and natural nutrients it uses to build, repair and renew the body versus the unusable, dead matter it will expel and eliminate. The body recognizes, counteracts, neutralizes and expels these toxins through channels in a manner which cause the least wear and tear to the body. The body selects the organs to act on the toxin.

There are other laws inherent to the living organism, but the above ones encompass most of them.

4.2 Dr. Mike's C.L.E.A.N. Living

Now that we know the laws, the question becomes: what do these laws mean and HOW do we apply them? HOW do we respect them?

The laws clearly and overwhelmingly tell us that the body can take care of itself and heal itself when necessary. The body knows what it needs, how to build, repair, renew, rejuvenate, regenerate. The body knows what nutrients to use in which amounts, what material is usable and what material is harmful and needs to be expelled. The body knows how to perfectly manage these trillions of cells with their even more trillions of chemical reactions per second. The body knows what processes and functions are the most important and knows how to deal with emergencies. The body adapts to constantly changing conditions, external and internal.

The body is a perfect creation. The body knows nothing else but to strive for perfect health and would be in perfect health for 120 years if cared for properly.

In a healthy body, when we disrespect the laws of human life occasionally (for example one drink of alcohol at a party) no long-term harm is done because the body will neutralize the toxin by using some vital energy from the energy reserve. However, with habitual use the energy reserve will deplete and toxemia starts.

We learned that the body will continue to do the best it can to preserve life as long as it can, but it shouldn't have to do this. The body shouldn't utilize its energy to attend to these habitual emergencies. These laws are there to protect you in times of a real need, they are not there to be abused.

So HOW do we simply comply with these laws of human life and respect them? By putting and keeping our body in the RIGHT CONDITIONS. Besides protecting oneself from direct physical harm and trauma and given the provision of shelter, below are my 5 main rules or principles:

Dr. Mike's 5 MAIN PRINCIPLES – C.L.E.A.N.

1. We need to inhale CLEAN AIR, drink CLEAN WATER and consume CLEAN FOOD while trying to avoid environmental toxic exposure and man-made foods.

2. We need to provide our body with ENOUGH REST & SLEEP & SUNSHINE so that it can recuperate power and energy, and build up and maintain an energy reserve.

3. We need to CONTROL our emotions and feelings, and keep them balanced.

4. We need ACTIVITY, but in moderation and in balance with adequate rest.

5. We need to LISTEN to the warning signs of our body, and also AVOID overstimulation, overexcitement, and overindulgences.

REMEMBER them this way:

C.L.E.A.N.:

Control emotions and feelings.
Listen to the warning signs of your body: avoid overstimulation, overexcitement, and overindulgences.
Enough rest, sleep, and sunshine.
Active lifestyle
Natural and clean air, water and food.

The rest of the book will now expand on these 5 rules or principles and provide the knowledge, understanding and skills to implement these 5 rules. It won't be easy, but it will be worth it. You will most likely have to change some habits in order to succeed and you need to be WILLING to change those habits. You need to be WILLING to SACRIFICE what you want now for what you want later!

The Health 4 Life Action Plan is set-up in phases to allow for gradual improvement and successful implementation.

4.3 What do Animals in the Wild do?

The best way to find out how Mother Nature wants us to respect and comply with these natural laws and implement the 5 rules is to look at animals in the wild. Their instincts make the RIGHT decisions for them and put them in the RIGHT CONDITIONS all the time. They are in perfect health and don't know of any disease. So whenever you don't know the answer on what's best for your body in a certain situation or with any given stimulus, ask yourself:

WHAT DO ANIMALS IN THE WILD DO?

This will give you the ONLY correct answer. After you know what's wrong and what's right, you can make a choice.

Let's put this to the test and ask the following questions. Make sure you think about each question for a few minutes. Try to find some rationale with the knowledge you acquired so far. Ask the WHY question.

- Do animals in the wild drink milk?

- Do animals in the wild eat 3 meals per day and snack in between?

- Do animals in the wild rest after they feed?

- Do animals in the wild combine their food?

- Do animals in the wild drink with their meal?

- Do animals in the wild overeat and become fat?

- Do animals in the wild eat when not hungry?

- Do animals in the wild party and overindulge?

- Do animals in the wild have sex for pleasure?

- Do animals in the wild fast?

- Do animals in the wild use mouthwash?

- Do animals in the wild shop for man-made food?

- Do animals in the wild go on diets?

- Do animals in the wild have diabetes, heart disease, stroke, cancer?

- Do animals in the wild have rotten teeth?

- Do animals in the wild get enough physical activity?

- Do animals in the wild use microwaves?

- And so on…

I'm sure you got most of them answered correctly. Do you understand WHY it is what it is, WHY animals in the wild with their instinct make the best choices, and WHY they are in perfect health?

The next chapters will go in detail and will explain the HOW and WHY. Have fun!

4.4 Key Points

Just like the law of gravity, the laws of human life are unwavering and solid. No matter what your idea or thought or opinion is about them, they won't change.

The laws of human life tell us overwhelmingly that we don't have to understand the complexity of our body, and that there is no need to interfere with its unique and complex workings. To interfere with your body is to be so arrogant to think you actually understand the body and wrongly assume it needs help. In order to preserve life and stay in perfect health for 120 years we just have to put our body in the RIGHT CONDITIONS.

Besides protection from violence and the provision of shelter, we need to live C.L.E.A.N.:

Control emotions and feelings.
Listen to the warning signs of your body: avoid overstimulation, overexcitement, and overindulgences.
Enough rest, sleep, sunshine.
Active lifestyle.
Natural and clean air, water and food.

If you are uncertain on what response you should choose in certain situations or conditions, ask yourself: WHAT DO ANIMALS IN THE WILD DO? This will give you the one and only correct answer. YOU are responsible for then making the RIGHT CHOICE.

Chapter 5 – Feeding versus Feasting

While the first few chapters painted a good picture of your current 'health' condition at this current time, the next chapters will show you what it takes to be in perfect health.

You will see a huge gap between where you are right now and where you should be. Even though the advice and recommendations presented sometimes may seem 'crazy' or 'extreme', it all makes sense if you think about it. They are all simple truths.

So don't get bent out of shape thinking you will never be able to do all this, and make these 'crazy' or 'drastic' changes. I know you can, but you don't have to do all of this overnight. The Health 4 Life Action Plan will guide you through several stages in order to get closer to that perfect health. You will never reach perfect health, but you can reach optimal health (near perfect) by taking steps in the RIGHT direction.

Over the centuries, our eating habits have deteriorated so much that not only the prime purpose of eating is overlooked but also that overeating has become an epidemic.

I'm not just talking about the outrageous number of overweight and plain fat people, but also about the unnecessary excess burden the average person places on his or her digestive system. This excess burden depletes vital energy reserves quickly and initiates the disease process. Symptoms may not be noticed for decades to the untrained eye of the individual and the conventional doctor.

The digestive process is so elaborate that in normal circumstances it will utilize approximately 80% of all vital energy available at the time.

5.1 Hunger versus Appetite

It seems that we are holding on to the popular idea that we can eat anything and as much as we want as long as no immediate discomfort is produced. This is in violation of several natural laws and we are simply oblivious and ignorant to the impact of this habit.

Appetite is defined as the DESIRE for food or drink, a desire to satisfy a taste or craving. Appetite is psychological, dependent on memory and associations. Appetite is fake hunger. It's a creature of habit and cultivation. It is stimulated by the sight, taste, smell or thought of food, the arrival of habitual meal time, condiments and seasonings. This stimulation is accompanied by the flow of saliva in the mouth and gastric juice in the stomach.

None of these stimuli can arouse true hunger. Hunger is only physiologically aroused when there is an actual need for food, and is accompanied by 'watering of the mouth'. It arises spontaneously, without the help of any external factor.

One may have an appetite for alcohol, tobacco, coffee, tea, opium, drugs etc. but one can never be hungry for these because they never serve any real physiological need. The hungry person is able to eat a simple crust of bread and be satisfied while the person who has only an appetite must have one's food spiced and seasoned to enjoy it.

Food has become the number one ADDICTION, no doubt. This food addiction is far worse than any other addiction, including drugs and alcohol or tobacco. It's just not recognized as an addiction because appetite and feasting are confused for hunger and eating. Desire is mistaken for need. Only the food manufacturers seem to know as they load up their

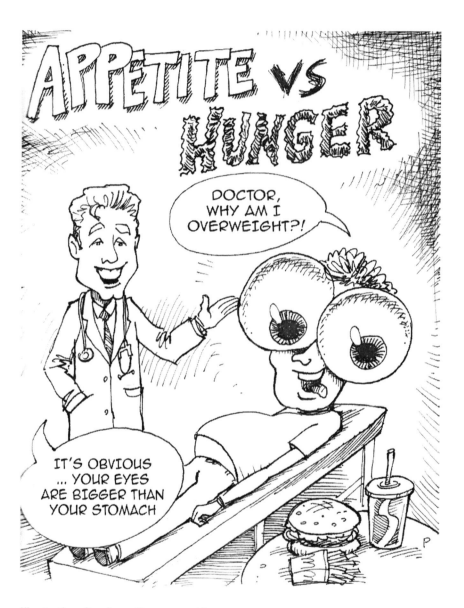

Illustration 8 – Appetite versus Hunger

products with sugars and other addictive substances. Did you know that Coca-Cola actually had put Cocaine in its coke products? True, look it up.

5.2 Back to Basics

Nutrition is a major factor in one's health. As human beings, we will eat and drink whatever is put in front of us while carefully checking the type of oil we put in our car. We give no value to health until we lost it. We are odd creatures. We will do anything to preserve life, only to kill it slowly at the dinner table.

In order to stop overindulging on foods and drinks and in an attempt to relieve the burden on our digestive system and body, we must listen to the needs of our body and go back to basics.

The following rules apply:

EAT ONLY WHEN HUNGRY

Hunger is simply the voice of our body and nature telling us that food is required. There is no other guide to tell us WHEN to eat. Rules or habits of society such as the 'three meals a day' habitual meal time are not guides. Likewise our children are forced to eat at a certain set time in school rather than when they're hungry.

Eating when not hungry only burdens the body. This activity uses unnecessary power and vital energy, depletes energy reserves, produces unnecessary toxins, and causes unnecessary wear and tear on our tissues.

For more than thousands of years civilized nations consumed only one meal a day. The time was set after a day of work so man could rest and food digest. The Romans, the Greeks and even the Jews from Moses till Christ only ate one meal a day.

What do animals in the wild do? Their instinct makes them eat only when hungry, one time per day. Rest follows to allow for proper digestion.

How did we humans turn feeding into feasting?

Commercialization and industrialization turned food and drinks into an addictive commodity. Eating has become a social event, a feast, a pleasure. Our addiction now has to satisfy that pleasure.

We turned hunger into appetite and are exposed to the sight, false tastes, false smells of foods and drinks constantly. The addiction not only satisfies the appetite (not hunger) but fills voids when emotions and feelings are out of balance. Many people eat just to comfort themselves when lonely, depressed, irritated, worried etc. Food eaten during these mental states is not digested and causes the food to ferment and poison the body. Why? Because the body needs all the energy to meet the mental stress and cannot meet the needs for effective digestion at this time.

All so called scientific evidence, thoughts or ideas about "3 meals a day" or "5 meals a day" or "lots of snacks during the day" or "breakfast is the most important meal" are all senseless, useless propositions.

Overeating just overworks the body and also poisons it. The 'light' eater has more power and energy reserve because he does not expend his power and energy in excessive physiological activity. This person is much stronger and healthier and lives longer.

NEVER EAT DURING, IMMEDIATELY BEFORE OR AFTER PHYSICAL OR MENTAL ACTIVITY

All parts and products of the body are manufactured from the blood which carries all the material supplies throughout the body. The blood is manufactured from the air, water, food and sunshine. The body cannot supply every part of the body with extra blood at the same time (law of distribution).

We established that digestion consumes a great deal of energy. If we would eat during the performance of physical activity or work or mental activity, then digestion would be halted. The muscles and brain need all the extra energy. Digestion will not start. Food will rot and ferment in the stomach, and once digestion can start after the activity, not nutrients but toxins are released in the blood.

What do animals in the wild do? They all rest or sleep after a meal. They don't eat while running or hunting, and they don't eat before physical activity either (because they rest after a meal).

So WHEN do we eat then? Society has forced us into a schedule more or less, and therefore we should eat at night. Here's the logic:

First, one needs to know that normal digestion takes 4-8 hours to complete, depending on the type of food ingested. If we work (physical or mental) that digestion will take much longer.

Second, food supplies energy but only after it has been digested and absorbed. Therefore, food taken in the morning – *breakfast* - can never supply the energy for that day's work. Quite the opposite holds true: food consumed during breakfast will take away from the energy for the day's work. I challenge you to put this principle to the test by skipping breakfast for a few weeks and note the difference.

Furthermore, rest and sleep do not produce hunger. Eating breakfast then would violate the first rule: eat only when hungry. I know what you are thinking now: "but I am hungry in the morning". Well, you think you are hungry in the morning because you confuse hunger with appetite AND you are conditioned into the bad habit of breakfast. Breakfast is best omitted altogether. One piece of fruit or some fresh vegetable juice can be taken (fast and easy digestion).

Lunch then should be skipped or very light for the same reasons as one goes back to work. We all know that tired and weak feeling we have immediately after lunch when we go back to work. Now you understand why. Your body withdraws some blood from the muscles and brain to start digestion, but digestion is slow and sluggish also because your body needs energy for work. Result: two half-ass jobs.

Dinner or the evening meal should be the one and only meal. Ideally one takes a little rest after work and then eats this 'heavier' meal. The digestive system can now utilize all extra energy to effectively digest and assimilate the food during the evening. During this period, there should be no physical and mental activity (even emotions should be at rest) as blood is withdrawn from muscles and brain. Digestion is uninterrupted.

Ideally, one should have 3-4 hours of uninterrupted digestion prior to going to sleep.

During sleep, there is no active physical or active mental activity, and digestion has hopefully and mostly completed. This is necessary so that the body can focus on recuperation, renewal and replenishment during sleep. Eating just prior to going to sleep will cause fatigue and restless sleep since the digestive system is at work. Refer to chapter 8 for more information on rest and sleep.

Furthermore, in the morning one is ready for the work day, full of energy from the foods digested and absorbed during the evening prior. This is why one should not be hungry in the morning.

Note: if you plan to work-out or play sports after work you don't eat before, you eat after. You may consume only one piece of fruit or fresh vegetable 30 minutes to 1 hour prior to the work-out. This principle will maximize your work-out and maximize your digestion of your meal after the work-out.

NEVER EAT WHEN SICK, IN PAIN OR IN MENTAL DISCOMFORT

This is common sense. When the body is in a state of emergency it requires energy to solve this emergency. When sick or in pain, pathogens need to be expelled. When in mental discomfort such as fear or worry, the brain consumes much vital energy to deal with the discomfort and balance our mental status.

Eating only would worsen sickness, pain and mental discomfort. Energy is taken away from the emergency for digestive purposes.

When sick or in pain the desire for food is absent. Conventional medicine labels this natural, normal symptom as 'poor appetite'. When the desire is absent, don't eat. The body is telling you it needs its energy to heal. Listen to your body and its warning signs. Don't listen to the ill advice of doctors or others.

You may wonder: would that sick person not become weak without food? No. That sick person would become weak when consuming food. The digestion of food would further deplete energy reserves and worsen the sickness. So how long would one not eat then? For as long as the body has no desire for food.

What do animals in the wild do? Even your pet? They omit food when sick.

PROPERLY MASTICATE AND INSALIVATE ALL FOOD

You heard it before but it's true: digestion starts in the mouth. Biology and physiology shows that the flow of gastric juices of the stomach is largely dependent on the taste of food.

In order to really taste food, one has to properly chew and insalivate (mix with saliva) the food. In fact, the longer one keeps food in the mouth the more one tastes. Try it!

Not only do you promote proper digestion when tasting your food, but chewing breaks down the food prior to entering the stomach so the digestive juices can go to work immediately. When chunks are swallowed, the stomach needs extra energy to break them down prior to digestive action.

This habit of eating fast and swallowing food also causes overeating. When the body received enough food it sends a message to stop eating. When we eat too fast, that message comes late. When we chew and taste our food it allows the time for our body to stop the hunger feeling and give us a feeling of satiety.

Furthermore, our saliva contains digestives enzymes which then help and accelerate the digestive process.

Much vital energy is saved when one masticates and insalivates all food.

What do animals in the wild do? I have never seen them being in a hurry to eat. They take their time, they chew and they salivate... that is if they are mammals and have teeth. I know snakes and others swallow the entire pray but their anatomy and physiology is different. They do rest though after the kill to allow digestion to complete.

DO NOT DRINK WITH MEALS

This rule should be followed strictly. Any fluid, even water, ingested during a meal leaves the stomach in approximately 10 minutes. Unfortunately, it carries the diluted digestive juices with it and therefore seriously impairs digestion. Digestive juices are weakened and more juices need to be secreted.

Some obstructed minds would argue that water stimulates the flow of gastric juices and thus enhances digestion. First, there is no need to stimulate the flow of digestive juices as this is a natural process. In the long-term, this only will impair the secretion power of the glands. Second, there is no value to increase secretion if the water with the digestive juices leave the stomach before the food is acted upon.

We already established that digestion takes 4-8 hours. So we must not drink 1, 2, or 3 hours after a meal since that fluid would impair digestion drastically.

So WHEN do we drink? Drink either 10 to 15 minutes before a meal or 4 hours after a meal.

Drinking also leads to the swallowing habit, not chewing and insalivating the food. When we drink during a meal we merely 'wash our food down'.

Drinks always should be room temperature. Cold drinks further impair digestion because cold stops the action of the enzymes. The stomach then has to use more vital energy to raise the temperature of the stomach again. The same holds true for ice cream.

Hot drinks reduce the tone of the stomach and weaken the mechanical part of the digestion.

What do animals in the wild do? None of them drink when feeding.

DRINK ONLY WHEN THIRSTY

We established that we only eat when hungry, so why would we drink when we are not thirsty? We have been told over and over again that we don't drink enough water lately. The doctor says we are dehydrated. The personal trainer or fitness guy or wellness expert on T.V. tells us we need to drink more water. What do they base these assumptions on? Not sure. It's just another dogma of modern science.

So how much do we drink then you may ask? No hard rules can be set. The intelligent person will not attempt it. Drink as much as nature calls for. There is no exact number because it depends on a number of conditions and circumstances, including age, climate, amount and type of work performed, amount and type of food eaten etc.

The more one eats (overeats), the more water one needs. The person who eats mainly fresh fruits and vegetables receives large quantities of pure water through his food and consequently will have little thirst. We need more water in summer than in winter, and we need more water after labor than rest.

But be aware, appetite for drinks does not equal thirst. Irritation caused by the ingestion of spices, condiments, greasy foods, and dairy usually mimics thirst. Drinking will not solve this irritation and one keeps drinking more and more.

Too much water literally water-logs the system. The power of the blood to absorb oxygen and carry oxygen is weakened and inhibited. One sweats more when he drinks more. The one that drinks more suffers more from summer heat.

What do animals in the wild do? They find a river or pond to drink out of when thirsty. Their instinct brings them there, but they don't stay. They drink and go. They don't drink all day long like we do. We are addicted again to the sight, false taste and smell of these drinks. We wrongly assume irritation equals thirst.

NEVER CONSUME FOODS THAT ARE TOO HOT OR TOO COLD

The temperature of our stomach is approximately 104 degrees. Consuming cold foods or beverages therefore would prolong digestion and result in rotten foods, and toxemia. Consuming hot foods or beverages usually results in quickly swallowing the foods without proper mastication and insalivation. Furthermore, the taste buds are unable to signal the start of digestion.

In short, cold is a NO-NO. Hot food can be consumed but needs to be masticated and insalivated properly. Hot drinks are ok, but one needs to respect the rules of drinking prior to a meal or 3-4 hours after a meal.

5.3 Food Combining

Besides the basics on eating already discussed in this chapter, there's another major basic principle of healthy eating: proper food combining. Food combining is nature's logical way to feed or consume foods in such a way that optimal and effective digestion is assured.

The purpose is to facilitate digestion, maximize the nutrient value from digestion and reduce the burden on the digestive system.

We obtain NO value from undigested food. To the contrary, undigested food ferments (rots) and is converted into alcohol and other poisons which wreak havoc in the stomach and digestive tract. When food combining rules are not followed, many poisons are produced and toxemia results.

Even when consuming healthy fruits and vegetables, but combining them wrongly and therefore leaving them undigested, causes more harm than good. Instead of obtaining vital nutrients from these fruits and vegetables, poisons are generated and absorbed.

The absolute best rule for combining food: DON'T DO IT.

By understanding how our body and digestive system work and respond to different kinds of food, we can put our body in the right conditions for proper digestion.

Each food has its own chemical composition. Our digestive system employs different enzymes, each designed to break down specific foods. Furthermore, each stage of the digestive process also requires a different enzyme. Each of these specific enzymes requires a different acidity level to effectively carry out its function.

The greater the variety of foods consumed during a meal, the greater the burden on the digestive system.

For example, when we eat a burger with a bun or a steak sandwich, we combine carbohydrates with protein. The digestion of carbohydrates starts in the mouth with an enzyme called 'ptyalin' present in one's saliva. Saliva is an alkaline medium. The action of ptyalin in the mouth would be destroyed if we consumed acid food with that carbohydrate.

In the stomach, pepsin acts upon proteins and amylase (secreted by the pancreas) acts upon carbohydrates. However, pepsin requires an acidic environment so the stomach pours much hydrochloric acid into the stomach, while amylase requires little acidity.

Combining the starch or carbohydrate with protein causes great confusion and results in an overburdened digestive system. The stomach first excretes enough acid so that the proteins can be broken down. This process takes several hours.

Meanwhile the starch or carbohydrate is fermenting. Once the protein is digested and the acidity of the stomach adjusts to digest the starch, the starch has rotted. The body will absorb toxins instead of the nutrients it should have.

FOOD	TRANSIT TIME (minutes)
Water	0-15
Juices	15-30
Fruit	30-60
Melons	30-60
Sprouts	60
Wheatgrass Juice	60-90
Vegetables (majority)	60-120 (1-2 hours)
Grains & Beans	60-120 (1-2 hours)
Meat & Fish	180-240 (3-4+ hours)
Shell Fish	480 (8+ hours)

Illustration 9 – Transit Times

Another point of view is that when acid and alkaline substances are mixed, they neutralize each other. In this case, digestion is greatly impaired. Undigested proteins will putrefy while undigested starches ferment.

Digestive disorders such as gas, bloating, acid reflux, heartburn etc. are the result. Only removing the cause (combining the wrong foods) will cure these digestive disorders.

Not only does this process of food combining require much more vital energy, it robs the body of nutrients and produces toxins instead.

What do animals in the wild do?

I have never seen any animal combine different foods in one meal, you? That would be a circus act! Some birds may eat seeds one meal and insects another, but they would never combine seeds and worms. A wild lion may kill its prey and consume the meat but I have never seen one put some starch or a fruit with it. Yet again their instinct tells them not to combine foods.

Besides common sense and the example of Mother Nature, straight forward biology and physiology give us the same facts.

To minimize energy expenditure and maximize digestion and nutrient absorption, we must follow the following rules:

DO NOT COMBINE PROTEIN WITH CARBOHYDRATES

Carbohydrates and proteins require different acid levels for digestion. Combining proteins and carbohydrates results in fermentation and putrefaction.

Proteins include meats, eggs, dairy, nuts and seeds.

Carbohydrates include bread, potatoes, rice, cereals, and pastry.

DO NOT COMBINE CARBOHYDRATES WITH ACID FOODS

The acids of fruits such as lemons, limes, pineapples, grape fruit, sour apples, sour grapes, oranges, berries, tomatoes etc. destroy ptyalin in the saliva and suspend the digestion of carbohydrates.

DO NOT COMBINE PROTEIN WITH ACID FOODS

The digestion of proteins in the stomach, as established earlier, requires an acidic environment. One may assume that the addition of acid fruits would facilitate the digestion of protein but the contrary holds true. The acid foods inhibit the excretion of acid gastric juices and thus interfere with the digestion of proteins, plus the enzyme pepsin is destroyed in excess acidity.

DO NOT COMBINE PROTEIN WITH ANOTHER PROTEIN

Proteins of different character and different composition call for different modifications of the digestive system. The timing and concentration of the gastric secretions varies based on the type of protein. Combining different proteins therefore results in putrefaction and burdens the digestive system.

So don't combine meat with eggs, meat with nuts, meat with cheese, eggs with nuts, cheese with nuts etc. You may combine 2 different types of meat.

DO NOT COMBINE PROTEIN WITH FATS

Fat has an inhibiting effect on the excretion of gastric juices. Foods that contain fat need a longer time to digest: nuts, cheese, milk, fatty meat. If fat is combined with protein, digestion is slowed down.

Avoid cream, butter, oils, gravies, fatty meats when consuming protein.

Since an abundance of green vegetables neutralizes the inhibiting effect of fat, one should always eat these vegetables when consuming fat.

DO NOT COMBINE PROTEIN WITH SUGAR

All sugar has an inhibiting effect upon the secretion of gastric juices and the mechanical movement of the stomach. When taken alone, sugars pass the stomach fast and are digested in the intestines.

When sugar is combined with other foods, this sugar is held up in the stomach and causes acid fermentation.

DO NOT COMBINE CARBOHYDRATES WITH SUGAR

The same holds true for sugars and carbohydrates. When combined, the sugar ferments in the stomach.

Jams, jellies, commercial sugar, honey, molasses, syrups are added to cakes, cereals, pastries, breads, potatoes etc. They all cause acid fermentation in the body. Sweet fruits with carbohydrates such as dates, raisins, figs, bananas etc. in breads, or syrup on pancakes are dietetic abominations.

EAT MELONS ALONE

Melons undergo no digestion in the stomach. They are digested in the intestine. If melons are combined with other foods, they get stuck in the stomach and quickly decompose resulting in indigestion and gas.

ALWAYS EAT JUICY FOODS PRIOR TO CONCENTRATED FOODS

Juicy foods are digested faster than concentrated foods. If one would consume the concentrated foods first, the juicy foods would rot while waiting to be digested.

So eat a salad prior to your protein or carbohydrate meal, eat acid fruits prior to seeds and nuts, and eat sub-acid fruits prior to sweet fruits.

DESERT DESSERTS

Ice cream, cakes, pastries, puddings, even fruits all wreak havoc in the stomach if taken shortly after a meal. They serve no purpose.

Now that we know what foods NOT to combine, what foods can we combine? How should we take them?

Protein foods are best combined **with green leafy vegetables and/or non-starchy vegetables** such as spinach, broccoli, cauliflower, corn (sweet), asparagus, green beans, string beans, celery, onions, cucumber, lettuce, kale, fennel, leeks, mustard greens, collard greens, turnip greens, cabbage, Brussels sprouts, alfalfa sprouts, artichoke, summer squash (except Hubbard squash), radish, rhubarb, eggplant, bell peppers, parsley, endive, okra, chard, dandelion, bamboo sprouts and shoots etc.

Carbohydrates are better combined with the more **starchy vegetables** such as peas, carrots, beans, winter squash, beets, corn (field), dried beans, lima beans, potatoes and sweet potatoes, beets, turnips, pumpkins etc. Don't add tomatoes or acid foods to your salad.

Beans and peas are carbohydrate-protein combinations in themselves and therefore are better eaten as a carbohydrate OR a protein, and not combined with one or the other. They should be eaten with green vegetables.

Potatoes are mostly starch and therefore should be the starch part of a starch meal.

So avoid burgers on buns, steak or meat on a sandwich, spaghetti with meatballs etc. Eat your protein with a large salad and eat your carbs with a large salad or veggies.

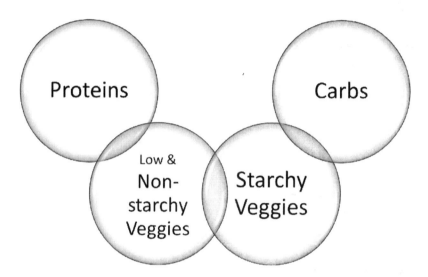

Only combine if circles touch, do NOT combine if circles do not touch.

Illustration 10 – Food Combining 1

Fruits are awesome mixtures of vitamins, minerals, and pure rich food elements. Some are blends of acids, while others are not. Few are rich in protein, avocado and olives being the exceptions. Many fruits are loaded with sugar.

Fruits NOT high in sugar include lemons, limes, bell peppers (green, yellow, red), avocados and tomatoes.

Fruits should be eaten **alone as a fruit meal**, not in between meals. If eaten between meals, fruits would hamper digestion and rot. So will the ingestion of all kinds of fruit juices.

Do not combine sweet fruits with acid fruits. So don't eat dates or figs or bananas with pineapple, oranges or grapefruit. Don't use sugar or honey on acid fruits such as grapefruit. Combine sweet fruits with sweet fruits and acid fruits with acid fruits.

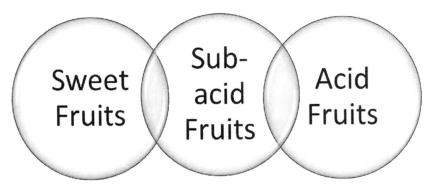

Only combine if circles touch, do NOT combine if circles do not touch.

Illustration 11 – Food Combining 2

I suggest eating fruit daily. Replacing breakfast with some fruit would be good. Consume a majority of acid fruits. Limit your intake of sweet fruits since they contain lots of sugar. Don't eat too much. Don't eat if you are not hungry.

If you can, eat fruits in season, when ripe, and grown as locally as possible. Have you ever seen an Eskimo eat water melons?

Botanically, *nuts* are considered fruits. Nuts (protein) can be combined with acid fruits but not with sweet fruits. Nuts do combine best with green vegetables.

Avocados (protein and fat) are best combined with acid fruits (not sweet fruits or nuts or other proteins).

An example of a fruit salad with protein would be: lettuce, celery, nuts, avocado, apple, orange, pineapple, and grapefruit. A salad made out of sweet fruits such as dates, raisins, bananas, prunes, etc. would be quit sugary. I suggest eating just one piece of sweet fruit.

An example of a nice spring fruit salad could be a combination of lettuce, celery, peach, plum, apricot, cherry, nectarine.

<u>Some guidelines for salads:</u>

Make your salad big. The salads in restaurants are too small.

Do not add salt, pepper, vinegar, or any dressings. A very small amount of oil or cream is allowed when combining the salad with a carbohydrate meal, but not if combined with a protein meal. When a salad is eaten by itself, lemon juice or oil may be added.

Do not use tomatoes in your salad when the salad is eaten with a carbohydrate or protein meal. You may add tomatoes when your protein comes from nuts or avocado.

Bitter foods such as onions, radishes, watercress etc. are better avoided all together, not just in salads.

Salads are best made simple. An example may be spinach, tomatoes and celery. Maybe add a bell pepper and some parsley. Lettuce, celery, cucumber and fresh peas make a nice combo.

Note: You can download **Dr. Mike's FOOD COMBINING CHART** for FREE at www.Health4Life.info. You will also find easy to use lists of foods, properly categorized (fruit protein, seed protein, nuts, legumes, grains, green leafy vegetables, starchy vegetables, non-starchy vegetables, fruit vegetables).

INDIGESTION

Overeating, eating when not hungry, eating just because of an appetite, eating for comfort, combining foods, eating in between meals, drinking during or immediately after a meal... impairs digestion.

Not only is half of the food consumed by people passed out undigested, but the digestive system is overburdened, energy depleted, nutrient depleted, and toxins build-up.

Drugs to relieve indigestion (antacids such as Nexium) are all frauds. They do not aid digestion. They do not improve in any way, shape or form the functional powers of the digestive organs. These drugs further impair the digestive system.

The only remedy to indigestion is to respect the biological and physiological limitations of our body. I personally have helped many people with digestive problems and acid reflux in as few as 2 to 3 weeks by simply teaching them proper food combining practices.

MY DAY

I personally eat a sweet fruit in the morning or an acid fruit salad or I drink a veggie juice. If I don't feel hungry, I don't eat anything at all. I may drink a glass of water or fresh orange juice, but only if I'm thirsty. This morning for example I drank 2 glasses of fresh veggie juice, blended with my 'Vitamix' (a commercial grade blender). I mixed fresh spinach leaves with cilantro, kale, collard greens, sweet bell peppers, and celery. I added clean, pure water, one piece of fruit (apple, banana, or a few berries) and some concentrated lemon juice to improve the taste.

I often skip lunch, but if I feel hungry I may either eat a veggie salad (or drink more of my breakfast veggie juice which I left in the refrigerator). I do NOT combine the salad with a protein or carbohydrate. I drink water or water with lemon 20 minutes prior to my lunch if I feel thirsty.

For dinner I used to combine a protein or carbohydrate with a large salad or slightly cooked or steamed veggies. Examples are a fish (salmon, grouper, trout) with steamed asparagus and a large salad, OR a lean chicken breast with cooked spinach (lightly cooked) and a large salad, OR a sweet potato with steamed veggies (broccoli and spinach, or a combo of garlic, carrots, green and red bell peppers), OR a brown rice bowl with veggies, Or a turkey or chicken burger (without a bun or bread) and a large salad will do for a healthy dinner. Now, I'm not consuming any DEAD meat anymore.

Dinner is best eaten late, and after all physical and mental activity. When my daughters have soccer practice or any other activities after school (early evening), I try to make them dinner after their practice session and ideally a few hours before they go to bed. However, they are 'hungry' coming home from school at 4pm and don't want to wait another 4 hours to eat something. So they make themselves a fruit salad. In this case, it works out fine because their timely forced school lunch at 11am has been digested already, and their fruit salad only will take approximately 1 hour to digest. Soccer practice is at 5:30 or 6pm.

5.4 Alkaline Model

In order to fully understand the alkaline way of living or the alkaline food model, one needs to be familiar with pH, alkalinity and acidity and their effects on the body. So let's get started with clarifying these terms.

The body, as you know, continuously strives for balance and perfect health. In the medical profession, they call this balance: homeostasis. A good example is that of our body temperature. Our body always strives to maintain a pretty constant body temperature of approximately 97 degrees F. When the heat hits us on a summer day, we start sweating and a trip to the ice skating rink without proper clothing causes shivering. Sweating and shivering are the attempts of the body to normalize body temperature. Sweating cools the body down when too hot and shivering produces energy and heat when too cold.

Another example of homeostasis is the pH of our body. Just like a swimming pool or a fish tank, the pH or acid-alkaline balance needs to be normal for optimal functioning. If not, problems arise quickly. If the pH of your fish tank is off, you better add some alkalizing liquid. If not the water gets acidic, it will turn green and your fish will be swimming backstroke on the surface pretty soon while bacteria infest the tank and start the party. The same happens with a chemical imbalance in a swimming pool. Once the chemicals are off, the water turns greenish and if not corrected, trouble starts. The filter system becomes slow and sluggish and if continued, the pump will blow.

The same holds true within our body. Unfortunately we don't have a window on our stomach to take a peek once in a while and check for the color. Our blood has a normal pH of 7.35 – 7.55. The pH values differ based on where and how they are measured. For example, the pH measurements of urine are slightly more acidic than those of saliva. Regardless, our body constantly strives to keep these pH values within a normal range. When acid nutrients or toxins enter the blood stream, our body needs to buffer the blood and neutralize these acids. The body depends on free forming alkalizing minerals such as calcium, potassium, magnesium etc. from our diet to neutralize the acids and buffer the blood.

The pH scale goes from 0 to 14. A normal blood pH range is 7.35 – 7.55, urine approximately 7.2, saliva approximately 7.7. A pH measurement below normal values indicates excess acid in the body while a pH measurement above normal values suggests catabolic illness. The former is usually the problem while the latter is not.

Our Standard American Diet (S.A.D.) results in excess acid production. When foods high in fat, protein and sugar are metabolized, acid products remain. The body of course will link these acids with alkaline minerals (calcium, magnesium, potassium, zinc, iron and others) to buffer and neutralize them, thereby reducing the acid burden.

Over time, when this process continues, free-form minerals in the body deplete and acid builds-up in our cells and tissues. This acidic environment impairs function and reduces the effectiveness of normal metabolic activity. Symptoms include lack of energy, fatigue, pain and illness.

When the body runs out of free-form minerals (obtained from a healthy diet), it's forced to do two things:

1. The body actually parks acids in our fat cells so that these

acids cannot float around and damage the system. This causes weight gain.

2. The body is forced to leach alkalizing minerals from its own organs and bones.

The body will leach calcium from the bones, resulting in osteopenia and osteoporosis. It will also derive calcium from our muscle tissue causing muscle cramps and restless leg syndrome. Besides calcium, the body also takes magnesium from the muscles causing weakness.

The body will take iron from the red blood cells which in the long-run could cause anemia and leukemia. The body also has to produce excess amounts of cholesterol to bind to the acids.

This state of acidity then burdens our immune system. Our immune system responds to this distress with an increase in cortisol, adrenaline and insulin (our chemical messengers of distress). The physiological response to these distress messengers is also acid enhancing, thus per-petuating the situation and increasing the acid burden. A vicious cycle is put in motion and only can be stopped by taking away the cause: acid forming foods in excess of alkaline forming foods.

While acid forming foods are a great contributor to an acidic body, excess acid can also accumulate as a result of distress, toxins, and immune reactions.

In order to regain and maintain an acid-alkaline balance, we then need to incorporate more alkaline forming foods in our diet and reduce the intake of acid forming foods. Simultaneously, we need to reduce toxin build-up and avoid distress.

Acidity & Germs

Guess who thrives in an acidic environment? You got it: microforms such as germs, pathogens, bacteria, yeast and fungus.

Bacteria, yeast, fungus and other pathogens simply can NOT survive in a normal, alkaline environment. It's that simple. When your body is alkaline, you cannot catch a 'bug' or sustain a bacterial infection or yeast infection... Impossible!

It comes down to the same old stuff: eating the things that Mother Nature gave us in their purest form sustains alkalinity of the body. An alkaline body has a normal, strong immune system which not one single germ has a chance to beat.

Meat is nothing but DEAD animal FLESH, loaded with microforms. First, the animals are slaughtered and gutted. The contents of their intestines (including bacteria, yeast and mold in the feces) literally spill all over the meat. Then the carcasses hang in the meat locker for days before they are cut up, washed with bleach, and shipped to the distribution centers. If you think this is a clean process, think again. The meat is infested with bacteria; after all bacteria multiply exponentially.

You could cook this meat at high temperatures and kill all these bacteria, but then you also killed all essential nutrients and denatured the proteins. The meat has no longer any nutritional value at all. It only burdens our digestive system.

And of course, meat is highly acid. Meat contains a lot of uric acid. Even a single, average piece of meat contains more uric acid than the body can handle. This uric acid leaches calcium from the bones, again. That's why meat eaters have the weakest bones.

It's best to just skip meat. Humans should get their protein from vegetables. I know what some of you are thinking: we are omnivores! We have canines! We are supposed to eat meat! Not to blow your bubble, but here are some straight-forward facts:

1. Real flesh eaters take nourishment from parts of the whole prey, not just the muscle meat as men tends to eat.

2. Real flesh eaters immediately consume their prey after the kill, maximizing the nutrient and protein value of the meal. Our meat is as dead as it can be prior to consumption...

nutrient and protein value: close to zero or zero, especially when cooked.

3. Men seldom consume raw meat and they cook the meat as to disguise it from the dead corpse it really is.

4. Flesh eaters have long, sharp teeth while men have the teeth of grain eaters (grains, nuts, seeds, fruits and vegetables). Men can grind with their jaw, flesh eaters can only move the jaw up and down.

5. Flesh eaters secrete into their stomachs 10 times the amount of hydrochloric acid that humans and other non-flesh eaters do. That's because our stomach shouldn't have to cope with the digestion of meat, bones, feathers, tendons, etc.

6. Flesh eaters are equipped with a short bowel to enable them to expel the putrefying flesh rapidly and avoid toxemia. Men have a long bowel and rather complicated digestive tract to allow for effective digestion of plants and vegetables.

7. Flesh eaters have a different type of intestinal bacteria than men and other non-flesh eaters.

8. The saliva of flesh eaters does NOT contain the enzyme ptyalin (which initiates carbohydrate digestion), while men do.

9. The liver of flesh eaters is much larger in comparison with men.

10. Flesh eaters sweat through their tongue, while men and most non-flesh eaters all sweat through their skin.

Simply stated, we are not meant to eat the meat of animals, birds and fish. Nature provided us with plenty plants and vegetables containing complete proteins. Complete proteins are proteins that contain all essential amino acids. As you already know, there are 22 known amino acids, 8 of which are essential.

These essential amino acids cannot be manufactured by our body and therefore need to be obtained through our foods. Amino acids have many vital functions and play a key role in building and repairing muscles, tendons, nails, skin, hair, blood and internal organs such as the heart and brain.

Here are you best sources of proteins:

Fruit proteins: avocados, olives and coconuts.

Legumes: yellow peas, lentils and peanuts.

Seeds: flax, pumpkin, chia, sesame, sunflower and quinoa (a gluten-free grain/seed).

Nuts: almonds, cashews, macadamia, pecans, pistachio, walnuts, pine nuts, brazil nuts, candle nuts, hickory nuts, pignolia nuts, filberts, pinon nuts, beech nuts.

Yeast products are another category of poisons. Common expressions are Candida and yeast infections. These yeast products not only contain yeast but also the little creatures' waste products. With breads, pastries, and other bakery goods, the dough rises because of the gasses that are produced by the yeasts when they ferment sugar into flour. But the yeasts, which are resilient buggers, survive the baking process and end up in the bread and bakery goods along with their toxic wastes. Yummy! So cut out these breads and pastries, and choose yeast-free ones if you have to.

When drinking beers and brewed drinks, you are not only ingesting the sugars and alcohol, but you are also consuming the yeasts and their toxic and acidic waste products (yes, their feces) produced by fermenting the sugars.

<u>Fungus and molds</u> are often inhaled but these are also plenty in algae, cheese and mushrooms. All mushrooms contain various amounts of a toxin named amanitin. In large amounts, amanitin kills a human immediately. In smaller amounts it just takes a little longer to kill that human. Research shows that all mushrooms contain at least 5 nutrients that are carcinogenic. There is no good reason to consume mushrooms, as there is no reason to consume cheese or any diary product, period.

When it comes to mushrooms of any kind: don't eat them.

Acid – Alkaline Food List

The following is an acid-alkaline forming food list. I organized the foods alphabetically in 6 categories: highly alkaline, moderately alkaline, slightly alkaline, slightly acidic, moderately acidic and highly acidic forming foods.

Note that we are talking about HOW these foods act in the body, whether they are acid forming or alkaline forming in the body, and to what degree. We are not talking about their pH level or acidity prior to ingestion.

A question I always get and confuses many people is: How is it that a lemon or lime is alkaline forming in the body? Aren't they very acidic fruits?

True, they both are acid foods or fruits. They taste acidic because of the citric acid in them. However, both lemons and limes are loaded with all kinds of minerals which have not much taste and are overpowered by the acid taste of the citric acid. Once ingested, digested and assimilated though, both the lemon and lime have an alkalizing effect in our body because of the majority of minerals, antioxidants and other nutrients.

The list thus categorizes foods by how they act within the body, after being digested.

Certain foods may be listed as slightly acid forming, but this fact doesn't necessarily mean they are bad for your health. They may have other health benefits.

THE ACID – ALKALINE FORMING FOOD LIST

HIGHLY ALKALINE FORMING FOODS

Alfalfa grass, barley grass, black radish, cucumber, dandelion, dog grass, jicama, kale, kamut grass, shave grass, soy sprouts, sprouted seeds (all kinds), straw grass, wheat grass.

MODERATELY ALKALINE FORMING FOODS

Alfalfa, avocado, baking soda, cabbage lettuce, cayenne pepper, celery, cilantro, endive, green beans, garlic, ginger, lima beans, oregano, sorrel, spinach, red beat, red radish, white navy beans.

SLIGHLY ALKALINE FORMING FOODS

Almond, almond butter (raw), artichokes, asparagus, banana (ripe), basil, bee pollen, bell peppers (all), bok choy, borage oil, Brussels sprouts, buckwheat, caraway seeds, carrot, cauliflower, cherry (sour), chives, coconut, coconut oil, comfrey, cumin seeds, eggplant, evening primrose oil, fennel seeds, figs (raw and dried), flax seed oil, ginseng, green cabbage, green tea (herbal), horse radish, kamut, lamb's lettuce, leeks, lentils, lemon, lettuce, lime, mustard greens, olive oil, onion, pine nuts, parsnips, peas, peppers, potatoes, pumpkin, red cabbage, rhubarb (stalks), royal jelly, savoy cabbage, sea salt, sea vegetables, sea weed (all), sesame oil, sesame seeds, spelt, squash, thyme, tofu, tomatoes (all), turnip, yams, water (clean), watercress, white cabbage, white radish, zucchini.

SLIGHTLY ACID FORMING FOODS

Acai berry, agave nectar, apple cider vinegar, apples, apricot, banana (not ripe), barley, barley malt syrup, beans (mung, adzuli, pinto, kidney, garbanzo), blackberries, blueberries, brazil nuts, bread (rye and whole grain), brown rice syrup, butter, cantaloupe, cashews, cherry (sweet), clementines, cranberry, cod liver oil, cooked vegetables (all), corn oil, couscous, cream, currant (black, red), dates, flax seeds, fructose, fruit juice, goji berries, gooseberry, grapefruit, grapes (ripe), hazelnut, honey, hummus, kiwi, liver, macadamia nuts, mango, maple syrup, margarine, nectarine, nutmeg, oats, orange, organs (as meat), oysters, papaya, peach, pear, plum, popcorn, pumpkin seeds, spring water, strawberries, sunflower oil, sunflower seeds, sweet potatoes, tangerine, tempeh, walnuts, watermelon, whey protein powder, yeast.

MODERATELY ACID FORMING FOODS

Alcohol, sugars (saccharides such as xylitol), beet sugar, bread (white, sourdough), brown rice, buffalo meat, canned foods, cereals, cheese (all kinds), chicken, chocolates, corn tortillas, duck, egg (whole and egg whites), fish (fresh water and ocean), jams, jellies, ketchup, mandarine orange, mayonnaise, microwaved foods, milk (pasteurized), miso, molasses, mushrooms, mustard, olives, pasta (wheat), peanut butter, peanuts, pineapple, pistachios, pomegranate, raspberry, rose hips, salmon (wild), soda pop, sourkraut, soy sauce, sugar (white), sugarcane, vegetables (canned and frozen), water (sparkling), wine, wheat, wheat kernel.

HIGHLY ACID FORMING FOODS

Artificial sweeteners, beef, beer, black tea, coffee, drugs, flour (including pastries and cakes), fruit juice (sweetened), liquor, pasta (white), pork, rice (white), sardines (canned), tobacco (if you consider this a food), tuna (canned), veal, vegetables (pickled), vinegar (white).

More about some of the highly acidic foods and beverages

<u>Coffee</u> is one of the most acidic liquids. With a pH of 4.2, coffee is several thousand times more acidic than neutral water. Do you have any idea how much minerals need to be used (or leached from bones, tissues and organs) to buffer this acid onslaught? WOW!

Coffee is the most toxic substance for the liver to metabolize (yes, worse than alcohol).

Another myth is that coffee burns fat and assists in weight loss. This misconception is based on the fact that the caffeine in coffee causes a short-lived 'high' or 'jolt' and stimulates the sympathetic system (increase in heart rate, vasodilation etc.). We know that this is just an attempt of the body to purge the toxin and is only an expenditure of energy and not the addition of 'external' energy. Coffee actually blocks weight loss efforts by forcing the body to deposit acids in the fat cells and slowing down metabolism (depleting energy reserves).

Besides the extreme acidity of coffee as a disturbing health hazardous fact, coffee contains caffeine. Caffeine is the cousin of nicotine and both are depressants (an initial 'high' or 'jolt' followed by weakness, fatigue and impaired function). The same is true for other products containing caffeine such as tea, chocolate, sodas, and many over-the-counter medications.

It's time to completely STOP your coffee consumption, it's a terrible habit. You should not do it gradually to reduce withdrawal symptoms (because this significantly lowers your success), and you should drink pure, alkaline water (with lemon or lime) instead.

Vinegar is created by allowing bacteria that produce acetic acid to convert wine, cider, or alcoholic beverages to vinegar. The pH of vinegar is approximately 2.9, even more acidic than coffee. This is an immense acid load coupled with the fact that you also will be ingesting all the bacterial toxic waste. Substitute vinegar with lemon or lime juice.

Soy sauces are created the same way as vinegar. These products are fermented and loaded with yeast waste products (yes I mean feces). Soy sauces are not only extremely acidic but they are loaded with high levels of sodium (even the "low-sodium" ones) and most of them contain MSG. If you like the taste of these soy sauces, replace them with Bragg's Aminos which you can buy at health food stores. This product is loaded with amino acids instead of waste.

Sodas are poison cocktails without doubt. They are a combination of strong acids (citric acid, phosphoric acid etc.), artificial food additives (benzene, aspartame etc.), excessive sugar and caffeine. Sodas receive the gold medal for acidity. They are a death sentence.

Did you know that coke is so acidic that it dissolves a T-bone steak in less than 2 days and a nail in 4 days? Easily removes stains from china? Cleans toilets? Removes rust spots on car bumpers and drive ways? Cleans corrosion from a car battery?

Did you know that a commercial truck transporting Coca-Cola syrup must use the hazardous material place cards? These cards are used only for highly corrosive materials. Did you know that the distributors of coke use coke to clean their trucks? Did you know that in many U.S. states the highway patrol carries 2 gallons of coke to remove blood from the road after a car accident?

It's all true. Try some of it. Now give me one good reason why you would swallow that highly acidic, poisonous, corrosive man-made addictive cocktail? If it dissolves a nail and T-bone steak, what does it do inside your body? Yes, soda wreaks a lot of havoc. Every can of soda con- sumed is an emergency that has to be dealt with by your body in an attempt to keep homeostasis and stay alive. Regardless the short-term solutions of the body, long-term use takes its toll and degeneration and disease emerge with no mercy.

Practical Application

So what do we do with this list? Here's my strategy:

First, let's determine what our current acid level in our body is. Let's measure the pH. This is what I like about this alkaline model. It allows us to objectively measure progress. Of course, one should feel much better once the body recovers from an acidic state and becomes nor- mally alkaline again. This would express itself in more energy, less fatigue, more clarity, along with a restoration of normal bodily functions and normal health, and a resolution of many ailments. But being able to measure at certain intervals and making sure your body sustains an alkaline environment is a plus. It's also a motivating factor and allows us to chart progress.

These measurements are not always or necessarily precise and accurate, but when performed in a consistent and reliable manner, decline and improvement can be observed.

You will need to buy some pH strips at the health food store. Preferably, ask for pH strips that can measure both urine and saliva pH.

On day 1, you will take a total of 6 measurements (3 urine and 3 saliva). The first 2 measurements (1 urine and 1 saliva) are first thing in the morning, before breakfast. The next 2 measurements (1 urine and 1 saliva) are after lunch, and the last 2 measurements are after dinner. If you opt not to eat breakfast and/or lunch, just measure at a set time. Try to be consistent regarding the exact time you perform these measurements.

The instructions on how to execute these measurements will be on your pH strips package. Usually, the pH strip is placed in the urine (or held under the urine stream) for 3 seconds or placed under the tongue for 3 seconds. Of course, do not use the same strip more than once. The strip will show a color and that color corresponds with a pH value found on a chart.

On day 2, do exactly the same as on day 1. Now you have a total of 12 measurements (6 urine and 6 saliva). Total up the 6 urine measurements and then divide by 6 so you have an average urine value. Do the same with the 6 saliva measurements. Record both values.

At first, repeat the 2-day measurement protocol every 2 weeks. After your pH has normalized, repeat monthly.

Now that you know how to do these pH measurements, we need to transform our acidic body into an alkaline one. How?

Use a yellow marker and high-lite all the foods on the ACID – ALKALINE FORMING FOOD LIST that YOU LIKE TO EAT.

You can use the list above but you also may download the **ACID – ALKALINE FORMING FOOD LIST** with instructions for **FREE** at www.Health4Life.info.

Next, make a shopping list of the marked foods within the HIGHLY, MODERATE and SLIGHTLY ALKALINE FORMING FOOD categories. Go shop for them. I'm sure you haven't eaten many of them in a long time. Eat lots of them, and use them in your salads and with each meal.

Next, buy less of the marked foods within the SLIGHTLY and MODERATELY ACID FORMING FOODS and STOP consuming foods listed in the HIGHLY ACID FORMING FOODS category.

Initially consume 80% ALKALINE forming foods and 20% ACID forming foods. No need to measure this, just look at your plate. You will need a large amount of veggies and large salads with a smaller portion of protein (fish and meat) or carbohydrates (pasta, potatoes etc.).

Once your pH indicates your body has returned to a normal, alkaline state you may change your food intake ratio to 60-70% Alkaline and 30-40% acid forming foods. This ratio should sustain and maintain a healthy alkaline environment.

What if your pH doesn't increase to within normal limits? You will have to be more stringent and consume even more alkaline forming foods while reducing or omitting acid forming foods and drinks. Furthermore, you may need to add a high quality nutritional supplement to boost alkalinity in your body. Please refer to the SUPPLEMENTS chapter in this book.

Another reason why your pH is not rising to within normal ranges may be due to excess stress and distress, and excess toxins. You will learn HOW to cope with stress, emotions, overstimulation, and overindulgences later.

5.5 Organic Foods

It wasn't but a few years ago that only farmers' markets and health food stores carried organic foods, but today most supermarkets want to take advantage of the fast growing market for these products. Over 5 billion USD of organic products are sold yearly in the U.S. and the industry is growing at a steady 20% each year. So consumers are obviously not only aware of these organic products but they are also willing to spend the extra money for them.

What does 'organic' really mean?

Simply stated, organic produce and other ingredients are grown without the use of pesticides, synthetic fertilizers, sewage sludge, genetically modified organisms, or ionizing radiation. Animals that produce meat, poultry, eggs, and dairy products do not take antibiotics or growth hormones.

The USDA National Organic Program (NOP) defines organic as follows: "Organic food is produced by farmers who emphasize the use of renewable resources and the conservation of soil and water to enhance environmental quality for future generations. Organic meat, poultry, eggs, and dairy products come from animals that are given no antibiotics or growth hormones. Organic food is produced without using most conventional pesticides; fertilizers made with synthetic ingredients or sewage sludge; bioengineering; or ionizing radiation. Before a product can be labeled "organic," a Government-approved certifier inspects the farm where the food is grown to make sure the farmer is following all the rules necessary to meet USDA organic standards. Companies that handle or process organic food before it gets to your local supermarket or restaurant must be certified, too.

However, organic foods can be grown with pesticides, just not synthetic ones. An example is 'Bacillus thuringiensis' which is a natural bacterium found in soil. This particular bacterium is toxic to the larvae of several insects but harmless to animals and humans. But not all of these organic pesticides are harmless, including copper compounds (toxic) and pyrethrins (possible allergic reactions).

Furthermore, organic foods may be contaminated with chemicals that persist in the soil or are carried by the wind from other fields. Still, the pesticide levels are approximately 70% less than conventional foods.

The farmer who wants to convert his land to organic status has to go through a three-year process. There is a two-year conversion process consisting of building up the fertility of the land. Produce grown in the first year cannot be stated as organic. In the second year produce may be stated as "In Conversion". It is not until the third year that produce may be stated as fully organic. Soil and natural fertility building are important parts of organic farming.

Organic Labeling

Since 2002, all foods that are sold as organic in the U.S. have to be certified in accordance to federal standards. When approved these organic products receive the USDA label.

The USDA Organic seal assures consumers of the quality and integrity of organic products. Organic-certified operations must have an organic system plan and records that verify compliance with that plan. Operators are inspected annually, and in addition there are random checks to assure standards are being met.

Be aware that this USDA label has 4 different meanings:

1. "100% Organic" means that all ingredients are organic. These products MAY carry the USDA Organic seal.

2. "Organic" means that at least 95% of the ingredients are organic. These products may carry the USDA Organic seal.

3. "Made with organic (ingredients)" means that at least 70% of all ingredients are organic. These products can NOT carry the USDA Organic seal but may list up to 3 organic ingredients. There are strict restrictions on the other 30% of ingredients, e.g. no GMO's (genetically modified organisms).

4. "Organic (ingredients)" means that the product contains less than 70% of organic ingredients. These products can

NOT call themselves organic on the front panel and they can NOT carry the USDA Organic seal. However they can list the organic ingredients on the side panel.

Important note:

The label 'Certified Organic' thus indicates the percentage of ingredients not grown with synthetic pesticides and chemicals but does NOT mean that these foods are less likely to be contaminated with pathogens that may cause food-borne illness. 'Organic' chickens and eggs for example still can be contaminated with salmonella, just like conventional chickens and eggs.

Organic Products & Safety

Even though so called researchers conclude that eating conventional foods loaded with pesticides, herbicides, insecticides, fungicides and other chemicals can have adverse health effects on the farmers who grow the foods, the evidence on the effects on the consumer's health is inconclusive. The reason why the evidence is inconclusive is because these silly researchers do not take into account the long-term effects of the intake of these chemicals. We already know that a daily onslaught will slowly but surely give rise to toxemia and degenerative disease, including cancer. These chemicals are not direct killers, they are silent killers.

The government does have some safety guidelines on the levels of certain chemical compounds. Even though the established margins are wide, children consuming conventional compounds are found to have levels of organophosphate pesticides in their urine higher than these safety margins. This is really alarming.

Knowing that organic foods do not carry pesticides, or in the worst case scenario carry at least 70% less pesticides than conventional foods, does make a significant difference.

Are Organic Products Healthier?

At this time, there is no definitive research that makes this claim. It is extremely difficult to conduct studies that would control the many variables that might affect nutrients, such as seeds, soil type, climate, post-harvest handling, and crop variety.

However, many recent studies, published worldwide in peer reviewed journals, have shown organic foods to have a higher nutritional value. The most important variable here is the soil in which the foods are grown. Many times if the soil is depleted of nutrients, so will the foods. The soil in which organic foods are grown is usually more balanced and contains more nutrients than the soil in which conventional foods are grown.

Even if the nutritional value of organic foods is only slightly higher than conventional foods, the fact remains that these organic foods are certainly much healthier because they aren't loaded with pesticides and other chemicals.

Are Organic Products worth the extra Money?

One assumes that organic foods are more expensive, and while meats and produce are more expensive than their non-organic counterparts, some items such as cereal, bread, and even hamburger, may cost the same or even less. As the demand for organic foods continues to grow, the cost will continue to come down.

The reason why organic produce and meats are more expensive is the following:

1. Organic farming is more labor and management intensive.

2. Organic farms are usually smaller than conventional farms and therefore do not benefit from the economies on the same scale as the larger farms.

3. Organic farmers don't receive federal subsidies like conven-

tional farmers. The price of organic food reflects the true cost of growing them.

4.   The price of conventional food does not reflect the cost of environmental cleanups that we pay for through our tax dollars.

But here's the REAL STORY. Even though some organic foods are pricier than conventional food, the health conscious person will SAVE MONEY. Here is why:

1.   Healthy people consume far less food than un-healthy people:

Conventional, man-made foods are deprived from essential nutrients. So when you consume a burger with fries and a soda or when you eat a large man-made meal, you will feel hungry again just a few hours later. Why? Because your body will send you the "I'm hungry" signal again since it didn't receive the nutrients it really needed from your previous meal. The body is still deprived of natural nutrients and begs for them so it can carry out its normal functions.

So now you consume even more 'dead' food or indulge in snacks all day long, and the cycle continues. End-result being that the digestive system is overburdened, toxins continue to pile up, and the body stays deprived of the nutrients it needs. One becomes overweight and obese, slow and sluggish, fatigued and diseased.

When consuming normal portion size, organic and natural foods the body doesn't send signals to receive more foods. The body received in one normal, healthy meal all the essential nutrients it needs. Healthy people are far less hungry and need to consume far less food to maintain normal bodily functions. Consuming far less food means having to buy far less food. Buying far less food saves lots of money.

2.   Healthy people will end-up with far less medical bills:

Sick people not only make regular doctor visits and are responsible for deductibles and co-pays but they also pay for over-the-counter drugs and prescription medicines, allopathic treatments, diagnostic tests etc.

Besides these regular out-of-pocket expenses, these unhealthy people will eventually end-up in and out of emergency rooms and hospitals, and the medical bills become astronomic. Often, medical bills ruin people's retirement and shatter dreams.

So you tell me if organic products are worth the money? Of course they are. Unlike the common misconception that they cost more, they are actually a great investment with a direct ROI (return of investment) and an indirect ROI.

The direct ROI are the immediate savings on shopping expenses because you buy far less conventional food and man-made snacks, comfort food, etc. The indirect ROI are the absence of future medical and hospital bills.

The true savings are the savings of your health and your life.

5.6 Clean Foods

We now have a better understanding about what I mean with CLEAN FOODS as part of my 5 Rules of C.L.E.A.N. living.

In short:

ALWAYS choose organic, natural foods and drinks.

ALWAYS choose wholefoods.

ALWAYS choose fresh, local, seasonal and ripe fruits and vegetables.

ALWAYS listen to your body and only eat and drink when you are hungry or thirsty. Shop in advance and make a meal plan. Organize your meals to allow for optimal digestion.

ALWAYS opt for alkaline forming foods, while avoiding most acid forming foods. Omit coffee, sodas, vinegar, soy, yeast products, fungi and molds.

ALWAYS respect the food combining rules for maximum absorption of nutrients and minimal energy expenditure of the digestive system.

ALWAYS REMEMBER:

Raw is better than lightly steamed, lightly steamed is better than cooked, and cooked is better than overcooked, and overcooked is better than microwaved.

Fresh is better than frozen, frozen is better than canned and processed.

Organic is better.

Local is better than imported.

ALWAYS wash your produce with pure, CLEAN water. Rinsing your fruits and veggies under tap water merely defeats the purpose.

ALWAYS cook with the proper utensils. Aluminum pots and pans may leach aluminum into your food while Teflon surfaces may flake. Use stainless steel and cast iron pots, pans, and utensils.

ALWAYS AVOID:

SALT: salt is an inorganic substance and contains NO organic minerals, vitamins, or any other essential nutrients. Therefore salt is toxic to our system. It's wrong to assume that we need salt as a mineral. The best sources for minerals are fruits and vegetables, of course.

When we chemically break down salt, we have sodium chloride, a lethal poison. That's WHY one feels really thirsty after consuming salt because the body tries to wash the poisons out of the stomach via the kidneys.

Salt is a major contributor to heart and kidney (so called) diseases, high blood pressure, osteopenia and osteoporosis (it robs the bones from calcium); and salt waterlogs the tissues and irritates the nervous system, among others.

Salted foods are everywhere, but commonly found on potato chips, nuts, pretzels, crackers etc.

ENRICHED FLOURS: these flours are deprived, depleted, incomplete grains that have been bled white. White grains do not exist in nature. Enriched flours are very acidic and the particular acids they form within the body are extremely difficult to neutralize by the secretions of our body. Furthermore, it's safe to say that enriched flours are the number one contributor to constipation. Therefore, use ONLY local or home-made whole grain flour.

REFINED SUGAR: too many books and articles have already been published on the countless health hazards of excess sugar. The list of the health destroying effects of sugar is extensive and includes: increases blood sugar levels, overstimulates insulin production, injures the pancreas, causes diabetes, interferes with digestive juices, interferes with the absorption of protein, calcium and other minerals, leaches calcium from bones (including teeth) and blood, causes tooth decay, causes stress, depletes all the B-vitamins, causes arteriosclerosis, mental illness and loss of memory, inhibits the growth of vital intestinal bacteria etc. In short, a poison to avoid at all cost!

Refined sugar is commonly found in jams and jellies, ice cream, cakes and pastries, cookies, candy, commercial fruit juices, canned fruits, puddings, chewing gum, soda, preserves etc.

DAIRY: The misconception about milk and dairy products is further explained in chapter 15, but it's worth mentioning already that milk and dairy products are great poisons, causing all kinds of allergies, digestive problems, abnormal calcium deposits, arteriosclerosis, obesity and so much more. These DAIRY poisons contribute to toxemia: the ONE AND ONLY CAUSE of ALL so called DISEASE.

Milk drinkers have significantly more headaches, colds and flus, and produce far more mucus than non-milk drinkers. The only type of milk one should drink is mother's milk, and I kindly suggest that only infants drink it. Adults may consume coconut milk or almond milk, since both of these are just the respective juices of coconuts and almonds, and are not dairy.

The PLAIN and SIMPLE FACTS on milk and dairy are laid out in Chapter 15.

HYDROGENATED OILS: butter, margarine, peanut butter, canned foods packed in oil, fried foods, lard, shortenings and many other food items contain these poisonous oils. Our body is UNABLE to break down these oils because it takes a temperature of 300 degrees to do so (and our body is only 98.3 degrees). It's plain stupidity to even think about eating these. Besides the fact that our body can't produce enough heat to break them down, these hydrogenated oils coat the stomach walls and prevent the digestives juices from doing their job. The digestive process is prolonged and incomplete which results in poisoning, malnutrition, obesity and any so called disease. Better choices would be cold pressed, natural oils such as olive oil, sesame oil, avocado oil, walnut oil, almond oil, peanut oil, apricot oil, sunflower oil etc. READ the LABEL on your food products and avoid these hydrogenated oils like the plague.

OTHERS: besides salt, all other condiments should be avoided. They are hiding the taste of the real food and cause a false sense of hunger (appetite), besides being totally unnatural and poisonous of course. Condiments include ketchup, mayonnaise, mustard, all salad dressings and sauces, pickles, green salted olives etc.

Avoid commercial dry cereals such as cornflakes, avoid fried foods, peanut butter containing salt and hydrogenated oils, meat and lunch meats (lunch meats are dead meat but also contain sodium nitrate or nitrate), canned soups (they usually contain salt, sugar, white or wheat flour, preservatives etc.), canned food of all kinds, bleached and unbleached white flour products (white bread, or mixed wheat bread and rye bread, biscuits, sandwiches, noodles, spaghetti, pizza pie, cakes, pastries, ready-mix bakery products etc.), pre-mixed salads, dried fruits (they contain sulfur dioxide as a preservative), cottonseed oil, white rice, and anything else that MOTHER NATURE DOESN'T RECOGNIZE.

5.7 Key Points

The digestive process is so elaborate that in normal circumstances it will utilize approximately 80% of all vital energy available at the time.

Appetite is defined as the DESIRE for a food or drink, a desire to satisfy a taste or craving. Appetite is psychological, dependent on memory and associations. Appetite is fake hunger. It's a creature of habit and cultivation. It is stimulated by the sight, taste, smell or thought of food, the arrival of habitual meal time, condiments and seasonings.

Hunger is only physiologically aroused when there is an actual need for food, and is accompanied by 'watering of the mouth'. It arises spontaneously, without the help of any external factor.

Back to Basics:

EAT ONLY WHEN HUNGRY.

NEVER EAT DURING, IMMEDIATELY BEFORE OR AFTER PHYSICAL OR MENTAL ACTIVITY.

NEVER EAT WHEN SICK, IN PAIN OR IN MENTAL DISCOMFORT.

PROPERLY MASTICATE AND INSALIVATE ALL FOOD.

DO NOT DRINK WITH MEALS.

DRINK ONLY WHEN THIRSTY.

To maximize nutrient absorption and minimize digestive efforts, combine foods properly:

- Fruits are best eaten as a meal. Don't combine sweet fruits with acid fruits.

- Protein meals are best combined with low and non-starchy veggies while carbohydrate meals are best combined with starchy veggies.

Your body can only function optimally in a normal, alkaline environment. Pathogens and bacteria cannot survive in this normal, alkaline environment.

Consume a majority of alkaline forming foods while reducing your intake of acid forming foods to regain and maintain normal body pH.

Organic foods are more nutritious and contain far less agricultural chemicals. There's a misconception that eating healthy is more expensive but the contrary is true.

RAW, FRESH, ORGANIC, LOCAL foods are the best choice for CLEAN eating.

Chapter 6 – Clean Air
& Clean Water

Our ancestors didn't have to worry about air pollution and toxic water. We do. We don't live in nature anymore, we live in cities and villages in which air and water pollution is rampant.

6.1 Clean Air

You could go days without food and water, but you would last only a few minutes without air. On average, each of us breathes over 3,000 gallons of air each day. We obviously need air and oxygen to survive. But inhaling polluted air promotes toxemia and sickness.

Air pollution, chemicals that form acid rain, and ground-level ozone can damage trees, crops, plants, wildlife, lakes and other bodies of water.

In addition to damaging the natural environment, air pollution also damages buildings, monuments, and statues. It not only reduces how far you can see in national parks and cities, it even interferes with aviation.

According to the EPA (Environmental Protection Agency) the health, environmental, and economic impacts of air pollution are significant. Each day, air pollution causes thousands of illnesses leading to lost days at work and school. Air pollution also reduces agricultural crop and commercial forest yields by billions of dollars each year.

The problems are well documented. Nitrogen oxide, diesel fuels, sulfur dioxide, dioxins and furans, methane gasses and many other particles cloud the air in our cities. Researchers at the New York City School of Medicine determined a significant increase in lung cancer deaths with an increase in air pollution.

Inhalation of polluted air sets off many allergies, irritates eyes, nose and throat, and may cause breathing difficulties, asthma, respiratory problems and heart disease.

Some toxic chemicals released in the air such as benzene or vinyl chloride are highly toxic and can cause cancer, birth defects, long term injury to the lungs, as well as brain and nerve damage. And in some cases, breathing in these chemicals can even cause death.

Other pollutants make their way up into the upper atmosphere, causing a thinning of the protective ozone layer. This has led to changes in the environment and dramatic increases in skin cancers and cataracts (eye damage).

And then we have the methane gasses from our landfills. Thousands of tons of garbage dumped daily and releasing toxic gasses. A real shame because the technology to convert any type of waste (including municipal, solid, medical, radioactive and nuclear waste) into a green by-product such as electricity, hydrogen or a bio-fuel is not new and is commercially available. We could easily clean up all our land-fills, stop dumping our waste and produce clean energy. We wouldn't need to buy any energy from the middle-east nor would we have to drill in our own oceans and put aquatic life at risk. We would be able to turn all our garbage and trash into energy. I must assume that politics and bureaucracy hold us back from doing so. Not to mention the millions of dollars it costs to transport garbage to landfills and build these landfills.

The bottom line remains that all these pollutants are toxic and the inhalation of them contributes to the toxic load in our body and therefore toxemia.

In 1970, Congress created the Environmental Protection Agency (EPA) and passed the Clean Air Act, giving the federal government author-ity to clean up air pollution in this country. Since then, the EPA, states, tribes, local governments, industry, and environmental groups have worked to establish a variety of programs to reduce air pollution levels across America.

OXYGEN

It's not news when I share with you that each and every cell in our body depends on a sufficient supply of oxygen. Knowing that our health depends on the proper functioning of many trillions of cells, it seems to me that oxygen is quite important. Studies have shown a direct correla-tion between the levels of oxygen and someone's health and vitality.

When a cell receives sufficient oxygen, it not only carries out its own functions effectively but it also produces ATP (adenosine triphosphate) to fuel the body. Our energy levels thus depend on oxygen levels in our body. We feel energetic when sufficient oxygen is present and we will feel fatigued and weak with low levels of oxygen.

Furthermore, sufficient oxygen in our blood alkalizes our body. So besides using the alkaline model to normalize your pH, proper oxygen-ation will also help to this effect.

INDOOR AIR QUALITY

Even though many studies and statistics are available in reference to outdoor air quality, not much information is available on indoor air quality. Due to our social lives and work, the majority of people spend countless hours indoors; usually more hours indoors versus outdoors.

Offices and buildings these days don't allow for fresh air because they have been insulated to conserve energy. We are forced to breath in recirculated, lifeless air all day long. On top of that we are exposed to volatile organic chemicals from building materials, office furniture and equipment, carpets and paint. If that's not enough, we also have molds circulating in the heating and ventilation systems.

I'm sure you can see the problem. We breathe in poor quality air which means we supply our cells with low levels of oxygen.

What can we do to improve this situation (at your house and at the office)?

1. Vacuum often, ban smoking indoors (you shouldn't be around smokers anyway), minimize the use of candles and wood fires, and use the exhaust fans in the kitchen, bath, and laundry areas.

2. Test your home for radon gas, which can cause lung cancer (test kits cost about $15). This is usually only necessary when you live in an older construction home.

3. Minimize the risk of deadly carbon monoxide gas by properly maintaining heating equipment, wood stoves, fireplaces, chimneys, and vents. Install carbon-monoxide alarms on all levels of your home.

4. Don't idle your car, run fuel-burning power equipment, or light a barbecue grill in your garage, basement, or in confined spaces near your home.

5. Don't store chemicals, solvents, glues, or pesticides in your house.

6. Use natural household products versus chemical ones, including detergents, soaps, cosmetic products etc. Many of these products release toxic gasses, e.g. hairsprays.

7. Consider a commercially available air filter designed to improve the quality of air indoors. It may be a great investment since your health, and the health of others, is priceless.

8. Most of us are air conditioning junkies. Air conditioning in the house or office, or the car is yet another bad and (most of the time) unnecessary habit. Lifeless, reused air - cold

or hot - doesn't serve any good purpose. If you use the system, make sure you replace the filters regularly. Save some money and only use your A/C when extremely cold or hot. Open those windows in your house or office, and when driving a car open the roof, sunroof or windows and have the fresh air circulate.

9. Keep some green plants indoors. As you know plants and trees exchange CO_2 (Carbon Dioxide) for O_2 (Oxygen). Therefore, a few green plants in your home or office provide you with some fresh oxygen.

10. Open windows if you can, as much as possible, and let fresh air circulate. If you open a few you really get some circulation of fresh air (unless you live right by a busy highway or next to an industrial plant of course).

11. Spend more time outdoors. Go and eat your lunch (if you have any) outdoors, go for a short walk during a break or lunch time. Don't stay indoors.

12. If you exercise, maybe consider outdoor activities or suggest to your yoga instructor to do some outdoor classes.

13. On your days off or in the evenings, go sit outside to read a book or to relax or to have dinner with your family. The kids will love it also. Make some trips to parks and springs (lots of fresh air from trees and plants), or go to the beach if you are close (fresh ocean air).

14. Learn to breathe properly and maximize oxygenation (find instructions below).

15. Activity stimulates the circulation and therefore proper and timely distribution of oxygen to the cells and tissues.

AIR PURIFIERS

Pollutants that can affect air quality in a home fall into the following categories:

1. Particulate matter includes dust, smoke, pollen, animal dander, tobacco smoke, particles generated from combustion appliances such as cooking stoves, and particles associated with tiny organisms such as dust mites, molds, bacteria, and viruses.

2. Gaseous pollutants come from combustion processes. Sources include gas cooking stoves, vehicle exhaust, and tobacco smoke. They also come from building materials, furnishings, and the use of products such as adhesives, paints, varnishes, cleaning products, and pesticides.

Air filter systems and in-home air purification systems and cleaning devices are available, each designed to remove certain types of pollutants.

I'm not a technician and I don't want to write several pages on these. There are so many available and based on your needs and the size of your home and rooms, and the type of pollutants that need filtered or purified, there's a system out there for you. I recommend you do some diligent research by studying some consumer reports or visit the EPA website: www.epa.gov. I also have some useful links listed on our website www.Health4Life.info, under the 'free downloads' section.

Air purifiers are an excellent tool in the fight against indoor allergens and pathogens. However, you should pay close attention to the technology the air filter uses. Ionizers and UV-lights used with these systems have potential dangers and clean air is not worth damaged lungs. So conduct some diligent research if you opt for an air purification system.

I personally don't have one. If you live C.L.E.A.N the pathogens in the air don't have a chance against your healthy body. However, clean and fresh air is a must if one wants to be healthy. Spend more time outdoors, ventilate your rooms by opening the windows, practice diaphragmatic breathing, and incorporate the above recommendations to improve indoor air quality.

EFFECTIVE BREATHING

Oxygenating your blood not only depends on the quality of the air but also on your breathing. We breathe, involuntarily, all day long. But the majority of people are not aware on how they breathe and how they should be breathing to maximize oxygenation.

Most of us are what we call 'shallow chest breathers'. Just take a moment and notice how deeply you are breathing at this very moment. You are breathing pretty shallow, right? And now try and notice which part of your body moves when you breathe? Does your chest slightly move up and down or does your stomach move in and out? Most likely it's your chest moving. Hence, most of us are 'shallow chest breathers'.

Shallow breathing only fills about 20 – 30% of the lungs and this is actually enough to carry out basic metabolic functions. However, when we work or exercise or need more energy we need lots more oxygen. In order to alkalize the body, we also need more oxygen.

The part of the lungs that is filled with oxygen during shallow breathing is the upper lobes, not the lower lobes. Many health problems thus arise because of poor blood flow in the lower lobes of the lungs. Chronic fatigue, anxiety, panic attacks, digestive problems (reflux, heartburn, bloating, gas), chest pain and palpitations, muscle cramps (neck and back), numbness and tingling in the extremities, headaches and migraines, disturbed dreams and hallucinations may all be caused by insufficient oxygenation.

Proper breathing or deep breathing is done by contracting the diaphragm, a muscle located horizontally between the chest cavity and stomach cavity. Air enters the lungs and the belly expands during this type of breathing. This deep breathing is marked by expansion of the abdomen rather than the chest during inhalation.

How do we do this deep or diaphragmatic breathing?

Place one hand on the chest and the other hand on the stomach. Breathe in slowly and deep as to fill up your lungs from the bottom all the way up. If done correctly you will feel your stomach push your hand up while your chest just moves a little bit with your stomach. This deep breathing fills up the lower lobes of the lungs and the diaphragm contracts. This contraction makes your stomach stick out.

This breathing technique not only maximizes oxygen intake into the lungs with each breath but also stimulates contraction of the diaphragm which enhances circulation.

Start practicing this technique 3 to 5 times per day, and prior to any activity or when you feel fatigued and tired, stressed or just need physical or mental energy. Just take 10 breaths each time. Your inhalation should take about 1 second, then hold 3-4 seconds, and exhale for about 2 seconds.

CONCLUSION

You may be of the opinion that you cannot do much yourself to improve the outside air quality, but that would be a wrong assumption.

You could start to make sure you don't buy any unnecessary plastics which would end-up in the land-fills. You need to recycle for sure, but you also can reuse many items within the house. For example, don't buy any plastic bottles of water or other drinks. Just get some glass bottles and continue to refill them with clean, alkaline water (see below). You will save lots of plastic and money. The plastic won't leach in your drinking water either.

When you go shopping, don't have the baggers put your stuff in a plastic bag. What a waste. Get a regular bag (or use our Health 4 Life tote bag) and use it over and over again to go shopping. I'm sure you can think of many other ways to recycle and reuse.

If you can walk or drive the bicycle instead of being lazy by jumping in the car all the time, you will exhaust less toxic fuels into the air. Have you ever thought about carpooling? With a colleague that lives in the neighborhood maybe? One of our friends has 2 children that go to the same school as my 2 daughters, so we alternate bringing them to school. Not only do we save time and gas but we also help minimize air pollution. We also carpool to soccer games etc.

If you have a yard, plant some more trees. Maybe you can help planting some trees in your community. Trees and plants provide oxygen.

Your indoor air quality can be improved with the 15 recommendations presented earlier in this chapter.

Trust me, it will make a big difference in how you feel and perform.

Even though we cannot avoid the constant onslaught of these air pollutants, we can minimize the intoxication of them as much as possible. Just the awareness of this toxic onslaught should urge one to not only take action and prevent breathing in polluted air as much as possible, but also emphasizes the importance of a simple and effective detoxification program.

6.2 Clean Water

Just like air, water is vital to life. With 2 parts hydrogen and 1 part oxygen, water is the most abundant substance in our body.

When we are born, 80% of our body is water and only 20% is matter. As adults, approximately 65% is water. As seniors our body dries up to hold only 50% of water reflecting in stiff joints, dry and wrinkled skin, reduced saliva flow (dry mouth) etc.

Our brains consist of 75% water, our blood 80-85% and our bones 25%. Water provides for all essential bodily and cellular functions including respiration, elimination (removes wastes, alkalizes and detoxifies), perspiration (regulates body temperature), digestion (saliva and digestive juices) and absorption, circulation and nutrient transportation and many other chemical processes.

Water is also the base for building all body tissues and organs, and is the base of all blood and fluid secretions (tears, saliva, sweat, gastric juices, synovial fluid that lubricates our joints etc.).

Therefore a loss of 5 to 10% of body water results in significant dehydration while a loss of 20% results in death.

WATER RETENTION

When the body receives an inadequate amount of water it will start holding on to water as a means of survival (remember the first law?). This water is stored in the spaces outside the cells (extracellular space) and presents itself as swollen ankles, feet, legs, and hands along with of course some significant weight gain. This gain in weight is due to water retention plus the storage of fat that has not been metabolized by the liver. The natural feeling of thirst is also inhibited during this process.

Our conventional, western medicine solution is the prescription of... yes, diuretics. As usual, just the opposite of what really should be done. It's almost a given. If you really want to know what the answer is to any given problem, just look at what conventional medicine does and then do the opposite. That's how you get healthy, and not sicker.

Oops, did I go off track again? I apologize. Well, diuretics force the stored water out of our body along with some essential nutrients. Yet again our body will react by storing water as a means of survival. The short-term 'results' (better called adverse effects) of the diuretics are corrected by the body. More diuretics need to be swallowed and so on.

The ONLY WAY to overcome the water retention is to consume more water. As soon as the body receives sufficient water to carry out its normal functions, it releases the stored water.

Excess salt (sodium) intake is a prime contributor to water retention. The more salt is consumed, the more water the body needs to utilize to dilute these salts. Watch your salt intake (or omit salt altogether), but more importantly consume enough water.

DEHYDRATION

While *water retention* is a sign of dehydration (yes that is correct) there are other signs that indicate lack of bodily water:

Dry skin is a sign of dehydration. The skin is not only the largest organ but it's also the organ that reflects the conditions of the internal organs. This is not only a diagnostic tool in TCM (Traditional Chinese Medicine) but simply a fact. If the skin is dry, the internal environment is dry. If the skin exhibits break-outs and pimples it reflects toxicity in the body. How is that you may ask? The skin is an organ of excretion. It expels toxins. These toxins come from inside your body and show up at the skin as a variety of skin conditions: rashes, dermatitis, eczema, rosacea, oily skin etc. Any or all cosmetic products or topical agents designed to improve these skin conditions produce no or very limited result. Why? Because the cause of these skin problems is internal, and temporarily masking the superficial symptoms can't be the solution. The internal toxicity needs to be addressed if one wants to obtain lasting results. Normal skin has a healthy, vital complexion and is flexible, soft, and odorless.

Dark urine with odor indicates excess toxins in the urine accompanied with little water for their excretion.

Constipation or difficult stool is also a result of lack of water. Water is the main force behind normal elimination. When water in the body is limited, the body will halt elimination since using the available water for survival is more important. As we continue to eat more, food and toxins pile up and we become constipated.

A normal stool is soft (but not loose) and floats, doesn't require straining during elimination, is painless and has no foul odor. In a state of perfect health, one wouldn't even need to use toilet paper... I'm not kidding, really! Do animals in the wild wipe their butt? It's not necessary because their diet is normal and therefore there stool is normal. If your stool is hard and sinks right to the bottom of the toilet, you are dehydrated and if not resolved soon you will be constipated.

Dryness of lips and dry mouth are other signs of dehydration. Many of us would eat to overcome this dryness as thirst is mistaken for hunger. Another reason people overeat unnecessarily.

Fatigue and weakness are common signs of dehydration. If our body lacks sufficient water all bodily and cellular functions become sluggish resulting in physical and mental weakness.

A quick note about water and WEIGHT LOSS:

First off, water reduces appetite (not necessarily hunger). We already discussed when to drink and when not to drink. We only drink when thirsty and preferably 15 to 20 minutes before a meal or 4 hours after a meal. When we drink before a meal, we reduce appetite and help prevent overeating.

Second, it has been proven that water helps metabolize stored fat. Here is how. If the kidneys receive insufficient water they can't function optimally and a part of the work load is then dumped onto the liver. One of the liver's prime functions is to metabolize fat but when preoccupied with helping the kidneys, some of that fat will be stored instead.

Drinking enough water thus is the catalyst in losing weight (fat) by promoting metabolism of stored fat in the body. It also is crucial in keeping that weight (fat) off. More will be discussed about sensible weight loss later in this book.

HOW MUCH WATER SHOULD WE CONSUME?

This is a topic of controversy and we all have been led to believe in false thoughts and ideas, false assumptions, and wrong habits... including myself. But nature yet again will tell us the truth.

Here is the dilemma and the confusion. Let's clear it all up. In **NORMAL** circumstances, meaning in optimal health, we only would drink when thirsty. We would only have to listen to the warning signs of our own body. Our body will tell us when it needs water.

If we would simply follow these 'instincts' or 'warning signs' of the body, we wouldn't have to worry about all these questions: how much do I drink? When do I drink etc.

Confusion arises here however. Man has adopted many perversions. **Perversion** is a concept describing those types of human behavior that deviate from those which are understood to be orthodox or normal. Perversion is behavior or habits that are antagonistic to the normal, natural laws of human life.

The cause for our perversions stems from our ability to choose our response. When we decide to place our body in the WRONG conditions for optimal health (eat man-made foods, overeat, overburden the digestive system when eating at wrong times, drinking during a meal, consuming contaminated water or inhaling pollutants, lack of rest and sleep, lack of sunshine, overstimulation, mental and emotional stress etc.), toxemia occurs and the disease process starts and progresses unless the cause is taken away and the body is placed under the RIGHT CONDITIONS.

After a time period of ignoring the RIGHT CONDITIONS, the warning signs of the body are no longer there. This creates confusion. We mistake appetite for hunger and appetite for thirst. We mistake symptoms of healing for disease and interfere with the healing process of the body. We live life by overindulging and overstimulating our senses.

A simple example is that of alcohol or other stimulant. The first time one consumes the toxin, the body reacts with a headache, vomiting, nausea etc. in a successful attempt to expel the toxin from the body. This should have been a warning sign NOT to ever consume the alcohol again, right? We tend to ignore these warning signs and we violate the natural laws over and over again. After consuming the alcohol a few more times, the body does not react with vomiting anymore. The energy expenditure is too high and the reaction too violent. The body warned you but you ignore the warning signs. The body stops warning you and is now forced to deal with this regular intoxication differently. It will continue to deal with it by expending countless vital energy and essential resources, all in an effort to preserve life.

Now you can understand WHY there no longer are any warning signs and the body just has to deal with this situation of habitual intoxication as long as it can in order to preserve life. After years of abuse, disease finally shows up and one wonders what went wrong. 'Why me?' one wonders.

The habitual ignorance is called a perversion, a deviation from normal. The body is not functioning in normal circumstances and is not functioning in a normal environment.

So when the normal and natural sense of thirst is messed up (as in most of us, believe me) we need to look for these other signs of dehydration: water retention, dry skin, dry mouth, dry lips, constipation or hard stool, dark urine, fatigue and weakness, weight gain. THESE are NOW - in our perverse situation – the WARNING SIGNS of the body.

To overcome these dehydration signs and provide the body with sufficient water, we will need to drink more water even when not having the sense of being really thirsty. When we have signs of dehydration we need to force ourselves to drink, or force others who show these signs. Even when not thirsty, keep in mind WHEN you should drink!

How much should we drink?

In normal, healthy circumstances: until we feel no longer thirsty. Imagine a herd of wild cattle drinking from a pond in the African desert lands. They drink a lot of water. They wait until their body tells them to stop. They don't drink all day long, like we do. It's because they don't confuse thirst with appetite. We drink because of appetite: the sight, taste, smell, habit of toxic, sugar-loaded, man-made, addictive toxic cocktails.

So how much do we drink then in this perverted, abnormal situation in which our sense of true thirst is messed up? That's arbitrary and depends on the individual's condition. But a guideline to start is to drink the amount of ounces of water equal to half of one's body weight in pounds. For example, if one weighs 140 pounds, he or she should drink a minimum of 70 ounces of pure, alkaline water per day. I think that's a good start but one would have to adjust this amount based on the warning signs of the body. Are the signs of dehydration improving, or not? What about the circumstances? What is the external temperature? What is the activity level? What other emergencies is the body dealing with? Etc.

Be sure not to drink all day long in a forced effort to consume this water. Just like the animals, drink a huge amount only a few times per day. For example, you may drink a huge amount 20 minutes before breakfast or just drink that water and skip breakfast. You can drink lots of water 4 hours after breakfast or about 20 minutes before lunch, or 4 hours after lunch, or 20 minutes before dinner. I don't have to explain why. You already understand.

Drinking more water will make you go to the bathroom quite more often, and that's ok. Your body is used to being dehydrated and is not used to this amount of fluid intake. As your body becomes more hydrated, frequency of urination will lower.

Be careful not to consume too much water. Drinking too much water quickly can lead to water intoxication. Water intoxication occurs when water dilutes the sodium level in the bloodstream and causes an imbalance of water in the brain. Water intoxication is most likely to occur during periods of intense athletic performance, but some people force too much water into their system in an attempt to hydrate. Again, watch for signs and gradually increase your intake.

Over time, the skin, mouth, and lips will be moist again, the urine will be clear (no color) and free of odor, the stool will be normal, soft and frequent and water retention, fatigue and weakness will be no longer. At this time the sense of thirst returns and becomes, once again, your warning sign indicating when to drink.

Be aware that in order for this to happen and normal thirst to return, other perversions need to be returned to normal as well. In other words, normal eating needs to replace feasting, food needs to be combined properly to allow for effective digestion and absorption of nutrients, emotions need to be balanced, rest and sleep need to be sufficient, as well as sunlight etc. ONLY in the RIGHT CONDITIONS can HEALTH BE RESTORED.

SHOULD WE ONLY DRINK WATER?

Yes. Do animals in the wild drink anything else but water? No. Only the calves or the young drink mother's milk to grow strong. As humans, our baby's should do the same: only drink mother's milk. As children (after 1 year of age) and adults we also should do the same as animals: only drink water.

It's yet another, and really sick if you think about it, perversion of us humans (excluding me and hopefully you soon) to consume not only milk as adults, but even consume milk from a different species... perverted, right? We will discuss milk and dairy later but already know that there is no nutritional value to consuming any dairy product.

And then we have juices. As long as the juices of fruits and vegetables are all natural and contain no colorings, additives, preservatives, added sugars etc. you may certainly consume them. However, be aware that even most of the natural juices are very sugary since they are made from sweet fruits. So, limit your intake. Maybe consume just a glass of orange juice in the morning.

The amount of fruit juices consumed, especially by our children, far exceeds what is needed. Remember that sugar induces acidity. We can also look at animals in the wild again and observe nature. Most of nature is vegetation consisting of plants and trees, not many fruit trees in relation to green vegetation. While fruits are loaded with a variety of essential nutrients, fruit is Mother Nature's candy and needs to be consumed in moderation. Some animals eat fruit, but not in excess.

Also, just as with fruit itself, don't mix sweet and acid fruits in fruit juices.

Any other man-made substances should be omitted from your diet, including all soda's and carbonated drinks, man-made fruit juices, milk, coffee, alcoholic beverages and anything else. All are just a burden on our body, robbing us of energy (yes, also the so called stimulants) and increasing the toxic load in our body, while providing no essential nutrients or benefit to our body. We do not have a physiological need for these drinks. We merely created a perversion or appetite for them.

OUR DRINKING WATER

We understand the major importance water holds in our lives but many of us know very little about the water we use each day.

We drink and use tap water and enjoy the convenience and cost-effectiveness of this practice. However, we fail to recognize the serious threat this water poses to our health. Those who are willing to forgo the convenience of tap water and indulge in bottled water often know very little about the contents of that water. They simply assume that bottled water is better than tap water. Even conscientious consumers, who wisely attempt to treat their own water in an effort to ensure the healthfulness of that water, often know little about the many home water treatment options now available.

In this age of information, with so many resources immediately at our fingertips, there is no reason why anyone should remain so ill informed about our drinking water.

Tap water, is it safe? There are more than 2100 known drinking water contaminants that may be present in tap water, including several known poisons.

Besides the occasional episodes of waterborne illnesses, our drinking water becomes increasingly polluted by pesticides, chemical and radio-active wastes, nuclear wastes, industrial wastes, fertilizer etc.

Common contaminants are the following:

Chlorine: as part of the process to treat our drinking water chlorine is added to destroy bacteria. This comes with a price though. Chlorine itself is not just a toxin releasing toxic fumes, but it can combine with other organic matter and form CDBP's (Chlorinated Disinfection By-Products). The long-term exposure or consumption of these CDBP's increases the risk of cancer (bladder and colon cancer).

Lead: mostly coming from the erosion of pipes and holding tanks through which the water comes to your tap, lead build-up in the body causes damage to blood cells and organs. According to the EPA, lead in drinking water contributes to 480,000 cases of learning disorders in children each year in the United States alone. It is especially important for pregnant women to drink pure water as lead in drinking water can cause severe birth defects. A common recommendation would be to run the water for a little bit before using it so the lead is flushed, but it's much wiser to not use tap water at all.

Arsenic: mostly coming from the industrial wastes and as a result of burning fossil fuels such as coal, but also from rocks or mineral deposits containing arsenic and dissolving into the water. Even though the amounts in our drinking water may be minimal and below so called safe levels, it's the chronic accumulation that causes cancer and heart disease.

You could test your water for lead and arsenic, but again I wouldn't use tap water.

Aluminum: most water treatment facilities add ALUM, a clarifying chemical agent (making water clear) to the water. As a result aluminum is left in our drinking water.

Fluoride: both natural and added fluoride is found in our tap water. The common notion that we need this toxin to protect our teeth is pure ignorance. Do animals in the wild brush their teeth with fluoride paste? Our teeth are in bad shape because of the toxic, man-made foods and drinks we consume, and it's the acidity that breaks down our enamel.

Cadmium: another heavy metal commonly found in our drinking water is also responsible for adding to the toxic load and causing all types of cancers.

Microorganisms: as a result of the suspension of matter such as clay or decaying plants in our water, disease causing micro-organisms escape disinfection by adhering to these matters. They usually cause gastroin-testinal illnesses.

Parasites: mostly through sewage and animal waste parasites living in the intestines of humans and animals end up in our water. They can cause gastrointestinal symptoms including diarrhea, nausea, vomiting, poor appetite, dehydration, and even infection and death.

You can request a report from your city (or download it from their website) and get information on the contaminants and their levels in your drinking water, or have your water tested. And that's a good start: create some awareness for yourself.

Bottled water, is it safe? There's no direct answer to this question since there's various types of bottled water. I would omit all of them just because of the fact that a plastic bottle can leak plastic into your water and expose you to various toxic chemicals. So regardless the purity of the water, having it sealed in a plastic bottle concerns me.

Bottled water can come from a municipal water supply or from a spring. The water is then treated by one or several various processes: distil-lation, deionization, reverse osmosis etc. An estimated 25% of bottled water is just filtered tap water.

Mineral water is spring water containing a minimum of 500mg of minerals per quart or liter. Mineral water is often high is sodium and while some are naturally carbonated (they contain CO_2) others are being carbonated.

Carbonated water is not considered water, it is considered soda.

Spring water comes from a natural underground spring source and must have the same properties as it did underground. In theory, this water is better protected from contaminants and pollutants than lake and river water. Some of the more expensive brands actually have an alkaline pH because of the minerals and trace-elements in them, including Fiji™

and Evian™.

Distilled water may be contaminant free (if the distillation process was followed by a carbon filtration) but it is 'dead' and doesn't contain nutrients or minerals.

So whether bottled water is safer than tap water is hard to tell. It depends on the quality of your tap water and the type of bottled water. Bottled water is much more expensive and burdens the planet with plastic. In my opinion, both options are very poor and detrimental to health.

HOME FILTRATION SYSTEMS

This is definitely the way to go. A wide variety of systems is available on the market, ranging broadly in cost and effectiveness. Whether you just need an inexpensive pitcher or unit to attach to your faucet, or a more expensive under-the-sink unit depends on the quality of your tap water.

But there is more to know:

Merely avoiding drinking tap water by purifying the tap water is not an effective means of protection against dangerous water contaminants. It's a great start preventing direct ingestion of all these toxins but it's not enough.

The EPA has stated that every household in the United States has elevated levels of chloroform in the air due to chlorine released from showering water. Tap water often contains at least as much, if not more, chlorine than is recommended for use in swimming pools.

More chlorine enters the body through dermal absorption and inhalation while showering than through drinking tap water. The chlorine in showering water has harsh, drying effects on skin and hair and can cause rashes and irritation when absorbed. Skin pores widen while showering, making dermal absorption of chlorine and other chemicals possible.

Chemicals in showering water vaporize at a much faster rate than the actual water. Thus, the steam in a shower contains a much higher concentration of chemicals than the water itself.

Inhaled chemicals make their way into the bloodstream much more quickly than ingested chemicals, without the added filtration benefits of digestion.

More water contaminants are released into the air of a home from the shower than from any other source. But harmful chemicals not only constantly escape into the air in a home from the shower, but also from the dishwasher and the toilets. The release of water contaminants into the air results in poor air quality in a home. This poor air quality is a leading cause of asthma and bronchitis, as we discussed earlier in this chapter.

Many skin rashes and other irritations are a result of chlorine and volatile organic chemicals (VOCs) that have become embedded in clothing washed in chlorinated water.

Chlorine is a suspected cause of breast cancer. Women suffering from breast cancer are all found to have 50-60 percent more chlorine in their breast tissue than healthy women.

The use of a *whole house water filter* is the only way to ensure pure, filtered water from every water source in the house. A whole house water filter purifies water efficiently and cost-effective, making it a viable solution to drinking water contamination and all its uses in the house.

You will need to do some homework. You will need to test your water or look at the reports of your city and see what contaminants are of concern. Then, you will need to educate yourself on the various systems and select the one that best removes the contaminants of your drinking water. To make things much easier for you, I did most of the homework already and therefore I suggest you visit our informational website at www.Health4Life.info. Use the FREE information and links available to make an informed decision as to which system you should purchase. This is very important. You want to spend your hard earned money the right way and assure that this relatively small investment REALLY benefits your health and that of your loved-ones. Agree?

You will learn that the carbon filters used in the popular water pitchers and tap or faucet systems such as Brita™ and Pur™ will remove chlorine, organic compounds, odor, bad taste and color from your water but they are ineffective in removing metals and inorganic pollutants. Another concern is that bacteria and molds grow within the filter (that's why they tell you to replace the filter every so often). Even more importantly, these filters ONLY treat your drinking water and don't protect you against the contaminants from other water sources such as the shower, toilet, dishwasher, washer etc.

Other systems are reverse osmosis systems and KDF home purification systems. In my house I have a centaur carbon filter and a reverse osmosis system. The centaur carbon filter removes the chloramine (my city uses chloramine and not chlorine) and the reverse osmosis system purifies my drinking water. But again, you may be better off with another system, based on the contaminants in your water.

Remember that water filters offer the last line of defense between the body and the over 2100 known toxins that may be present in drinking water.

CONSERVING WATER

There are literally 100's of ways to conserve water. Too many to list here, but you could find them on our website, for FREE.

It's important to realize that even though most of the earth's surface is water, less than 1% can be used as drinking water. That's because most of earth's water is either salty or frozen.

We established that pure, clean water is vital for life and therefore we need to cherish it. But it's not drinking the water that wastes the water.

Water is used as a raw material in many processes. For example, it takes 1500 gallons of water to process one barrel of beer, 120 gallons of water to produce one egg, 12 gallons to process one chicken, almost 10 gallons to process one can of fruit or vegetables, 6,800 gallons of water is required to grow a day's food for a family of four, 1,850 gallons of water to refine one barrel of crude oil, and manufacturing one new car uses 39,000 gallons of water.

We use more and more water each year, with Americans using five times the amount of water that Europeans do. We use about 50 gallons of water daily.

Less than 1% of the water treated by public water systems is used for drinking and cooking. Two thirds of the water used in a home is used in the bathroom. To flush a toilet once we use an average of 5 gallons of water and only a five-minute shower uses 25 to 50 gallons of water. Brushing your teeth uses 2 gallons of water while the automatic dish-washer uses about 10 gallons, and so on.

Don't you think it's time to start paying attention and be more aware and conscious about the use of water? With the help of the information on our website, make a list of the things you can do to conserve water and discuss it with your family members. Make some simple rules, and inform them WHY we need to help conserve water. You also will see a drop in your water bill!

Some examples to conserve water in the home:

When washing dishes by hand, don't let the water run while rinsing. Fill one sink with wash water and the other with rinse water.

Some refrigerators, air conditioners and ice-makers are cooled with wasted flows of water. Consider upgrading with air-cooled appliances for significant water savings.

Adjust sprinklers so only your lawn is watered and not the house, side-walk, or street.

Run your clothes washer and dishwasher only when they are full. You can save up to 1,000 gallons a month.

Install covers on pools and spas and check for leaks around your pumps.

Use the garbage disposal sparingly. Compost your vegetable food waste instead and save gallons every time.

Wash your fruits and vegetables in a pan or pot of water instead of running water from the tap. Collect the water you use for rinsing fruits and vegetables and reuse it to water houseplants.

Use a broom instead of a hose to clean your driveway and sidewalk and save water every time.

If your shower fills a one-gallon bucket in less than 20 seconds, replace the showerhead with a water-efficient model.

Shorten your shower by a minute or two and you'll save up to 150 gallons per month.

Put food coloring in your toilet tank. If it seeps into the toilet bowl without flushing, you have a leak. Fixing it can save up to 1,000 gallons a month.

When running a bath, plug the tub before turning the water on, and then adjust the temperature as the tub fills up.

Install a rain sensor on your irrigation controller so your system won't run when it rains.

Don't use running water to thaw food. Defrost food in the refrigerator for water efficiency and food safety.

Turn off the water while brushing your teeth and save 25 gallons a month.

Reuse the water left over from cooked or steamed foods to start a scrumptious and nutritious soup.

Turn off the water while you wash your hair to save up to 150 gallons a month.

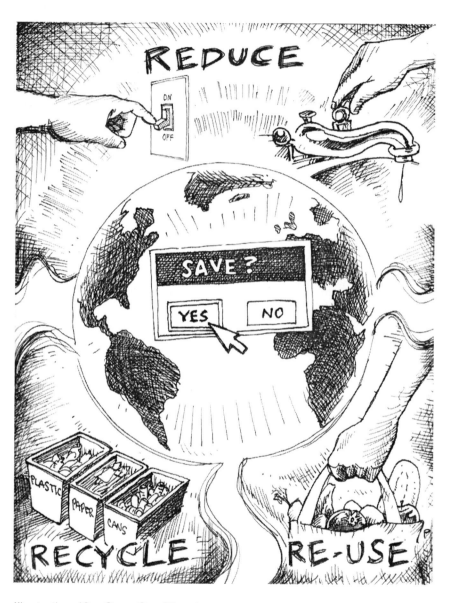

Illustration 12 – Save Our Planet

When you give your pet fresh water, don't throw the old water down the drain. Use it to water your trees or shrubs.

Do not rinse your dishes before putting them in the dishwasher. Even better, don't use the dishwasher (uses too much water compared to hand washing the dishes).

And you can find many more ways to conserve water on our website or online!

CLEAN WATER

Knowing that one of the major roles of water in our body is to expel toxins, it doesn't make sense to consume water loaded with toxins, does it? So we simply can't go without a home purification system.

We need to drink pure, alkaline water. How do we make our water alkaline? After purification, our water may be neutral or alkaline. Just measure it by using one of your pH strips.

Simple and cheap ways to alkalize your drinking water are to add a lemon or lime (squeeze it) or just a dash of baking soda. There are potent alkalizing supplements on the market also, but they require a small investment.

The purest water we can consume actually is contained in our organic, natural fruits and vegetables. Be aware that as you start a healthier, greener diet and consume more alkaline foods (which are the majority of vegetables and certain fruits) you will notice that you will be less thirsty and consume less water. That's because these live veggies contain lots of pure, alkaline water!

Most veggies contain over 90% of water while most fruits contain over 75% of pure water. For a FREE list of water-rich foods, please visit the website.

I hope you can see the importance of consuming pure, alkaline water. It doesn't take much effort and it will drastically affect your health in a positive way. Even though a home purification system is a monetary investment, it's a good investment with a positive ROI (Return of Investment). No need to buy any more bottled water or any other drinks for that matter, along with conserving water in the house will save you money.

6.3 Key Points

Both air and water are vital not only for our survival but for optimal health.

Today both our air and water is severely contaminated but we can take some action to reduce and control much of this contamination.

Recycling and reusing reduces waste and therefore air and water pollution.

Improving indoor air quality is important and easily done, while proper breathing and exercise both maximize oxygen levels.

Conserving water and installing a home water purification system is certainly worth the effort and investment.

Both clean air and clean water in sufficient amounts help alkalize the body and expel toxins.

When providing your body with clean air and clean water, you drastically reduce the toxic load in your body in two ways: (1) by reducing the amount of toxins ingested and inhaled and, (2) by increasing the effectiveness of the elimination process.

Sufficient clean water and clean air are crucial to providing the RIGHT CONDITIONS for your body in an effort to regain, sustain and maintain optimal health.

Chapter 7 – The Power of Sunlight

Dr. Oswald (Nature's Household Remedies, 1885) said: "Life is a sun-child. Nearly all species of plants and animals attain the highest forms of their development in the neighborhood of the equator. Palm trees are tropical grasses, the python-boa is a fully developed black snake, the tiger an undiminished wild cat. With every degree of a higher latitude, Nature issues the representatives of her arch-types in reduced editions: reduced in beauty and longevity, as well as in size and strength".

It's not news to anyone's ears that sun and sunlight are vital to development and health, but we have become a species that lives indoors and overprotects oneself against sunlight. Healthy organisms live and excel outdoors and are in their real element when exposed to sunlight while sedentary, often underdeveloped creatures live in the dark.

The importance of sunlight is so profound that life wouldn't even exist on planet earth without it.

The beneficial effects of sunlight were recognized as early as 600 BC. Heliotherapy (treatment with sunlight) was used by Herodotus to stimulate bone growth, and by the Romans, Greek, and Egyptians to treat a wide variety of conditions including pain, arthritis and asthma.

In the 1660's, Newton discovered the visible spectrum and in the 1800's man was able to increase the effectiveness of insolation (incoming solar radiation) with the use of devices such as lenses and glass boxes.

At the end of the 19th century, scientists investigated the photobiological effects of sun radiation and discovered the bactericidal action of sun-light, which still finds its application today in the use of UV-radiation for sterilization.

In 1903, Dr. Nils Finsen from Denmark received the Nobel Prize for introducing the first recognized therapeutic application of an artificial light source (treatment of surgical TB, rickets and lupus).

As a result of Einstein's vision and his Theory of Relativity, lasers were developed in the mid 1900's. Lasers are used in a wide variety of medical applications today, including its use in ocular surgeries, cancers, dermatology (aesthetics, warts, port-wine stains, cancers etc.), and diagnostics (Doppler-flow, spectroscopy etc.).

Even though artificial light and lasers are used as therapeutic devices, we established that therapeutic intervention is not wise and we will learn that real sunlight is far superior to artificial light.

Our skin:

Our skin is not only and by far our largest organ but it's the only organ in direct contact with the external environment. The skin provides a strong protective covering for the rest of the body and resists the intrusion of external and infectious matter.

A skin that is weakened by clothing and lack of sunlight becomes a less effective barrier and therefore becomes prone to infections, including all kinds of skin inflammations (dermatitis and 20 others), hypertrophies (about 40 varieties), atrophies (about 40 varieties), hemorrhages, neu-roses, parasitical infections, skin growths and cancers (about 70 variet-ies) and so on. So instead of supposedly 'protecting' our skin from sun-light we should make sure our skin receives plenty of natural sunlight to abolish the above mentioned conditions.

Cutting out infections, swallowing antibiotics, putting on chemical crèmes etc. only worsen the condition. Don't chase symptoms, correct the cause. The cause is still toxemia.

Our skin also plays a crucial role in the elimination of toxins and the regulation of our body temperature. We understand that toxemia is the cause of ALL so called disease so you can now understand the importance of a healthy functioning skin assisting in proper elimination of toxins.

Our skin can ONLY be healthy in the presence of abundant sunlight.

7.1 Man Was a Nude Animal

Man was a nude animal before he learned to make clothes, that's a given. But even in ancient times, nudity and sunbathing was practiced as a form of health and healing. Some even worshipped the sun.

It was Christianity and its extreme reactions against anything 'pagan' that ended the sunbathing so widely employed by as well the healthy as the sick.

I personally observed at first hand the use of sunlight in the treatment of arthritis in 1981. I was a 10 y/o boy on a swimming training camp in Romania. Older people rubbed in their whole body with black mud and would face the sun on a daily basis.

If we would run around naked (which I'm not advocating in public surroundings), our skin would be preserved, healthier and more vigorous AND it would carry out its important functions much better, including its function of elimination.

Without clothes, movement and respiration would be far less restricted, and bones would be stronger. The whole physical and physiological system would operate much more effectively and development would be much more symmetrical and anatomically correct. As a result, sensual appetites would be more of pure instinctive nature (as opposed to a perversion) and imagination would be deprived of its great powers to conduct evil.

Housing and clothing have deprived us of our normal supply of sunlight. Our skin cannot be clean and functioning optimally when its contact with air and sunlight is deprived. An example is that one of sweaty feet. Anyone (all of us) who has experienced sweaty feet before knows how disagreeable the odor is that exudes from the shoes when removing them. Now, when you run around bare feet all day, you still sweat but you won't get the odor, right? That's because the air and sun disintegrate and carry away the excretions from the skin and feet. In the same way a manual laborer sweats all day, his clothes saturated with sweat and odor while his hands and face do not give off such an odor.

Furthermore, weakened skin loses its power of resistance to atmospheric changes. Therefore, many of us suffer with a sudden change in temperature.

7.2 Light and Vitality

We know that we can't live without light. Plants can't either. Plants absorb carbon dioxide and emit oxygen during daytime (light) but during the night (no light) this process is reversed. Therefore sleeping in ill-ventilated spaces with lots of plants is not recommended. Plants, animals and humans alike would suffer without light and become debilitated. The tadpole wouldn't develop into a frog without light but instead would continue to grow as a tadpole or turn into a monstrosity; as specimen of humans in underground parts of large cities also develop to be abnormal.

Even today in larger cities where people spend their time in small apartments, backrooms, cellars and vaults (underground level), and ill-lit buildings in narrow streets we can observe unmistakable signs of imperfect development and deficient vitality.

Light stimulates activity of both body and mind, while dark promotes indolence and obesity. People tend to be more active when they live in warmer areas and are able to be more outdoors, exposed to sunlight.

Sunlight is also the cause of all color in the body. Light is entirely reflected by white and completely absorbed by black. Some plants thrive best when exposed to strong sunlight, others in moderate sunlight, and some when considerably shaded. However, they all require the influence of light to become firm and vigorous, without any exception. Many fish and insects are constantly luminous (rays of light are emitted from their bodies) such as the firefly, the glow-worm and many others. Light is vital.

Light is simply hygienic. Light stimulates all biological processes and functions and helps maintain optimal health and vitally, as do clean water and air.

Light has the power to destroy noxious vaporous bodies existing in the atmosphere.

Light has many nutritional functions. Some of them are listed here:

- Sunlight enables the body to assimilate calcium.

- Sunlight increases phosphorus in the blood, increasing RBC (red blood cell) count.

- Sunlight increases hemoglobin in the blood, increasing the oxygen carrying power. When circulation and oxygenation improve, the cell function in the entire body is improved. Healing is therefore stimulated and accelerated also. Muscles grow firmer and stronger, as well as all other tissues.

- Sunlight dominates the chemistry of blood. With light, the blood contains all elements it needs for life. Clean foods, clean air, clean water, and effective supplements are of poor value to the body without abundant sunlight.

- Sunlight stimulates growth and repair.

The list goes on. Actually the list is never-ending since an improvement in circulation and oxygenation positively affects every single cell and every single function in our body.

7.3 Therapeutic Application

It's very simple. To guarantee optimal health and vitality, ABUNDANT SUNSHINE is a major key factor. Real, natural sunlight cannot be replaced by cod liver oil or vitamin D supplements.

Our pale, white skin is a sign of disease, not health. We have become accustomed to this longstanding error.

The pale complexions, skin conditions, weak and flabby muscles and overall sick complexion of many of us and also witnessed in many young children is most likely caused by a lack of sunshine. A lack of sunshine in turn impairs health and promotes toxemia.

Newborns and children need plenty of sunlight, every day. Sunlight promotes normal development and optimal health. One example is that one of cartilage. Cartilage has to be transformed into strong bones. Without the aid of natural sunlight, the assimilation of calcium and phosphorus salts will be impaired.

The sun cannot be replaced either. Tanning booths and artificial light do not possess the same organic quality of real sunlight. Plants for example will grow under artificial sunlight, but will never be as strong, vital and sturdy as when grown under real sunlight. The same holds true for fruits, vegetables, animals and humans. Vegetation grown in the dark lacks color. Potatoes for example are pale and unable to produce leaves.

LIGHT versus HEAT

People get confused when we talk about sunlight and its benefits. The LIGHT is beneficial, no it's VITAL. The heat is not.

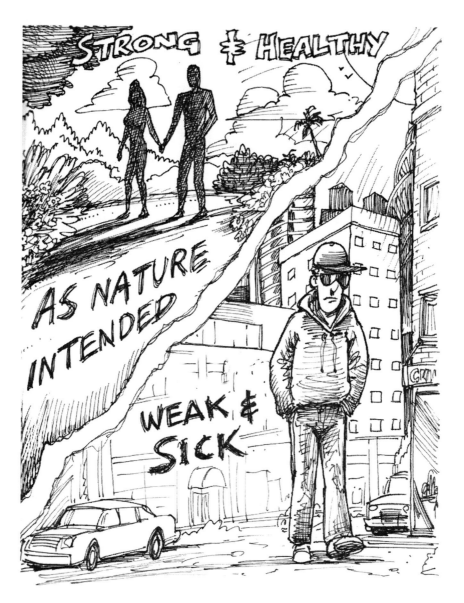

Illustration 13 – The Power of Sunlight

Animals seek the light of the sun, but avoid the heat. In other words, animals prefer to be in the sun in the cool part of the day and they seek shade during the warm or hot part of the day. Extreme heat robs one from energy and is depressing. The caveman and still today the natives or Indians of Peru, Mexico, South America, and the Africans follow this natural instinct.

<u>Practical Application:</u>

Gradually expose yourself more and more to natural sunlight. Start with 5-10 minutes per day and increase to 1 hour at least, while 3 hours or more would be ideal.

Avoid the heat, so expose your skin to natural sunlight in the morning or evening hours if you live in a warm part of the world.

Make sure to expose the largest possible area of your skin. I don't suggest you start running around naked on the street, but maybe you do that at home in your back-yard, or with minimal clothing just hiding the private parts (shorts for men, bikini for women). Wear shorts whenever you can as opposed to long pants or jeans, wear short sleeves t-shirts or none, walk bare-foot or opt for sandals etc. Clothes are not natural.

Ideally, present objections to nudity must be overcome. The idea that our body is ugly and vulgar, indecent and obscene is prudish... although many of us have ignored their body and it actually may be offensive to watch. Do something about it! But it's the machine-made morality, the thoughts of our neighbors, the laws of the land, and the prevailing customs that hinder nudity and therefore health. This attitude towards a nude body comes from a filthy mind, troubled with obscene suggestions, vulgarity and impurity.

Blond or pale types must be very cautious initially since they are more prone to overstimulation and burns. This is another reason to obtain sun exposure during the cool parts of the day.

And then we have to overcome another ridiculous misconception, that one of protecting the head and the eyes from the sun. We were created with a head and eyes and they adapt to sunlight as Nature intends. Just as for our entire body and mind, sunlight is beneficial to the eyes, head and hair. Sunstroke is NOT the result of an uncovered head or gazing into the sun; sunstroke is the result of excess heat exposure and subsequent exhaustion. Staring directly into the sun actually improves sight and aids in so called diseases of the eyes.

The co-reason for baldness and so called diseases of the eyes, including glaucoma, cataract, retinopathy, sensitivity to sunlight, and just poor vision is lack of sunlight. Nature did not intend us to wear clothes, hats and sunglasses.

I clearly remember a girlfriend. Her job demanded that she drive every day for work and she wore sunglasses all day long. Her vision was very poor to say the least, and she had come to a point where her eyes were so sensitive to light that she was practically unable to go out without wearing sunglasses, even on a cloudy day. Protecting the eyes from the sunlight was worsening and weakening the eyes, while a gradual increase in the exposure to sunlight would improve vision and abolish sensitivity.

Thus sunlight does not cure, nothing does. But sunlight is yet another hygienic agent that puts the body in the RIGHT CONDITIONS so that the body can heal itself, and regain and maintain optimal health.

7.4 Sunscreen

First of all, we don't need sunscreen because we shouldn't be out in the heat. We should enjoy the sunlight during the cooler parts of the day. However, many people living on the islands or in tropical places (or in Florida as myself) love to go and spend the day on the beach, on the boat or in the sun. The afternoon sun is way too strong for our skin. The extreme heat exhausts us and can damage the skin with all its important and vital functions.

We can still go out and have fun though, but ideally choose another time of the day and search for shade. Baking yourself in the sun to get that tan is plain stupid and self-destructive (carcinoma, melanoma etc.). Get that tan gradually by exposing yourself daily to adequate sunlight. This way you will have a constant tan! Pigment is healthy, pale is diseased. However, burnt skin is not an option. Would you let your heart or liver burn?

What about getting a nice tan with the use of sunscreen? First of all, the heat still exhausts your vital energy, and secondly your sunscreen is a chemical toxin. Rubbing that toxin all over your body and face causes an immense amount of toxins to be absorbed, then circulating in your entire body, adding to toxemia.

Are you really willing to smother the entire organ of the skin, its main function being elimination of toxins, with toxins? That would be self-destructive.

In short, avoid the heat. If you choose to have fun in the heat, at least look for shade. If you decide to have fun in the sun, with or without sunscreen, you will pay a huge price later. If you must use sunscreen occasionally, look for safer products at your health food store.

7.5 Key Points

Our skin is not only and by far our largest organ but it's the only organ in direct contact with the external environment. The skin provides a strong protective covering for the rest of the body and resists the intrusion of external and infectious matter.

Our skin also plays a crucial role in the elimination of toxins and the regulation of our body temperature. We understand that toxemia is the cause of ALL so-called disease so you can now understand the importance of healthy functioning skin assisting in proper elimination of toxins. Our skin can ONLY be healthy in the presence of abundant sunlight.

Housing and clothing have deprived us of our normal supply of sunlight.

Our skin cannot be clean and functioning optimally when its contact with air and sunlight is deprived.

Light is simply hygienic. Light stimulates all biological processes and functions and helps maintain optimal health and vitally, as do clean water and air.

Gradually expose yourself more and more to natural sunlight. Start with 5-10 minutes per day and increase to 1 hour at least, while 3 hours or more would be ideal. Avoid hats, sunglasses and (most) clothing.

Expose yourself to sunlight during the cooler parts of the day, including your eyes. Heat exhausts the body.

The use of sunscreen is obsolete since you shouldn't go out during the hot part of the day. Using sunscreen would increase the toxic load in your body and weaken the skin.

Chapter 8 – Sleep, Fasting & Detox

Besides the vital substances (clean air, clean water and sunshine) and the vital nutrients (clean food) the body needs to regain, sustain and maintain optimal health, the body also needs time to recover, repair, replenish and renew.

Only an abundance of vital energy guarantees a happy life full of energy, enjoyment, productivity and health. Energy production needs to exceed energy expenditure.

8.1 Rest & Sleep

The functions that sleep serves are well established as well as the fact that more and higher quality sleep improves our health and wellbeing.

What Is Sleep?

Sleep is a behavioral state that is a natural part of every animal's and every individual's life. We spend about one-third of our lives asleep. Nonetheless, people generally know little about the importance of this essential activity.

Sleep is vital and much more important than we tend to believe. We all recognize and feel the need to sleep. We typically remember little or nothing about the hours that have just passed. But after sleeping, we recognize changes that have occurred, as we should feel rested and more alert. Sleep actually appears to be required for survival. Rats deprived of sleep will die within two to three weeks, a time frame similar to death due to starvation.

A Dynamic Process

We wrongly assume that sleep is a passive activity. Rather sleep is a very dynamic process with a highly organized sequence of events that follows a regular, cyclic program each night. These events allow for essential physiological changes in the regulation of organs and tissues. Although some minor decrease in metabolic rate occurs, there is no evidence that any major organ or regulatory system in the body shuts down during sleep. To the contrary, many systems actually get to work. For example, the endocrine system increases secretion of certain hormones during sleep, such as growth hormone and prolactin. Also brain activity is found to be as pronounced as during awaking hours.

A Recovery Process

It's common sense that in order to preserve life and restore health, one must have an abundance of vital energy. Vital energy can be spent in various ways. It's spent to carry out one's daily activities and it should be spend to generate the powers of repair, renewal and replenishment. Sadly, it is often wasted to deal with emergencies such as excess digestive efforts, disease management, overstimulation, overindulgences, etc.

The more vital energy one spends, the more needs to be recovered. It's that simple. It's also pretty simple to understand that this vital energy can only be recovered during rest and sleep while we are not spending it.

If we spend more than we recover, we create a deficit in vital energy. A deficit in vital energy results in a deficit of powers, and therefore an inefficient functioning of the cells and organs in the body occurs. This causes toxemia and the whole disease process is yet again initiated or accelerated.

Be aware that the deficit continues to grow at a fast pace in the presence of a chronic lack of sleep and rest.

So now we have two ways to restore vital energy and reestablish optimal health:

1. Spend less vital energy: reduce the load on the digestive system by combining the right foods and eating at the right time, avoid overeating, avoid excess emotions and overstimulation etc.

2. Produce more vital energy: give your body enough rest and sleep so it can repair cells and tissues for optimal functioning, and replenish vital energy.

This is not just an issue of preserving life and living healthy. Sufficient vital energy allows for happiness, feelings of well-being, optimal performance on the job, enjoyment etc. It also sets one free of the bad habits and indulgences that have enslaved men.

The theory or idea that extra work or hard work, working out or exercising, and physical activity make us stronger or somehow increases vital powers is untrue. Activity only depletes us from vital energy and power.

If so called stimulants, or medicines, or food, or drinks, or air, or exercise would produce energy we would not need to rest or sleep. We would have plenty of energy to carry out all bodily functions effectively and feel vibrant and vital. Don't try this at home, but if you would omit rest and sleep for a few weeks you will cease to live.

The athlete thus cannot gain energy or power through exercise since exercise is an expenditure of energy. Exercise consumes energy and tears down tissue, and if prolonged causes exhaustion. Only through the regeneration of energy and power can the athlete become stronger and reap the benefits of exercise. This regeneration of energy and power can only be achieved through adequate rest and sleep.

It's the law of dual effect. This law doesn't know any exceptions. Just like the truth about stimulants, activity or exercise only give a false sense of increased vigor through the initial expenditure of energy. That's the first effect of activity. The second effect is fatigue or exhaustion. This is just the warning sign of the body telling you that rest and sleep is needed to recover for the energy expenditure. It cannot be ignored.

The opposite holds true also. Rest and sleep cause a false sense of weakness and laxity as their first effect. Nobody doubts that the second effects are increased vigor and energy.

Many of us believe that sleep is a waste of time, but now you can see it's just the opposite. The athlete will be weaker without proper rest and sleep, so does the party goer simply because an energy deficit is created.

For our kids, rest is essential for growth and development. Proof comes with the fact that a fetus experiences the period of most rapid growth and development while exhibiting the least activity.

But the importance of rest and sleep does not diminish as we age. One tends to believe that adults and older people require less rest and sleep than children. It all depends on your expenditure: the more energy you spend, the more you need to recover to keep a positive balance.

Generally speaking, we have extra expenditures because of our bad habits and therefore we don't need less sleep, but adults and older people often *get* less sleep. That's because the ability to sleep for long periods of time and to get into the deep, restful stages of sleep seems to decrease with age. But this has nothing to do with age of course. It has everything to do with the fact that our body is totally messed up, doing everything it can to preserve life.

Our perversions have led to abnormal functioning. Just as our normal feelings of hunger and thirst have been altered, so has our biological clock. We are more easily disturbed by light, noise, and pain. We have trouble falling asleep, staying asleep, falling back asleep etc. This rapidly becomes a vicious cycle in which symptoms of disease and 'medical problems' and medications contribute to sleep problems. Lack of sleep results in an increasing deficit of vital energy and thus results in less healing power for the body and so on.

A healing process

Rest and replenishment is the absolute FIRST STEP in healing. When sick, rest and sleep reduce function and restore health. The primary purpose is to shut down all waste-gates of vital energy and preventing an unnecessary expenditure of energy and power.

The rest we are talking about is COMPLETE REST. It's not resting in the couch while watching T.V. and eating snacks. Complete rest is only obtained when cutting off all sources of stimulation (light, sound, activity) and omitting food for a few days. In a state of non-perversion, a sick person would not have any appetite or hunger feeling anyway. So, it's resting in bed in a dark room without any noise or light or food. This type of rest secures complete rest of all the organs (and the mind), and secures absolute minimal expenditure of vital energy. All the energy is needed to heal, to repair, to recover, to renew and to replenish and expel the toxins.

To cease eating is so important! It ceases activity of the entire digestive system which not only frees up all that vital energy, but gives all the organs a chance to repair and recover and replenish. This allows the organs to return to their normal condition. You can look at complete rest as a RESET BUTTON.

Conventional medicine does recognize the importance of rest, but yet again doesn't understand it. The doctor will recommend rest but at the same time administer medicine, tonics or stimulants and recommend physical therapy, massage, electrical stimulation, hot or cold packs or baths etc. All of these promote activity and expend energy. Such patients do not rest. They are exhausted.

While rest and sleep are the ONLY means of recuperation, they cannot be expected to make you disease-proof.

Types of Rest

PHYSICAL rest is obtained by ceasing all physical activity. This can only be accomplished by going to bed and relaxing or sleeping. However, tossing and turning, rolling and curling up and contracting muscles are incompatible with rest. One must assure a comfortable bed, comfortable room temperature, full darkness and absence of noise, etc.

MENTAL rest is accomplished by relaxing the mind and removing all possible sources of disturbance and annoyance such as light, noise, and emotions such as worry, fear, anger, joy, etc. Most of us lost the ability and control to relax and repose our mind. We therefore must relearn and re-cultivate this poise and self-control (refer to our next chapter).

PHYSIOLOGICAL rest is achieved as a result of both physical and mental rest, combined with the absence of food, including any so called stimulant or medicine.

NOTHING can be more effective in promoting elimination, repair of tissue and organs, and restoration of health than PHYSIOLOGICAL REST.

Be aware that an aggravation of symptoms during this period of physiological rest does not mean that the patient is getting worse; it merely means the patient is getting better.

Biological Clock

An internal biological clock regulates the timing for sleep in humans (and animals). The activity of this clock makes us sleepy at night and awake during the day. Our clock cycles with an approximately 24-hour period and is called a circadian clock (from the Latin roots *circa* = about and *diem* = day). In humans, this clock is located in the hypothalamus of the brain.

The rhythm of this clock is linked to the light–dark cycle. The brain receives information about illumination through the eyes. The retina of the eye contains 'classical' photoreceptors ('rods' and 'cones'), which are used for conventional vision. But the retina also contains specialized ganglion cells which are directly photosensitive, and project directly to the part of the brain (suprachiasmatic nucleus) where they help in the management and proper regulation of this circadian clock.

There are also clear patterns of core body temperature, brain wave activity, hormone production, cell regeneration and other biological activities.

Just like our hunger and thirst feeling, our body precisely regulates thousands of biological and chemical functions based on the day and light pattern.

Ideally of course, we should be guided by our instinct when to rest and sleep but that only would be good if our instincts were normal. Most of us have a messed up biological clock. The so called stimulants keep us from knowing when we need rest or sleep.

These stimulants include food, drinks, drugs, overstimulation (light, sound, activity) and overindulgences (excess food, drugs, sex, etc.).

These habits interfere with the normal functioning of our biological clock, yet another perversion or abnormal functioning of our body.

So, just like with hunger and thirst, we will first have to ignore our messed up biological clock and give our body more rest and sleep at normal, dark-light intervals. While implementing the other RIGHT CONDITIONS (clean air, clean water, clean food, sunshine, balanced emotions, balanced activity etc.) a normal biological clock will slowly be reset. From that moment on, one can follow our instincts again and listen to the body.

How much sleep do we need?

The commonly accepted 8 hours per day for adults may be a guideline but I personally wouldn't know what to do with that guideline. It's so much simpler.

The more energy and power is used, the more sleep and rest one needs to recuperate this energy. In normal, healthy circumstances and with an intact biological clock our body would tell us when to rest by making one feeling tired and sleepy. In our current state of perversion, we need to just give our bodies more rest and sleep until our biological clock returns to normal.

The more work, physical or mental activity, exercise, and stimulation the more rest and sleep the body will require.

Keep in mind though that as you will improve your eating habits and thus waste a significant amount less energy on digestion, and as you start to control emotions and avoid overstimulation and overindulgences you will spend far less vital energy, and you may need not as much rest and sleep as you do now.

When do you know when the biological clock has returned to normal and you are giving your body enough rest and sleep? What do you think the answer is? Correct, when you have build-up an energy reserve, a positive balance of energy expresses itself as actual vitality, enjoyment, happiness, and health.

Lack of sleep not only causes the so called sleep disorders (insomnia, sleep apnea, narcolepsy, restless leg syndrome, parasomnias such as sleep walking and sleep talking, and bedwetting etc.) but more importantly is expressed by fatigue, lethargy, and poor performance (physical and mental).

Why? An energy deficit is the result of spending more energy than recuperating energy. Long-term, just like with any other perversions or bad habits, this contributes to the toxemia in our body and the chronic, degenerative disease process.

8.2 Fasting

Now that we fully understand the significance of rest and sleep, it makes sense we now discuss fasting.

In normal health, fasting is an instinct also. It's an instinct when we are sick or in less than optimal health. The body feels weak and there's loss of appetite. If we simply follow the warning signs of our body, we then should rest and sleep and omit food. Sounds like what we called COMPLETE REST earlier in this chapter.

It's said to be the oldest of all methods of healing, and it's obviously a strictly natural method also. What do sick animals do? They all will hide in a secluded spot and rest, while ceasing to feed.

Nature dictates in both animals and humans that in a state of acute disease food is omitted and water can be consumed, while in chronic disease the amount of food consumed should be less than when in normal health. If this simple, natural rule would be followed, an untold amount of useless suffering would be avoided and many would be rescued from an early death. Unfortunately, conventional medicine still has the delusion that the sick man must eat to keep up strength. We know better and understand already that eating only would consume unnecessary vital energy and worsen the sickness.

What is a fast then? A fast is a voluntary abstinence from food, except water. Restricted or limited diets are therefore not fasts. Be advised that during a fast, drinking lots of water is not indicated (unlike common belief). There is neither a need nor benefit from it. You already know the rule: drink when thirsty, don't drink when not thirsty, and only drink natural, clean, alkaline water.

During a fast, cells, tissues and organs can repair, rebuild, renew and recuperate energy. They can get back to normal and prepare for normal, effective functioning.

During a fast, some tissues are broken down. But the body follows the laws of self-preservation and vital economy and will therefore rid itself of the least important tissues first: fat, abnormal growths, exudates, deposits, effusions etc. Yes, that's correct. One of the most important functions of a fast is consistently overlooked. Fasting causes the breakdown and absorption of useless, even harmful deposits, including diseased tissue and tumors.

With a prolonged fast, other tissues will then be broken down in the order of least importance. The muscles would be next, followed by the organs (in order of importance to preserve life), the blood etc. The brain and the nerves don't sustain any significant losses, even upon death.

Not only is there a remarkable purification process taking place during a fast, resulting in the nourishment of all organs and the blood, but also mental faculties are vastly improved when fasting.

In general, fasting:

1. Allows the vital organs complete rest.

2. Halts toxemia or further poisoning of the body (no decomposition of food in the intestines).

3. Allows the organs of elimination to catch up with their work.

4. Promotes the break down and elimination of unwanted, dead matter including fat, deposits, exudates, effusions, diseased tissues, tumors and abnormal growths.

5. Conserves vital energy and builds up energy reserves and vital powers of all organs and tissues.

6. Clears and calms the mind, and strengthens the mind.

Some of the many positive and beneficial changes that have been observed during a fast include:

1. Increase in the number of red blood cells as a result of improved nutrition. How can nutrition improve while fasting, you may ask? Well, the abstinence of overeating definitely results in improved nutrition.

2. The liver, kidneys and spleen quickly see an increased effectiveness in their elimination efforts due to an increased amount of vital energy available during a fast. These organs can catch up during a fast since no food is consumed.

3. The stomach, intestines and colon are able to repair their damaged structures during a fast since these organs practically cease to function after just a few days. Colitis, gastritis, appendicitis, enteritis, typhoid fever (enteric fever) etc. would all recover quickly while fasting.

4. The stomach itself also repairs and resumes its normal size

and tone after being prolapsed and distended because of our perverse eating habits. Digestion improves and normal feelings of hunger start to restore.

5. The lungs seem to recover quickly during a fast and any lung or respiratory disease greatly benefits from fasting.

6. Sexual energies cease during a prolonged fast but return when hunger returns after a fast (sometimes with a slight delay). Both the male and female sex organs cure and repair during a fast, and menstruation is often brought on a week or more prior to regular time.

7. Gastric and intestinal hyperacidity are relieved within a few days of fasting since the stomach ceases to produce acid juices.

8. When the body is in a very toxic state, the secretion of bile is sometimes increased during a fast which results in nausea and vomiting. After such a crisis, the condition of the body significantly improves.

9. Saliva secretion is lessened and in some cases becomes more acidic, foul and un-tasty. After the fast, saliva returns to be alkaline.

10. Due to increased elimination and excretion during a fast, one may notice mucous secretions through nose and mouth, which may be slimy, yellowish, green or pussy. One may also notice acid secretions of the vagina and/or thick, dark, foul urine secretions, foul and profuse sweating, foul breath, etc. These are attempts of the body to eliminate toxins and acids. It's cleaning time!

11. In Chinese medicine, the tongue and breath indicate the condition of the internal organs and environment. So during a fast, one may notice a thick coated tongue, scalloped, greasy, yellow or white along with foul breath. The more toxic

the body, the more foul the breath and the more the tongue will be coated.

12. Heart rate or pulse varies greatly during a fast. Initially, the pulse tends to rise as a crisis is taking place. The heart itself greatly benefits from a fast for all the obvious reasons.

13. The body withdraws energy from the muscles during a fast, which often results in a feeling of weakness. But it's necessary to distinguish between actual weakness and a feeling of weakness. While fasting, vital energy is built up and the body is becoming stronger.

14. Fasting causes an initial loss of weight, but this is not muscle. The initial weight loss is simply the emptying of the alimentary canal of several pounds of food and feces which are not replaced. With prolonged fasts, one will continue to lose weight but less rapid that initially. And don't worry that weight loss can be harmful, it's not. The body will expel unwanted fat, cysts, exudates, tumors, toxins, and dead matter first.

15. Underweight people many times benefit from a fast also because often the reason for them to be underweight is an impaired digestive system and/or impaired assimilation of foods. A fast will restore these systems and the underweight person will become normal in weight again after the fast. Weight gaining diets are not indicated for these people.

16. During a fast, one has usually no appetite on the first day but a huge appetite on the second day which diminishes by the third day and disappears until the time the body must have food (natural feeling of hunger has returned). Meanwhile, during the period of fasting, nausea and vomiting may occur upon the sight and smell of food.

<u>Fasting is not starving:</u>

Fasting is a restorative and healing process. As long as there is no desire for food, the individual who ceases to consume food is fasting.

During a fast, the body lives on its reserves. Starvation does not start until the reserves are exhausted.

After the natural feeling of hunger returns, the individual who continues to cease the consumption of food is starving. Thus, the return of natural hunger (not the perversion of appetite) marks the dividing point between fasting and starvation.

<u>How long should one fast then?</u>

As long as nature calls for, meaning as long as it takes for normal, natural hunger to return. One must fast to completion since breaking a fast prematurely is not beneficial.

Since our feelings of appetite and natural hunger are messed up and unclear to the unhealthy body, what other signs indicate that the body is ready to break the fast?

1. Return of hunger is felt in mouth and throat, in absence of the sight and smell of food.

2. The breath becomes sweet and the bad taste in the mouth disappears.

3. Body temperature is normal.

4. Excretions become odorless (sweat, urine, feces).

5. Saliva secretion returns.

6. Tongue becomes clean (no coat or thin, white coat).

These signs indicate that the body has caught up with the elimination processes and has repaired and revitalized itself. Therefore the length of a fast is determined by these signs, and thus is very individual.

Breaking the fast should be done in proportion to the length of the fast. The recommendation is to break the fast on liquid food. An example could be:

Day 1: orange juice with water, fruit juice, tomato juice or a vegetable broth.

Day 2: fruit.

Day 3: raw vegetables and salads.

After day 3: normal diet. The longer the fast, the slower the introduction of food should be. In case of chronic disease, the introduction should be slower also.

Physical activity during a fast:

Ideally, for maximum benefits, one should not work or engage in any form of physical activity during a fast. Activity is an expenditure of energy and the purpose of a fast is to replenish energy.

Conservation of energy should be the guiding principle during a fast, but a light form of exercise daily (short, light walk) in the absence of work is indicated along with some diaphragmatic breathing. Although not much energy is spent on this light activity in the absence of work, it promotes circulation and oxygenation.

Although working and activity are contraindicated during a fast, it will not pose any danger to work during short fasts of 3-7 days. The abstinence of food during this period still has great benefits. However, working during longer periods of fasting can pose danger (fainting, exhausting, coma).

No enema:

The idea that the body would need help with its elimination process is just another perversion. When the body is put in the RIGHT CONDITIONS (complete, physiological rest), there is no more powerful tool than the body itself to expel and eliminate toxins and wastes. What makes one even think that interference would be beneficial? Normal bowel action is resumed much faster without an enema.

Fasting and Disease:

In acute disease, the body undoubtedly manifests its desire to fast. Symptoms include fever, increased heart rate, nausea, vomiting among others. Any acute disease would be simply cured with a fast. It's only when symptoms and warning signs are ignored, and when man interferes with medicine and treatment that simple, harmless symptoms turn into a complicated, serious condition and disease. All the textbook symptoms with all their textbook treatments are the CAUSE of disease by creating a mass pathology (that nature never builds) by drugging, feeding and squirting serum.

In chronic disease, the need for fasting is not the same as in acute disease. Nature probably asked for a fast many times (nausea, vomiting etc.) but never received it. Thus, giving the body a fast during chronic disease will be well perceived and beneficial.

Complications to fasting are very uncommon and the symptoms experienced during a fast are not to be confused with complications. These symptoms are part of the healing efforts of the body and may include fever, dizziness, headaches, cramps, nausea, vomiting, weakness, insomnia (don't worry if you can't sleep during a fast, a fasting person requires less sleep), etc. A fast should not be broken because of these temporary symptoms.

Crises can occur during the first days of a fast and wouldn't be any different from crises experienced at other times. Fasting often revives the symptoms of old problems that were suppressed and now need to be taken care of. In chronic diseases, a fast often starts with a worsening of the symptoms of that so called disease, but these are just temporary.

The most common misconception or objection to fasting would be that the person or patient weakens during a fast. The claim that the sick must eat to 'keep up their strength' is getting to be old news, right? Food is not nutrition. Digestion requires lots of vital energy. Fasting only can strengthen the person and a fast renews and rebuilds tissue and energy.

Another myth in regards to fasting is that fasting causes acidosis. This could only be true in the case of a prolonged fast in a chronic disease state.

In any other condition, the repair, renewal and replenishment activity of the body along with the elimination of acids and toxins only would promote alkalinity after the fast. If the body is acidic, a fast only would restore chemical balance and remove that acidity.

The only contraindications to a fast would be:

1. A person who fears a fast for whatever reason. Fear is a strong emotion and would eradicate any benefit from a fast. This person needs to be educated properly on what fasting REALLY is and HOW fasting would benefit him or her. Only when the fear is taken away would a fast be beneficial.

2. Extremely underweight people (extreme emaciation) should avoid prolonged fasting. However, they would benefit from short fasts or a series of short fasts alternated with longer periods of proper feeding.

3. Terminally ill patients or patients at the end-stage of disease will not benefit from a fast, except to relieve some suffering. Fasting is of distinct benefit in the early stages of chronic, degenerative disease and cancer.

4. Obese patients with kidney deficiencies or inadequacies will break down their tissues faster than the kidneys can eliminate them during a fast.

A successful fast needs a proper mental attitude. Any negative attitude or related emotion will rob vital energy and lessen the benefits of the fast.

Fasting does not cure disease but puts the body in the RIGHT CONDITIONS to help the body in healing itself and curing disease. Fasting allows the body to RESTORE itself: repair, renew, replenish; and allows the body to expel and eliminate unwanted toxins and dead matter. Fasting is house cleaning. Fasting is therefore a vital activity in our quest to obtain optimal health, and is implemented at regular intervals to sustain and maintain that optimal health.

8.3 Detoxification Practices

You may have heard or even been exposed to or participated in detoxification programs and products. And even though many nutrients have
detoxifying properties and could be of benefit, nothing is more effective in
eliminating toxins from the body than fasting. I'm sure we can agree on that.

The first and most effective step in detoxing the body (and mind) is a fast as
described above.

The effects and benefits of a fast are only temporary unless we live
C.L.E.A.N. and put our body in the RIGHT CONDITIONS for optimal health.

But even then, because of our extreme exposure to toxins in our industrial-
ized and commercialized environment, a toxic onslaught, and therefore a
toxic accumulation, is almost unavoidable. We MUST incorporate fasts at
regular intervals in order to assure that toxins do not accumulate and get
eliminated regularly. If not, toxemia occurs.

If we live C.L.E.A.N. and consume clean food, clean air, and clean water
we gather many natural nutrients that have detoxifying properties. In other
words, a clean diet consisting of mostly natural vegetables and some fruits
is loaded with alkaline, detoxifying nutrients that assist in the daily neutralization and elimination of toxins.

However, as we established earlier, even our natural and organic foods are
often deprived of essential nutrients because:

1. They are grown in soil that may be deprived of nutrients, and/
    or

2. They have been stored for several days prior to consumption
    and therefore lose many of the essential nutrients.

Therefore, knowledge of some specific nutrients that assist in detoxifying
the body or certain organs and tissues may be valuable. We can supplement with foods containing these specific nutrients or supplement with a
high quality product to assist in our detoxification efforts.

Please note again that it's not the nutrients or supplements that miraculously detoxify our body. A healthy diet and clean living optimize the function of our elimination organs which in turn effectively eliminate toxins from our body. Supplements or programs intended to detoxify the body don't work unless one lives C.L.E.A.N.

Only a body in good health can benefit from these programs or supplements since the healthy organs and tissues can utilize the nutrients correctly and effectively.

As stated earlier, there are many theories and programs out there to detoxify the body, but I like to think that the one described below makes most sense (that's because it's mine). The effect is optimal when executed while practicing C.L.E.A.N.

For effective detoxification, I suggest the following 5 phases:

PHASE 1 - SHORT FAST (DAY 1 - 3)

We start our detox with a 2 or 3-day fast. A fast is the best way to detox, but a fast should be done until completion, which is determined by the return of hunger or other indicators (breath, tongue, temperature, excretions and secretions). The purpose of this short fast is to stop overburdening our systems and promote elimination processes. Because our system is not operating effectively in a state of impaired health, we will prepare our body for proper elimination in Phase 2 and complete a 'real' fast in phase 5.

During this short fast, minimum physical and metal activity is advised, so scheduling phase 1 during a weekend is advisable.

PHASE 2 – DETOX PREPARATION (DAY 4 – 10)

In order to have an effective detoxification we need to prepare our body and open the pathways for elimination while simultaneously minimize the burden on our body and digestive system.

So, for one week I suggest to only consume vegetables and fruits, and add some pea protein (more about pea protein later). I personally juice a lot.

Omit meat, fish, pasta and junk food (of course). There is no need to be hungry at any time since you can eat as much good stuff as you want.

In addition, you need to add food sources rich in fibers, minerals, detoxifying herbs and vitamin C.

1. About Probiotics

Let's start by stating that the health of our GI-system (gastrointestinal) has a vast effect on the health of our body, mostly because everything we consume must pass through the GI-tract. All foods, beverages, and medicines pass through the GI-tract. A multitude of chemicals and toxins exist in or on these foods, beverages and medicines and must be neutralized and converted to harmless byproducts for elimination.

Our perverse eating habits obviously stress out our GI-tract, resulting in symptoms such as bloating, stomach upset, fatigue, achiness, reflux, heartburn, nausea, dizziness, bowel inflammation and IBS among others. Poor gastrointestinal health is a condition which lowers the overall level of good bacteria in the body.

So what are these 'good' bacteria or probiotics? The Joint FAO/WHO Working Group defines probiotics as "live microorganisms which when administered in adequate amounts confer a health benefit on the host."

In plain English, probiotics are a type of living, 'friendly' bacteria that act as balancing agents for non-friendly, pathogenic, gut-bacteria such as Candida or E. coli. When these probiotics or 'friendly' bacteria are lacking, the 'bad' bacteria wreak havoc and symptoms such as digestive upset, headaches, sluggishness, irritability, cadidiasis (an overgrowth of the bacteria Candida albicans), inflammation, anxiety etc. pop up.

Acidity, stress, and poor lifestyle choices destroy our natural amount of probiotics.

Food sources containing natural probiotics are the following:

One of the best probiotic foods is said to be live-cultured yogurt. Kefir is similar to yogurt as it's a fermented dairy product from a unique combination of goat's milk and fermented kefir grains.

Made from fermented cabbage (and sometimes other vegetables), sauerkraut is extremely rich in healthy live cultures. An Asian form of pickled sauerkraut, kimchi is an extremely spicy and sour fermented cabbage, typically served alongside meals in Korea and loaded with beneficial bacteria.

Probiotics are sometimes added to high-quality dark chocolate, up to four times the amount of probiotics as many forms of dairy.

Ocean-based plants such as spirulina, chorella, and blue-green algae have been shown to contain high amounts of these probiotics, while Miso as in miso-soup is one the main-stays of traditional Japanese medicine and is commonly used in macrobiotic cooking as a digestive regulator. Made from fermented rye, beans, rice or barley, adding a tablespoon of miso to some hot water makes an excellent, quick, probiotic-rich soup, full of lactobacilli and bifidus bacteria.

The dill pickle or green pickle is also an excellent food source of probiotics. A great substitute for meat or tofu, tempeh is a fermented, probiotic-rich grain made from soy beans. Kombucha tea is a form of fermented tea that contains a high amount of healthy gut bacteria and has been used for centuries. This tea is believed to help increase energy and assist in weight loss.

The above are food sources most abundant in probiotics but as you can see some of them are dairy products. Our body has no need for any dairy product (refer to Chapter 15, 15.2).

So we need to obtain our probiotics from fermented foods. Let's discuss briefly what fermentation really is...

Simply stated, fermentation is the breakdown of complex molecules in organic compounds caused by bacteria or micro-organisms.

An example of fermentation is when grapes are transferred or crushed into a press, and cultured yeast is added, the sugar in the grapes converts into alcohol.

In plain English, these bacteria start our digestion before we ingest our food. Therefore, we consider fermentation to be an act of external pre-digestion. This pre-digestion facilitates the actual digestion and assimilation of foods in our body. It's like having these 'little buggers' partially break down our food for us, prior to ingestion, in order to make it easier on our own digestive system.

When in a compromised state of health or in case of digestive/GI-problems these probiotics are vital for recovery.

Bacteria coexist in symbiosis with the human organism. Without these "little buggers", human life wouldn't exist. The onslaught of toxins and the extreme stress we impose on our digestive system warrants for more of these 'good' bacteria.

So what about probiotic supplements?

Assuming you select the right supplement (refer to Chapter 14; 14.2), these probiotic supplements can be of value in a compromised state of health. Recognizing that, the consumption of fermented foods on a regular basis has been shown to contribute greatly to the presence of healthy flora in the gut. Better to prevent than treat…

When probiotic supplements are indicated, just be aware that only few of those several billion cultures will survive the stomach (acid kills) and end-up in the intestines. Just know that these few 'lucky' bacteria will start colonizing (multiplying exponentially) in the intestines and restore the flora.

Antibiotics versus probiotics

As the adage goes, an ounce of prevention is worth a pound of cure. Probiotics, like most of the cornucopia of Complimentary & Alternative Medicine, so called "natural" medicine, is largely a "proactive" step toward the maintenance of health. Probiotics supplement and boost normal physiologic function allowing for inherent biological processes to take place, processes like immunity.

Antibiotics are a REACTIVE measure designed to deal with an exposure to a bug hell bent on killing us. They are like calling in the Marines to quell an invasion when local law enforcement is overwhelmed and faltering. They are equal opportunity killers, and often times our natural flora becomes a casualty of "friendly fire." Maintenance of our own probiotics may forestall the need to deploy more invasive countermeasures like antibiotics.

2. Fibers

Our S.A.D. (Standard American Diet) is deficient in plant fibers. Fiber is indispensable in maintaining a healthy colon and GI-tract, and will assist in complete, fast and easy bowel movements. Both soluble and insoluble fiber help to loosen the stool, absorb and eliminate fat and toxins, reduce transit time, and make elimination effortless and complete.

Most veggies and fruits contain fair amounts of fiber but the following sources are extra rich is dietary fiber:

Psyllium husk is the covering of seeds grown on a plant, named Plantago Psyllium, which flourishes in the Middle East. Psyllium husk has long been recognized as an excellent means of getting more dietary fiber into one's diet because it has a high fiber count in comparison to other grains. Oat bran, also a good source of fiber, has about five grams of fiber per 1/3 of a cup. Psyllium husk, on the other hand, contains approximately 71 grams of fiber for that same 1/3 of a cup.

This heavy dose of dietary fiber makes psyllium husk the choice of many who manufacture dietary fiber supplements and powders like Metamucil. For those suffering from constipation or diarrhea, appropriate daily dietary fiber intake can help improve these conditions. As psyllium husk travels through the human digestive tract, it absorbs water, but is not digested. This results in stool that is bulkier, but also softer, translating to fewer problems with passing stool.

Some studies have also suggested that regular use of psyllium husk supplements may help pass more fat in stools, translating to weight loss.

Possible adverse reactions may include diarrhea and flatulence if consumed in higher doses. Some people are severely allergic to psyllium husk.

The most important thing to remember when taking psyllium husk is to take it with lots of water.

Prunes are a dried type of plum. As a food, the health benefits of prunes are significant. They have long been used to maintain healthy bowel activity, and are particularly helpful in ending constipation. A ¼ cup serving of prunes contains a healthful 12% of one's daily dietary fiber needs. Prunes are also high in vitamin A, and potassium, and are known for their antioxidant benefits, containing a fair amount of beta-carotene.

Pectin is a soluble fiber from apples and citrus fruits, and is commonly used to make jellies & jams. Pectin relieves constipation by acting as a bulking agent, and protect against colon cancer.

3. Minerals

Minerals are plenty in fresh veggies and fruits and assist in alkalizing the body and neutralizing toxic and acidic compounds. Especially magnesium in this phase may be beneficial in relaxing the bowels and promoting normal (once or twice a day) bowel movements.

Great food sources for magnesium include dried herbs such as choriander, chives, spearmint, dill, sage, basil and savory. Great as a snack or in a salad are pumpkin, squash, and watermelon seeds. Other seeds packed with magnesium include flax seeds, sunflower seeds, and sesame seeds.

Cocoa powder and molasses (a good substitute for refined sugar) are also great sources of magnesium along with several nuts: brazil nuts, almonds and cashews.

4. Detoxifying herbs and plants

For the record, any and all natural herbs, plants, fruits and vegetables have detoxifying properties since they contain various essential nutrients, fibers, vitamins, minerals and so on. They are also rich in natural water and therefore all of them assist in detoxification of the body.

In this preparation phase however, especially beneficial can be artichoke, barley, pineapple (bromelain), celery, aloe vera and mint.

Aloe vera extracts have strong anti-inflammatory, antibacterial and antifungal activities and have been used as an immuno-stimulant. Aloe vera has been linked with improved blood glucose levels in diabetics, and is also associated with lowering blood levels. The consumption of aloe vera juice has also been traditionally used internally for healing and soothing of digestive conditions such as heartburn and irritable bowel syndrome due to its laxative properties.

5. Vitamin C

Vitamin C is a powerful antioxidant neutralizing free radicals and boosting the immune system.

Let's recap Phase 2:

Only consume vegetables and fruits (you may juice them), and add some pea protein. Omit meat, fish, pasta and junk food (of course).

Consume the following fruits for their fiber, mineral and vitamin C content: apples, prunes, citrus fruits and pineapple.

Consume the following veggies: artichoke, barley, mint, celery, aloe vera.

Add seeds and nuts high in magnesium.

Add psyllium husk and other dietary fibers (check out our FIBER MAX supplement).

PHASE 3 – LIVER DETOX (DAY 11 – 24)

The liver is our body's main detoxification organ and is responsible for removing all potentially detrimental molecules.

The liver detoxifies the blood in two distinct phases:

In Phase I, liver detoxification involves the conversion or transformation of fat-soluble and non-water soluble substances or chemicals into water-soluble chemicals. Specific enzymes during this phase 1 alter these non-water soluble chemicals which include inhaled petrol fumes, medications, recreational drugs, alcohol and other toxic substances. However, this conversion produces oxidants and other harmful compounds

In Phase II, the liver is responsible for neutralizing these toxic chemicals, a process called conjugation. During this phase, the liver binds water soluble molecules to these toxic chemicals and then they are passed on to the kidneys and excreted by the body as urine.

In this phase, the liver also produces bile, which assists the body in breaking down fats in the small intestine as part of the digestive process. Bile also breaks down toxins which travel through the intestinal tract and are expelled as feces.

Molecules used in Phase II in the liver include glutathione, sulfate, glycine, acetate, cysteine and glucuronic acid.

To promote liver detoxification and support the liver in its 2 phases of detoxification, we continue our only fruit and veggie diet for another 2 weeks, and we add the following nutrients:

1. To assist normal liver function and structure, and in response to environmental toxins we need to support methyl group metabolism. This is accomplished by consuming choline, betaine and methionine.

2. To stimulate both detoxification pathways of the liver, ITC's (isothiocyanates) found in cruciferous vegetables (cauliflower, cabbage, cress, bok choy, broccoli, kale, collard greens, turnip, and similar green leaf vegetables) are indicated. However, ITC's found in Wasabia japonica are 10-25 times more potent than those found in cruciferous vegetables.

Wasabi is a familiar green condiment in dishes that contain sushi. While many people are familiar with the condiment's spicy taste, most "wasabi" that is served in restaurants is often not true Japanese wasabi, but instead, American horseradish mixed with starch and food coloring. *Wasabia japonica* (true wasabi) is very different from American wasabi and is generally not found outside of Japan. Wasabia, a member of the cruciferous vegetable family, contains long chain ITCs (isothiocyanates). These long chain ITCs are unique to Wasabia and are not commonly found in other cruciferous vegetables.

The isothiocyanate (ITC) spectrum of *Wasabia japonica* contains long chain methyl isothiocyanates (6-MITC) not commonly found in our diet. 6-MITCs have been shown to be 10-25 times more potent at inducing Phase 2 liver enzymes than sulforaphanes found in cruciferous vegetables.

3. Sulforaphanes found in broccoli (powder) significantly increase the activity of phase 2 enzymes as well as sulfur-containing amino acids such as taurine, methionine and cysteine.

4. Glutathione is involved in DNA synthesis and repair, protein and prostaglandin synthesis, amino acid transport, metabolism of toxins and carcinogens, immune function, enzyme activation and prevention of oxidative cell damage. NAC (N-Acetyl-L-cysteine) is a biologically active precursor for glutathione synthesis.

5. Glutathione, sulfur and NAC support mercury detoxification.

6. Glutathione, B-vitamins, vitamin C and lipoic acid are potent antioxidants, scavenging free radicals.

More about glutathione:

Glutathione is regarded as a prime, if not the number one, antioxidant and detoxifier of the human body.

Glutathione is manufactured inside the cell from its precursor amino acids (glycine, glutamate and cystine). Therefore, glutathione levels cannot be increased by orally ingesting it. Hence food sources or supplements that increase glutathione must either provide the precursors of glutathione, or enhance its production by some other means.

The manufacturing of glutathione in our cells is limited by the levels of its sulfur-containing precursor amino acid, cysteine. Cysteine - as a free amino acid - is potentially toxic and is spontaneously catabolized or destroyed in the gastrointestinal tract and blood plasma. However, when it is present as a cysteine-cysteine dipeptide, called cystine, it is more stable than cysteine.

Consuming foods rich in sulfur-containing amino acids can help boost glutathione levels. Here are some food sources and dietary supplements that help boost glutathione levels naturally.

1. N-Acetyl-Cysteine (NAC)

   It is derived from the amino acid L-Cysteine, and acts as a precursor of glutathione. NAC is quickly metabolized into glutathione once it enters the body. It has been proven in numerous scientific studies and clinical trials, to boost intracellular production of glutathione, and is approved by the FDA for treatment of acetaminophen overdose. Because of glutathione's mucolytic action, NAC (brand name Mucomyst) is commonly used in the treatment of lung diseases like cystic fibrosis, bronchitis and asthma.

2. Milk Thistle (silymarin)

   Milk thistle is a powerful antioxidant and supports the liver by preventing the depletion of glutathione. Silymarin is the active compound in milk thistle. It is a natural liver detoxifier and protects the liver from many industrial toxins such as carbon tetrachloride, and more common agents like alcohol.

3. Alpha Lipoic Acid

   Made naturally in our cells as a by-product of energy release, ALA increases the levels of intra-cellular glutathione, and is a natural antioxidant with free radical scavenging abilities. It has the ability to regenerate oxidized antioxidants like Vitamin C and E and helps to make them more potent. ALA is also known for its ability to enhance glucose uptake and may help prevent the cellular damage accompanying the complications of diabetes. It also has a protective effect in the brain.

4. Natural Foods

    Asparagus is a leading source of glutathione. Foods like broccoli, avocado and spinach are also known to boost glutathione levels. Raw eggs, garlic and fresh unprocessed meats (good luck finding these) contain high levels of sulfur containing amino acids and help to maintain optimal glutathione levels.

5. Turmeric (curcumin)

    Treatment of brain cells called astrocytes, with the Indian curry spice, curcumin (turmeric) has been found to increase expression of the glutathione S-transferase and protect neurons exposed to oxidant stress.

6. Balloon Flower Root

    Changkil saponins (CKS) isolated from the roots of the Chinese herb named Jie Geng, commonly called Balloon Flower Root have been found to increase intracellular glutathione (GSH) content and significantly reduce oxidative injury to liver cells.

7. Selenium

    Selenium is a co-factor for the enzyme glutathione peroxidase. Selenium supplements have become popular because some studies suggest they may play a role in decreasing the risk of certain cancers, and in how the immune system and the thyroid gland function. However, too much selenium can cause some toxic effects including gastrointestinal upset, brittle nails, hair loss and mild nerve damage.

PHASE 4 – REPAIR (DAY 25 – 31)

The goal of phase 4 is to replenish nutrients used during detoxification and also provide specific nutrients to repair the GI-tract. These nutrients include vitamins, minerals, phytonutrients from organic fruits and vegetables, anti-oxidants, omega-3 fatty acids and glutamine.

Glutamine helps maintain normal intestinal permeability and mucosal cell regeneration and structure, especially during periods of physiological stress. Glutamine also transports toxic ammonia to the kidneys for excretion and helps maintain a healthy acid-alkaline balance.

Food sources rich in glutamine are lean meats such as chicken, pork, and beef but I don't recommend them as your primary source of glutamine for the obvious reasons. Beans also have a high-protein content making them a rich source of glutamine. Other good vegetable sources include cabbage, spinach and parsley.

PHASE 5 – FAST UNTIL COMPLETION

This phase would certainly put the icing on the cake and really guarantee effective detox, repair and replenishment. However, many of us won't be able to practically fit in this phase, which has to be executed until completion.

Instead, I suggest to fast 3-5 days with minimal physical activity. So, schedule it as to include a weekend. Complete rest is advised, but abstinence of food and minimal activity will do.

The following table summarizes my DETOX PROGRAM:

Please note that PHASE 1 and 5 are fasts, and only pure, alkaline water is consumed.

Some other nutrients proven effective for GI cleansing include:

Ginger has many health benefits. Most importantly, it is one of the most powerful, natural anti-inflammatories on this planet. Ginger is also used to cleanse the colon (bowel disorders), and stimulate circulation. It can relieve dizziness, sweating, nausea, headache, fever, cold/flu symptoms, and pain. Ginger is a strong antioxidant with antimicrobial properties (used to treat sores and wounds).

Fennel is a highly aromatic and flavorful herb with culinary and medicinal uses. Fennel is mainly used with purgatives to allay their side effects.

Fennel water has properties similar to those of anise and dill water: mixed with sodium bicarbonate and syrup, these waters constitute the domestic 'Gripe Water', used to ease flatulence in infants; it also can be made into a syrup to treat babies with colic or painful teething. For adults, fennel seeds or tea can relax the intestines and reduce bloating caused by digestive disorders. Essential oil of fennel has these properties in concentration.

The **licorice** plant is a legume (related to beans and peas), native to southern Europe and parts of Asia. Powdered licorice root is an effective expectorant, and has been used for this purpose since ancient times, especially in Ayurvedic medicine where it is also used in tooth powders. Modern cough syrups often include licorice extract as an ingredient. Additionally, licorice is also a mild laxative and may be used as a topical antiviral agent for shingles, ophthalmic, oral or genital herpes. It's also used as an aid for healing stomach and duodenal ulcers, and can be used to treat ileitis, leaky gut syndrome, irritable bowel syndrome and Crohn's disease as it acts as an antispasmodic in the bowels.

A common and affordable sweet for children in parts of the United Kingdom and Europe was a tender stick of **rhubarb**, dipped in sugar. Rhubarb is used as a strong laxative and for its astringent effect on the mucous membranes of the mouth and the nasal cavity. The roots have been used as an aggressive laxative for over 5,000 years. Therefore, rhubarb also has been used occasionally as a slimming agent.

Kelp compounds cleanse the digestive tract and eliminate toxins. They absorb toxins from the bowel and provide bulk for stool. Kelp is also an excellent source of calcium, magnesium, sodium and Iodine. As you may already know, iodine is crucial for thyroid function and increases

	PHASE 2	PHASE 3	PHASE 4
EMPHASIS	Prepare	Liver Detox	Repair
SPECIAL NUTRIENTS	Fiber Minerals Detox herbs Vitamin C	choline, betaine, methionine, ITC's, Glutathione, Sulfur, NAC	Omega 3, glutamine
VEGGIES	artichoke celery	Wasabia japonica and cruciferous vegetables (cauliflower, cabbage, cress, bok choy, broccoli, kale, collard greens, turnip, and similar green leaf vegetables), plus asparagus, avocado, spinach	ALL, especially beans, cabbage, spinach and parsley
FRUITS	apple pineapple prunes citrus fruits		Mostly non-sweet
HERBS	barley, mint, coriander, chives, spearmint, dill, sage, basil and savory	Turmeric, balloon flower root, milk thistle	
NUTS & SEEDS	Seeds: pumpkin, squash, watermelon, flax, sunflower, sesame. Nuts: brazil, almonds, cashews.		
OTHER		NAC, alpha-lipoic acid, selenium	
SUPPLEMENT	R3 Essentials, or Vemma, Fiber Max, C Max	Wasabia Detox, Glutathione Plus , Milk Thistle Max, Turmeric Max	Vemma, Pure Omega 3, Pea Protein, Glutamine Max

Illustration 14 – Dr. Mike's Detox Table

metabolic rate. Iodine strengthens connective tissues (hair, skin, nails) and is effective in the treatment of hypothyroidism, enlarged glands, debility, fatigue, eczema, psoriasis, arthritis & obesity.

Senna is a large group of around 250 species of flowering plants, native throughout the tropics. Senna is currently used in medicine as a laxative. Sennas act as purgatives and are similar to aloe and rhubarb in regards to their active ingredients, anthraquinone derivatives and their glucosides. The latter are called sennosides or senna glycosides. *Senna* acts on the lower bowel, and is especially useful in alleviating constipation. It increases the peristaltic movements of the colon.

Alginate (also referred to as Algin or Alginic acid) is a viscous gum, abundant in cell walls of brown algae. Alginate is effective in absorbing poisonous metals from the blood.

Cascara sagrada (Spanish for 'sacred bark') comes from the American buckthorn tree native to the western coast of North America. It is a laxative and one of the few herbs approved as an over-the-counter drug by the FDA. The main ingredients of cascara sagrada are anthraquinones, which stimulate the bowel.

This herb also provokes secretion of fluid and minerals into the large intestine and inhibits their reabsorption. It is therefore recommended for situations in which a soft, easily passed stool is desirable, such as with hemorrhoids or following rectal surgery.

Goldenseal is one of the most popular herbs on the market today. It was traditionally used by Native Americans to treat skin disorders, digestive problems, liver conditions, diarrhea, and eye irritations. Goldenseal is bitter and therefore stimulates the secretion and flow of bile, and can also be used as an expectorant. It also has strong activity against a variety of bacteria, yeast, and fungi, such as E. Coli and Candida. Goldenseal is used for infections of the mucus membranes, including the mouth, sinuses, throat, the intestines, stomach, urinary tract and vagina. Goldenseal was also the center of a myth in that it could mask a positive drug screen. This false idea was part of a novel written by pharmacist and author John Uri Lloyd.

8.4 Key Points

Only an abundance of vital energy guarantees a happy life full of energy, enjoyment, productivity and health. Energy production needs to exceed energy expenditure.

Rest and sleep are dynamic processes vital for healing, repair, recovery, renewal, and replenishment of energy and power.

Fasting is the absolute best way to provide the body and organs with complete physiological rest.

During a fast all organs of elimination can catch up on their work, and the breakdown of dead matter including fat, deposits, exudates, cysts, and tumors is promoted.

Physical activity and work should be avoided during a fast as these expend energy.

In both acute and chronic disease, fasting is beneficial and vital.

Fasting is the best detoxification method. However due to the industrialization and commercialization, the constant onslaught of toxins demands regular fasts and specific nutrients.

Dr. Mike's 5 Phase Detox program is a simple, easy-to-follow, common sense approach to prepare, detox and repair the organs of elimination.

Chapter 9 – Stress & Emotions

Addressing our body's physical needs is a clear cut task. Controlling stress and emotions is a more challenging task since it requires mental perseverance and input to achieve the proposed inner peace.

Inner piece begins the moment you choose not to allow another person or event to control your emotions. And this task is very obtainable since humans have the power to choose their response.

So let's dig into what stress is and how emotions and feelings affect our health.

9.1 Stressed out?

We all have stress... but what is STRESS? Dr. Stephen Fulder hit the nail on the head by stating: "Stress is not an illness in itself. Stress is change...our ability to adapt to all the changes that occur in life – moment to moment – whether emotional or physical. Stress can be from exercise, work, chemicals, drugs, food, radiation, bacteria, temperature, or simply too many late nights and too much fun."

Furthermore, due to the fast paced society we currently live in, job stress is increasing to worldwide epidemic proportions. It's affecting most people and this news is reported by the International Labor Organization of the United Nations. Sleep disorders are one of the main results of stress on the job and costs the U.S. economy well over $200 billion annually through reduced productivity, compensation claims, absenteeism, health insurance premiums, and direct medical expenses.

Stress has long-term, damaging effects on our bodies not unlike what happens to an automobile engine. After so many miles — especially *without* proper maintenance — it starts to wear out. It begins to burn more oil, loses power and starts to fall apart. *Stress* does the same thing to the human body.

Some simple examples of stress are the anxiety a person feels when their child is so sick they start to fear for the child's life. It's also the energy-draining fear when you feel you might lose your job. It's the *depression* many experience when divorce damages their self-image and their home. It's that heart-pounding, gasping-for-breath feeling when you narrowly miss a head-on crash knowing it would have killed you.

Stress comes at each of us in a never ending assault that changes our lives, damages us emotionally and, in ways we now understand, does extensive *physical* damage as well.

It's also agreed upon that 80% of all illness and disease is stress related. The 3 best selling drugs in the US: tranquilizers, pain killers, and gastro-intestinal remedies were developed to counter stress (I didn't say they work). Two-thirds of all visits to family physicians stem from stress. Stress is the root problem for many common ailments (which we know are just symptoms), including anxiety, irritability, alcoholism, headaches, hypertension, fibromyalgia, fatigue and many more.

How does that work then, you may ask? How does stress affect our body? Under stress, our body reacts by producing adrenaline. Adrenaline puts the whole body on a state of alert (chemical signals that prepare the body and mind for stress). This state of alert disrupts the body's metabolism, circulation and blood pressure; the body's resistance and immune system reduce drastically; productivity and per-formance suffer. We can go over all the physiological and biochemical details (but then this book would have been more expensive); but in short: stress undermines health and destroys well-being.

The solution would be to avoid the situations that cause our stress, or learn to control those situations. We first will have to recognize and acknowledge the situations that cause our personal stress and then acquire the skills to control these situations and neutralize the damaging effects.

There are many different ways to minimize stress and reduce stress. In order to minimize daily stress, time management and organization of work and activities are of utmost importance. If you are well organized and know how to prioritize your tasks, you are in control. When you are in control, you experience less stress. It's the daily uncertainties and unexpected emergencies that stress out the average person. Furthermore, in many families financial uncertainty causes major stress. Learn how to manage your money and save money, get in control of your financial situation so emergencies don't kill you.

Be proactive and start managing your work, life, finances, schedules etc. Most of us are not in control of their schedule, tasks, time or finances which induces major stress on all levels. Get help or help yourself by asking for advice and reading topic related books.

Sure, it will take some time to put these things in place and get in control. But it's time spent that will benefit you for years to come. No excuses!

It's not the purpose of this book to expand in detail on time management and management of your finances. Talk to a CPA or your representative at your bank in regards to managing your money and start saving for emergencies. A great book to help with stress and finances is "The total money makeover: a proven plan for financial fitness" by Dave Ramsey. You may think you don't have money to save, but you would be surprised how much money you spend on useless stuff and how much money you can save in many different ways, even without sacrificing daily indulgences. Just do it!

Personally, I prioritize my activities based on the 'four quadrants' model by Stephen R. Covey. I'm proactive with scheduling activities and organized when it comes to my work. I set deadlines, short term goals and long term goals. My CPA keeps me in-line and up-to-date on my finances. Less surprise equals less stress, and when prepared for emergencies, they hit less hard. The more control, the less stress.

Besides minimizing the sources of stress and avoiding stressful situations, one needs to employ means to relieve the remaining stress. Just as our body needs regular fasting to repair, recover, renew and replenish so does our mind. The same fast will accomplish that if the mind can relax and repose, without any stimulation (no light and sound, no stimulation such as TV, radio, reading a book etc.).

As we employ diaphragmatic breathing on a daily basis to improve circulation and optimize bodily functions, we need to employ a simple daily routine to repose the mind. Any form of mental relaxation will do, including meditation, Tai Chi, and yoga. Try them and decide which one(s) you enjoy and which one(s) accomplishes a relaxed, reposed mind. If time is restricting you from practicing mental relaxation, you need to redo your time management schedule and find some time. Prioritize your activities. If you think about it, I'm sure you must agree that your health and happiness are more important than many of your daily activities. In the worst case, learn to relax your mind and practice 5 minutes per day, maybe first thing in the morning? I know I freed up some time suggesting you don't need breakfast.

9.2 Our Mind

Clean food, clean water and sunshine do NOT cause health but are part of the essential conditions for normal, healthy living. The mind does not cause health either but can influence health.

I'm not going to spend pages on bashing the 'mind healers' of all kinds (including hypnotists, psychologists, psychiatrists, religious healers, priests, and other so called mind-curers). Just as doctors may have some book knowledge on pathology but no understanding of true health, these so called 'mind-healers' with their 'mind-cures' have no true understanding of our mind.

Even a child wouldn't believe that years of abuse of the body would potentially be cured by programming the mind or suggesting that the body will heal by the 'powers' of the mind. The mind is natural, not super-natural or extra-natural. The mind cannot cure. However, the mind will influence health, and stimulate or inhibit function if profound enough or prolonged enough. The mind therefore can contribute to 'disease' and can also contribute to the 'return' to normal health. The mind however can't cure 'disease' without taking the cause of 'disease' away. There simply is no short-cut.

Could one really believe that there is a short-cut (mind-cure) to wipe out all the years of bad living and overindulgences, neglecting and breaking the laws of nature and human life? Of course not! One would have to take away the cause in order to reverse health and therefore put the body in the right conditions so it can heal itself.

People with 'mental illnesses' may find short-term relief with any of these mind-cures because pills and talk (rationale, convincing, programming, modification etc.) can't work if the cause of this 'mental disease' is not addressed. As with physical illness, human interference only will worsen the condition.

Of all medical professionals (not sure we should use that term) the psy-chologist and psychiatrist are in my opinion the worst. Prescribing mind-altering toxic drugs that destroy brain cells and alter behavior in the most atrocious ways is nothing less than mental abuse and prolonged torture with lasting impairments. The last decades have seen a drastic increase in prescription of psychotropic drugs in children and teenagers, supposedly helping them with their ADD (attention deficit disorder) and ADHD (attention deficit and hyperactivity disorder) and other so called behavioral problems.

First, these fancy names and abbreviations are yet again made-up, unsubstantiated and so called diseases while in reality they are just symptoms. We already understand that it's impossible to cure 'disease' by chasing symptoms and that suppressing them only worsens that so called disease. The only cure is to take away the cause, as with any physical disease. And the cause is the same for all disease. That makes it simple, doesn't it? The mind-curers wouldn't be able to exploit our children and those with mind-symptoms.

You should have the understanding by now that no amount of stimulation or inhibition by whatever method (mental, physical, mechanical, chemical, electrical, thermal) can ever produce any state of health worthy of the name. The only legitimate approach to any mind-cure is the one of converting the destructive emotions of the mind with constructive emotions, and freeing the mind of false ideas. Fortunately, one doesn't need a mind-curer for this. All you need is the knowledge, skills and willingness to control your mind and emotions.

In short, the ones among us suffering from 'mental disease' need to address the cause, and there is only one: toxemia. There is only one cure also: put the body in the right conditions so it can heal itself. That's it, period. If you don't currently suffer from a 'mental disease' or when you recovered from one by applying the approach above and taking away the cause, you can be assured that stress and uncontrolled emotions are destructive to your physical, mental and spiritual health and therefore contribute to toxemia and impaired health. Your task is to learn how to control these emotions and achieve inner peace.

9.3 Feelings & Emotions

In Chinese medicine, several thousand years ago, emotions were already recognized as factors affecting health. The seven emotional factors in traditional Chinese medicine are joy, anger, melancholy, worry, grief, fear and fright. These emotions are considered normal emotional responses of the body to external stimuli and do not cause disease. However, intense or abrupt or prolonged emotional stimuli surpass the regular adaptability of the human organism and affect the functions of the body. These uncontrolled emotions are a major contributor to toxemia and the rise of all so called disease.

Some common examples illustrating the effect of emotions on the physiology of our body are the following:

The thought of food causing saliva to flow, fear affecting the heart by increasing heart rate and 'feeling the heart coming up in the throat', the effects of fear and worry upon digestion (for example a loose stool prior to an important performance or meeting), anxiety causing frequent urination. Joy, sympathy, sorrow can cause the eyes to tear and deep mental concentration suspends respiration.

These known effects of the mind are important enough to justify the need to carefully avoid any harmful and destructive effects our mind can produce. We must avoid fear, worry, anger, anxiety, envy, jealousy, self-pity etc. and cultivate love, joy, happiness, hope, faith, courage, contentment, gratefulness, self-respect etc.

How do we control emotions?

Step 1 – KNOWLEDGE

First, we need to know our emotions. What emotions do we feel and how do they affect us? There are thousands of different ways one can feel, but human emotions have been classified and the common ones are acceptance, anger, anticipation, disgust, fear, joy, sadness and sur-prise. Jealousy, for example, is then a manifestation of fear - fear that you're not 'as good' as someone else, fear of being abandoned because you're not 'perfect' or 'the best.'

You need to find out what kinds of situations cause which emotions, and be able to tell the difference between anger and fear. Sometimes multiple emotions can bubble up at the same time, and it may be difficult to distinguish between these different emotions.

How do we do this? Keep a 'JOE', a Journal Of Emotions.

1. Write down situations that caused an interesting or obvi-ous emotion in you. Record what the situation was and the emotion caused by the situation.

2. Recognize an emotion from the moment it materializes, as opposed to letting it build up and intensify. The last thing

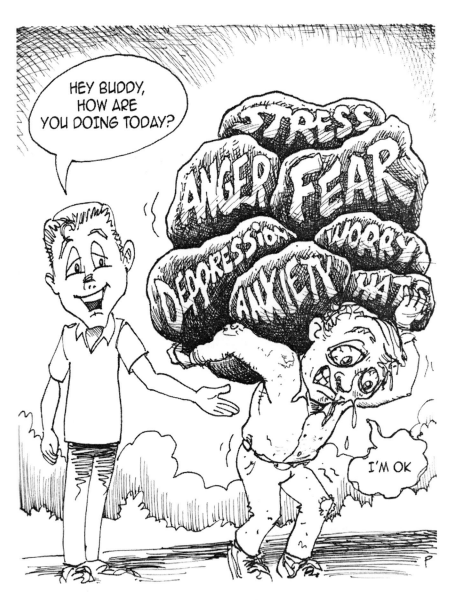

Illustration 15 – How are you doing today?

you want to do is ignore or repress your feelings. If you do, and you probably know this already, these feelings tend to get worse and erupt later.

3. Recognize that emotions don't just appear mysteriously out of nowhere. Many times, we're at the mercy of our emotions on a subconscious level. By recognizing your emotions on a conscious level, you're better able to control them. Ask yourself throughout the day: "How am I feeling right now"? Record interesting situations and the corresponding emotion.

4. Notice what was going through your mind when the emotion appeared. Stop and analyze what you were thinking about, until you find what thought was causing that emotion. Ask yourself whether this thought is reality or just an assumption. Explore all the different possibilities. If nothing else, thinking about other possible interpretations will alert you to many different scenarios, and prevents one from jumping to conclusions. Often, we make the wrong assumptions.

5. Another way to find out about your emotions and the situations that bring them on is to simply ask your loved-ones for honest input. I'm sure your spouse, parents, kids etc. can create a better awareness about your emotions.

Once you figure out what situations and thoughts elicit which emotions, we need to take ownership.

STEP 2 – TAKE OWNERSHIP

Don't blame others for your emotions. Take ownership of your emotions, after all you have the freedom to choose your response to any situation or stimulus. So if you decide to erupt in anger or frustration, or if you decide to worry or be fearful, that was your choice. You can't blame others for your own choices.

Recognize when you try to blame other people for your emotions and don't let your mind get away with that trick. Write down these situations in your 'JOE'. Taking full responsibility for your emotions will help you gain more control of them.

STEP 3 – CONTROL YOUR EMOTIONS

1. Choose your response

When deciding what to do or how to react to a certain stimulus or situation, it's important to make sure you make a conscious choice. Do not make a choice based on a reaction to another, competing emotion. For example, if someone insults you and you do nothing, is this your conscious decision or is it a response to your fear of confrontation?

You want to base your choices on your principles and some common sense. Your principles may guide you to make the right choices and therefore the right response. What are you moral principles and values? What kind of person do you want to be? What do you want the outcome of the situation to be? Which choice would you ultimately be proud of? Answering these questions may help you chose the right response.

Use your common sense in any situation. Which course of action is the most likely to result in the outcome you desire? For example, if someone wants to pick a fight at a bar because you accidently ran into him, and you want to walk away from the fight, there's a fair chance that the drunken man will feel insulted when you turn your back to him. So maybe it's better to apologize for the accidental bump and keep the conversation going until he calms down.

After you discovered what emotion(s) you're dealing with, think of more than one way you can respond. Your emotions control you when you assume there's only *one* way to react, but you always have a choice.

For example, if someone insults you, and you experience anger, your immediate response might be to insult them back. But no matter what the emotion, there are always one or more alternatives, and you can probably think of more.

Here are 4 common options you can choose from:

1. Don't react, don't do anything at all. This approach is especially good when you know that someone is trying to frustrate you on purpose or trying to get you angry. When you fail to show an emotional reaction, the person egging you on will become frustrated and eventually stop.

2. Relax. I know... easier said than done. But there are some ways to relax that do not require much effort, experience or willpower. When we are angry we tend to clench our jaws and tense up. Taking a deep breath (diaphragmatic breathing) is an easy and effective way to tamper down the emotional anger. It won't dispel the anger but it can dial it down just enough to keep us from saying or doing something we would regret after.

3. Do the opposite of what you would normally do. For example, if you get upset or frustrated when your spouse didn't put the trash out...again, instead of engaging in an argument, calmly take out the trash the second you notice it wasn't done. Then tell your spouse in a calm and collected way that you would appreciate help considering all you do in the household.

4. Remove yourself from the situation. Let's say that you are part of a recreational basketball team and your team mates are unfocused, negative and always show up late for practice. You invariably get upset when playing basketball. One strategy for dealing with this upset and frustration is to join a different basketball team. Basically, you remove yourself from a situation that you know will generate these strong, negative and unnecessary feelings and emotions.

2. Be Proactive

Many of us are reactive, meaning that we react to both situations we can and cannot control. This reaction elicits unnecessary emotions, affecting our health. Reactive people blame others and waste time worrying and complaining about things they don't have any control over or can't influence anyway. A simple example is people who get upset when it rains. Maybe they planned an outdoor barbeque for their friends.

Proactive people recognize the fact that certain situations can be influenced by them and other situations cannot. Proactive people won't blame the weather for their failed barbeque party. Instead, they recognize they can't change or influence the weather. Proactive people won't get upset with a change in weather, instead they act proactively and move the party indoors, or have a back-up plan in case of rain. The party is great, regardless the weather.

Proactive people recognize that they are able to choose their response to any given situation; they recognize this responsibility (ability to respond). They do not blame circumstances, conditions, or conditioning for their behavior. Their behavior and success is a product or direct result of their own conscious choice, based on values, rather than a product of their conditions, based on feeling.

Reactive people are often affected by their physical environment. If the weather is good, they feel good. If it isn't, it affects their attitude and their performance. Proactive people can carry their own weather with them. Eleanor Roosevelt stated: "no one can hurt you without your consent." And in the words of Gandhi: "They cannot take away our self- respect if we do not give it to them". It is our willing permission, our consent to what happens to us, that hurts us far more than what happens to us in the first place.

What has this to do with stress or emotions, you may ask? Well, we are talking about how you should be proactive and choose your response to whatever happens to you (other people's opinion, unpleasant situations at work, deadlines, raising your kids, a car accident, being sick, financial problems, etc.). You can have these circumstances knock you down, and let your emotions of anger, failure, and depression take over (this is how most people cope with the 'stresses' of life). BUT you have a choice! Be proactive, don't blame the circumstances and don't blame others, find a solution and ACT! Use your resourcefulness and initiative.

It's NOT what others do or even our own mistakes that hurt us the most, it's our response to those things. Chasing after a poisonous snake that bites us will only drive the poison through our entire system. It is far better to take measures immediately to get the poison out. Acknowledge that there are certain things that you won't be able to change. Those things aren't worth getting frustrated about. You're probably not going to change the way that some people drive their car, for instance. It's not worth getting upset over. What you can change is your reaction to people who drive recklessly and selfishly.

If you are a worrier, you will benefit from reading "How to Stop Worrying and Start Living" by Dale Carnegie, and "Don't Sweat the Small Stuff" by Richard Carlson, PhD. Worry sucks away energy, inhibits thinking and kills ambition, but worry can be conquered and controlled. I personally use several of the 100 pieces of advice in Carlson's book on a daily basis. I tend to sweat some of the small stuff, but now I'm able to catch myself and not engage.

One of the things that works for me is asking myself: "will this be important next year?". If it won't be important next year, it's not important enough to worry about or even think about it. I use one of the 4 options above (don't react, relax, do the opposite or remove yourself from the situation).

WORRYING DOESN'T TAKE AWAY TOMORROW'S TROUBLES, BUT IT DOES TAKE AWAY TODAY'S PEACE.

The illustration on the next page shows that there really is never a reason to worry or to get upset. Realize this truth and one day soon you may find inner peace.

3. The 'Self-fulfilling prophecy'

Change your perspective. The above steps show how to not let your emotions control your behavior on the spot. If you want to experience fewer negative emotions to begin with, change the way you see the world. If you learn how to be optimistic and change your perspective, you'll find that negative emotions make far fewer appearances.

Whatever you think or believe, you are right! If you think the world is a bad place, then you will unconsciously (reticular activator of your brain) look for all reasons (news on TV, war, another child missing etc.) to confirm your initial belief that the world is a bad place. If you believe you will fail a test, you will. But it also works the other way…If you truly belief you can regain your health or be the next millionaire, you will! How? You will recognize all the resources that will help you achieve your goals, and act upon them.

Being optimistic is important. Instead of letting emotions take over because you expect them to (being pessimistic), try believing in the notion that the world is essentially a good place and that people get what they deserve. Believe that you are a good person. You may soon find that your outlook changes your emotions.

Positive thinking and a 'yes' – attitude will contribute to an optimistic outlook and therefore promote a balanced emotional, mental and spiritual health…which in turn translates into better physical health. Your brain and your thoughts are your map, your blue print. Just as a house is not built without a blue print, a goal is not achieved without a blue print either. A faulty architectural blue print of a house results in a poorly constructed, less than worthy house just as negative thoughts result in poor health and unhappiness. A well planned, detailed, innovative, organized blue print of a house results in a masterpiece just as a positive, optimistic, organized, proactive brain and thoughts assist in achieving health and happiness.

4. Eliminate false core beliefs

Eliminate many of the selfish core beliefs which give rise to your disturbing thoughts and negative emotions. There are many irrational ideas that repeatedly upset us. They are all *false,* but many of us are inclined to believe at least some of them part of the time.

Here are some preconceived notions about the self that are wrong because people think of themselves too highly:

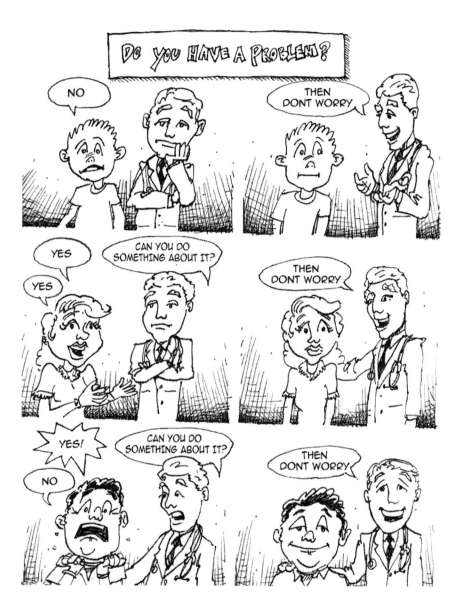

Illustration 16 – Don't worry

"I must be perfect in all respects in order to be worthwhile." Nobody can be perfect in *everything* that we have to do in life. But if you believe that you're a failure unless you are perfect in every way, you are setting yourself up for a lifetime of unhappiness.

"I must be loved and approved of by everyone who is important to me." Sometimes you just can't help making enemies, and there are people in this world who bear ill will to almost everyone. But you can't make your own life miserable by trying to please them.

"When people treat me unfairly, it is because they are bad people." Most of the people who treat you unfairly have friends and family who love them. People are mixtures of good and bad. Maybe there is something about you that displeases them.

"It is terrible when I am seriously frustrated, treated badly, or rejected." Some people have such a short fuse that they are constantly losing jobs or endangering friendships because they are unable to endure the slightest frustration. The world does not tick for only you. Be considerate of other people.

"If something is dangerous or fearful, I have to worry about it." Many people believe that 'the work of worrying' will help to make problems go away. They drive themselves crazy by making up things to worry about. "Okay, that's over. Now, what's the next thing on the list that I have to worry about?"

"It is terrible when things do not work out exactly as I want them to." Could you have predicted the course of your own life? Probably not. By the same token, you can't predict that things are going to work out exactly as you want them to, even in the short term.

There are people who do not think of themselves highly enough: Their self-esteem is essentially in the gutter, and their emotions are the result of not being able to love themselves adequately.

"Misery comes from outside forces which I can't do very much to change." Many prison inmates describe their life as if it were a cork, bobbing up and down on waves of circumstance. You can choose whether to see yourself as an effect of your circumstances, or a cause. Take responsibility for your actions.

"It is easier to avoid life's difficulties and responsibilities than to face them." Even painful experiences, once we can get through them, can serve as a basis for learning and future growth. It's childish to go through life thinking that difficulties won't ever affect us.

"Because things in my past controlled my life, they have to keep doing so now and in the future." If this were really true, it would mean that we are prisoners of our past, and change is impossible. But people change all the time and sometimes they change dramatically! You have the ability to be who you want to be, you just have to believe in yourself.

"I can be as happy as possible by just doing nothing and enjoying myself, taking life as it comes." If this were true, almost every wealthy or comfortably retired person would do as little as possible. But instead, they seek new challenges as a pathway to further growth. You're tricking yourself into believing that you'd be really happy doing nothing. People need novelty to stay satisfied.

<u>5. Recognize thoughts and ideas that worsen negative emotions</u>

Learn to avoid the cognitive distortions which make things look worse than they really are. Most of us have heard the expression, "looking at the world through rose-colored glasses." But when you use cognitive distortions, you tend to look at the world through *mud*-colored glasses! Here are some ideas that you should stop from rolling through your head if you catch yourself thinking them:

Avoid negative ideas that come from feeling inadequate. Inadequacy comes from low self-esteem, the idea that you aren't good enough to do something or deserve someone. Banish inadequacy from your emotions as much as possible, and you may find that it has been *keeping* you from accomplishing things.

All-or-nothing thinking: also referred to as 'black-and-white' thinking.

Everything is good or bad, with nothing in between. If you aren't perfect, then you're a failure. You procrastinate because "it's not perfect".

Disqualifying the positive: If somebody says something good or positive about you, it doesn't count. However, if somebody says something bad about you, you "knew it all along".

Personalization: You believe that you were the cause of something bad that happened, when you really didn't have very much to do with it.

Mind reading: You think somebody is disrespecting you and don't bother to check it out. You just assume that they are. You do this because you feel like you don't deserve respect, and so are overly sensitive to people whom you think might not respect you.

Avoid negative ideas that come from fear: Humans can be afraid of a lot of things; we let fear take over our rational brains because we're convinced something bad is going to happen, even when we don't have evidence or reason to belief that it will.

Overgeneralization: A single negative event turns into a never ending pattern of defeat. "I didn't get a phone call. I'll never hear from anybody again," or "She broke up with me. Why would anyone want to date me?" You generalize not because of a pattern, but because you fear the pattern.

Labeling and mislabeling: This is an extreme form of overgeneralization. When you make a mistake, you give yourself a label, such as "I'm a loser." When someone else's behavior rubs you the wrong way, you attach a negative label to him, "He's an idiot" Mislabeling involves describing an event with language that is highly colored and emotionally loaded.

The Fortune Teller Error: You think that things are going to turn out badly, and convince yourself that this is already a fact. You have no evidence for the prophecy, but you're convinced anyways. This is similar to the self-fulfilled prophecy.

Jumping to conclusions: You make a negative interpretation even though there are no definite facts that convincingly support your conclusion. You assume that preparing for the worst is better than hoping for the best, because you're afraid, not hopeful.

Avoid negative ideas that come from other complex emotions: Don't succumb to these defeatist emotional responses. Have faith in your ability to work things through. Believe in your own self-worth. If you catch yourself thinking any one of these thoughts, focus instead on a positive way of interpreting your worth.

Magnification (catastrophizing) or minimization: Imagine that you're looking at yourself or somebody else through a pair of binoculars. You might think that a mistake you made or somebody else's achievement is more important than they really are. Now imagine that you've turned the binoculars around and you're looking through them backwards. Something you have done might look less important than it really is, and somebody else's faults might look less important than they really are.

Emotional reasoning: You assume that your negative emotions reflect the way things really are: "I feel it, therefore it must be true." You want the world to be the way it feels to you because it will help you feel less powerless.

Should statements: You beat up on yourself as a way of getting motivated to do something. You "should" do this, you "must" do this, you "ought" to do this, and so on. This doesn't make you want to do it; it only makes you feel guilty. When you direct should statements toward others, you feel anger, frustration, and resentment.

6. Helping Others

And last but not least, we need to return to a basic human instinct and principle:

HELPING OTHERS

By helping others, whether it is your co-worker, your spouse, a loved-one, a neighbor, a stranger at the grocery store, or people and children in need....You Help Yourself!

How? You know that it feels AWESOME when you help someone, doesn't it? Even holding a door open for an older person makes you feel good inside. You know it, just admit it! This act of kindness makes you feel good and lowers your daily stress, it's a simple fact of life! So, why wouldn't you do more of that? Start helping people more often or all the time!

That doesn't necessary mean you have to donate money to the Red Cross or UNICEF (you can of course, even though these organizations waste most of your donation on administrative expenses and salaries, including a $250,000 salary for their CEO). I personally sponsor a child with CHILDREN INCORPORATED which helps children in need, locally and worldwide. I recommend you check them out. It's only $28 per month and you can communicate with your sponsored child.

And that's all good...BUT, it's the daily small things you do to help other people that will help heal you and combat the stress and negative emotions in your life! Don't believe it? Just try it for only 2 days and you'll see I'm right.

"You can get everything you want in life, if you just help enough other people get what they want."

Zig Ziglar.

Helping others also promotes the principle of 'Pay It Forward'. This principle suggests that when you help someone, you don't expect anything in return from that person but you hope and believe that this person will 'pay it forward' or in other words that this person will help someone else at some point in time.

When you do help someone, for example chip in some cash at the register when someone is a few dollars short, you don't want to brag about it or share the story with others. The satisfaction and internal kindness is unselfish and doesn't need rewarded or gratified.

Conclusion:

A positive, proactive ATTITUDE and a way of living in which you HELP OTHERS, REDUCES your stress and negative emotions, promotes inner peace and consequently promotes health and happiness, the purpose of life.

7. Final Recommendations

Don't let the fear from the past keep you from your future.

Some experiences like watching a film, hearing a sound or tasting a food (sensory input) can trigger or bring about good emotions. The more good ones you can recognize, pay attention to and be aware of, the easier it is to put yourself in that kind of a recognizable mood. It's far easier to get out of an angry or sad state of mind when you know what a happy or joyful state of mind is like.

Learn to recognize and anticipate 'triggers' that set you off.

No matter what you choose to do, it's important to continue acknowledging the emotion. Just because you're not reacting to an emotion doesn't mean that emotion doesn't exist.

When you see your mood changing, leave from whatever is causing it and take several deep breaths, and think about what was done or said to upset you. Figure out another way of dealing with it instead of getting upset! Also ask yourself: "is it worth it"?

Sometimes it's helpful to keep a binder with lined paper (JOE). Then at the end of the day when you're in bed you can write down all your thoughts and emotions.

Just try to calm down, don't panic.

Try making a list of a bunch of feelings you want to be aware of either feeling or avoiding. Each day leave a check or mark by them as you accomplish or fail to accomplish your goal.

Think about how you will see your reaction in 5 years from now. Will you be proud of yourself for walking away with your dignity intact or will you look back and remember falling apart ? Choose now.

To cultivate a YES-attitude, I recommend Jeffrey Gitomer's "Little Gold Book of Yes! Attitude". It's fun and effective, with practical tips and to-do's. The stuff in this book only works if you apply it of course. Don't be lazy. You can't afford not to be happy. Once you master some of the easy principles, you can share them with your loved-ones. They will love your new YES-attitude.

9.4 Nature's Answer to Stress

There is no elixir or magic bullet to control stress and emotions, and although stress and emotions don't cause so called disease directly, they do contribute to toxemia.

So reducing stress and controlling emotions are crucial in obtaining optimal health. Furthermore, the act of controlling emotions results in inner peace and happiness.

The above plan to control emotions and feelings is essential and one will only succeed with daily practice, commitment and willingness. Results can be seen and felt almost immediately but total control may take a long time. The short term results should act as a motivator to continue to work on controlling emotions and feelings, and reducing stress in the search for optimal health and happiness.

Having said that, derived from nature, we are provided with antidotes to modern stress. Grasses, grains, fruits and vegetables, and powerful herbs can provide every mineral, vitamin, enzyme, micronutrient, and omega fatty acid we need to combat stress and its damaging effects.

By providing our body with all essential nutrients, we balance our bodily systems. I will attempt to explain this but first a few refreshing facts. We already know that the cells in our body constantly replace/renew themselves, and that our body needs the RIGHT nutrients and tools to do so. Each and every cell in your body has about 10,000 receptors. The RNA (messenger) of the cell will tell the receptors (guards on look-out) what the cell needs. The receptors will 'stick out their neck' and look for the nutrients the cell needs. In most instances (due to the S.A.D. diet), the nutrients these receptors are looking for are not available and the cell has to settle for less.

The cell is forced to utilize inferior, unnatural materials in an attempt to rebuild itself. That's like making a copy of a copy of a copy (try it at home). The cell literally MUTATES (changes in structure) and DEGENERATES; its function impairs and disease rises and evolves (cancer, degenerative diseases etc.).

The essential nutrients and phytonutrients (nutrients from plants, and therefore nutrients from Mother Nature) can be recognized by our body. When we consume them daily, the receptors will almost always find the nutrients they need for the cell. The cell will successfully renew and replace itself and keep our organs and bodily systems function optimally.

Got it? If not, read it again, it's VERY important to understand!

Many of these ESSENTIAL and all natural nutrients have anti-inflammatory, anti-viral, anti-bacterial, anti-fungal, anti-arthritic, and antioxidant properties. They restore homeostasis to the different body systems, including the cardiovascular, digestive, immune, nervous and reproductive systems.

These nutritional super foods also VITALIZE the body. They rejuvenate, combat stress and fatigue (by relaxing the central nervous system), improve stamina and memory, boost the immune system (by increasing number of white blood cells), improve physical and mental performance and workload.

They help to strengthen the digestive system, promote liver function and detoxify the body (maintain healthy bowels and cleanse stomach and intestines), and help with a healthy metabolic function (help adjust blood sugar levels and reduce blood fat or hyperlipidemia).

Some of these natural nutrients are also useful in aiding neurological conditions, including anxiety, depression, and schizophrenia.

Studies into the anti-cancer activity of plants and herbs show that they may prevent cells from becoming cancerous. Duh! You already know how that can happen. Turn back a few pages if you forgot and read it all again! You need to understand that if the cells receive the nutrients they need, they will RESTORE normal activity and RENEW themselves (that's why it is possible to reverse cancer).

And if that's not enough, these awesome plants, herbs, grasses, grains, fruits and vegetables also contain many amino-acids, vitamins and minerals including calcium, iron, phosphorus, potassium, magnesium, selenium, zinc and more.

Am I implying that a combination of ESSENTIAL nutrients is the cure all? NO, NOT AT ALL! There is no 'Magic Bullet' and there is no 'Silver Bullet' either! What I'm stating is that they help balance your body and provide all the cells in your body the nutrients they need to function optimally. By balancing your body, you automatically resolve many issues and health problems that were the result of a dysfunctional organ or system. This doesn't mean it's going to cure all.

Essential nutrients are part of our C.L.E.A.N rule: clean food. Once you establish a healthy foundation by putting your body in the right conditions, you have given your body the tools it needs TO HEAL ITSELF.

NOTHING cures you. Prescription or OTC drugs don't and that's a given (they KILL you, slowly but surely). Natural medicines, herbs and botanicals, healthy nutrition and exercise don't either. **ONLY Your Body can!**

BUT the body can ONLY heal itself if it is in balance, placed in the right conditions. And in order to achieve and maintain balance, a healthy lifestyle (no prescription drugs, healthy nutrition, moderate exercise, effective nutritional supplementation, positive attitude, control over stress and emotions) is a MUST!

Adaptogens:

Adaptogens are by far the most studied and select group of plants that effectively assist in balancing and normalizing bodily functions, including adrenal gland function.

These unique herbs were first used by the Russian Cosmonauts and elite citizens, and later successfully employed to enhance athletic performance. Many Olympic athletes enjoyed the benefits of these adaptogens.

The plant adaptogens of significance include Schisandra chinensis, Bacopa monnieri, Rhodiola rosea, Eleutherococcus senticosus, Magnolia officinalis, Rhemannia glutinosa, Bupleurum falcatum, Panax ginseng, Coleus forskohlii and Withania sominfera.

How do these adaptogens function?

The response to chronic stress, first defined as occurring in three stages by Hans Selye as alarm, resistance and exhaustion, typically results in aberrant adrenal function and adrenal fatigue, as well as abnormal cognitive, metabolic, energy, endurance, immune and glycemic function. The consequences of intermittent stress, or episodic acute stress during resistance or exhaustion, interfere with recovery and also promote abnormal neuro-endocrine, metabolic and immune system function.

Adaptogens effectively address all stages of both acute and chronic stress, support the body's ability to adapt to stressors and help avoid the damaging consequences from those stressors. Collectively, plant adaptogens can help combat symptoms of fatigue and enhance endurance as well as support normal mental and emotional wellbeing. Plant adaptogens also can increase the body's ability to resist and recover from stress while providing an overall feeling of balance and normalization.

Next, I will go in a little more detail regarding the actions of these adaptogens. This info is not crucial so you may skip forward a few paragraphs if you are not interested in the details, and resume at 9.5. Bio-identical Hormones.

During acute stress, and the alarm stage of stress, Rhodiola rosea, Schizandra chinensis, Bacopa monnieri, and Eleutherococcus senticosus can support mental performance and physical working capacity, as well as promote the balanced response of the sympatho-adrenal-system (SAS) to the body's acute reaction to a stressor.

During the resistance stage Withania somnifera and Coleus forskohlii, are able to support the normal thyroid and gonadal function. In the exhaustion stage the Rehmannia glutinosa, Bupleurum falcatum and Withania somnifera act as primary agents to restore proper function of the hypothalamic-pituitary-adrenal axis and work synergistically with other plant adaptogens to support normal function of other body systems.

Adaptogens with adrenotrophic properties may also decrease adrenal atrophy seen in the exhaustion stage of chronic stress. The increased cortisol levels seen in various stages of stress are modulated by Schizandra chinensis and Magnolia officinalis. Rhemannia glutinosa can help restore normal function of glucocorticoid receptors that have been down regulated due to chronically elevated levels of cortisol. Bupleurum falcatum supports adrenal recovery and normalization of the hypothalamic-pituitary-adrenal (HPA) system by promoting the release of adrenocorticotropic hormone (ACTH), which is responsible for maintaining the normal size and function of the adrenal gland.

Stress induced elevations of catecholamines and adrenaline induced hyperglycemia can be modulated by Magnolia officinalis, Panax ginseng and Rehmannia glutinosa.

While the primary benefit of plant adaptogens is the ability to restore healthy, balanced adrenal gland function by supporting normal hypothalamic-pituitaryadrenal (HPA) axis function, the effectiveness of these adaptogens is in large part also due to their ability to protect and promote the recovery of neurocognitive, neuromuscular, cardiovascular, glycemic, hepatic, thyroid, gonadal and immune system health.

9.5 What About Hormones?

That's a fair question since the imbalance of hormones seems to cause a wide variety of physical and mental/emotional symptoms.

Of course, our perversions and poor lifestyle choices deplete our energy and essential nutrient supply, and affect every organ, tissue and cell in our body, including our hormones.

Hormonal balance is obviously crucial in obtaining optimal health (which includes losing weight for some of us).

<u>What are hormones?</u>

A hormone is a chemical released by a cell, a gland, or an organ in one part of the body that affects cells in other parts of the organism. Hormones are chemical messengers that transport a signal from one cell to another, and therefore crucial in every chemical reaction and bodily function.

Hormones have the following effects on the human body:

- stimulation or inhibition of growth

- mood swings

- induction or suppression of apoptosis (programmed cell death)

- activation or inhibition of the immune system

- regulation of metabolism

- preparation of the body for mating, fighting, fleeing, and other activity

- preparation of the body for a new phase of life, such as puberty, parenting, and menopause

- control of the reproductive cycle

- hunger cravings

- sexual arousal

A hormone may also regulate the production and release of other hormones. Hormone signals control the internal environment of the body through homeostasis.

Hormone History

Where did Hormone Replacement Therapy (HRT) start? Hormone Replacement Therapy (HRT) was born, in a sense, in 1942, when the Food and Drug Administration (FDA) approved synthetic estrogen alone, and later estrogen with progestin to relieve short-term menopausal symptoms including hot flashes and night sweats. In 1966, widespread use of HRT really took flight with the publication of Dr. Robert Wilson's book, *Feminine Forever,* funded by Wyeth-Ayerst, the leading manufacturer of synthetic hormones. Wilson characterized HRT as nothing short of a wonder drug and a fountain of youth for women who feared becoming dried-up, wrinkled, and sexless old hags in danger of losing their husbands. Negative side effects were not mentioned; in fact, Wilson claimed that *estrogen prevented* cancer and called women 'castrates' if they didn't take hormones. Also absent from books and magazine articles at the time were discussions of alternative therapies for menopausal symptoms.

Do You Want Pregnant Mare's Urine?

Synthetic hormones are made in a laboratory from nonhuman sources. For example, Premarin®, a drug commonly used in estrogen replacement therapy, is derived from pregnant mares' (horse) urine. In fact, there are more than 50 horse estrogens in Premarin®. Because horse estrogen is foreign to the human body, women lack the enzymes and co-factors to metabolize it safely.

Foreign estrogens, like those in Premarin®, are called *xeno-estrogens*. With potentially dangerous side effects, they are also found in insecticides and plastic bottles. Synthetic progestins (like ProveraTM, which is medroxyprogesterone acetate or MPA) can have negative side effects including possible blood clots, an increased risk of heart disease, headaches, fluid retention, weight gain, mood swings, and breakthrough bleeding. In addition, other chemicals that may produce adverse side effects must be added to the synthetic hormones to facilitate absorption and utilization by the body.

Once considered the 'cure' for menopausal symptoms, synthetic hormones do more harm than good. A portion of the widely publicized Women's Health Initiative (WHI) Study on HRT was stopped early when it concluded that risks including increased breast cancer, heart attacks, strokes, and blood clots exceed the benefits. According to the California Healthspan Institute, synthetic HRT "is not really true hormone replacement therapy since to be categorized as a 'hormone' the substance must naturally exist in the human female or male body." Plus, if every woman's body is different, common sense would dictate that a standardized dose could *not* be the appropriate treatment for an individual woman.

Bio-identical Hormones - A match made in heaven?

Sometimes called natural hormones or human identical hormones, biologically identical hormones are derived from plants, such as the wild yam or soybean plant, and are <u>chemically</u> and <u>functionally</u> identical to human hormones. The wild yam is rich in precursor molecules that can be converted in the laboratory into estrogens and other hormones whose molecular structure is the same as those produced in the human body. The key in distinguishing what is 'natural', is *not* where the hormone originated, but whether it's <u>chemical</u> make-up *matches* the one it is intended to replace.

Biologically identical hormones are believed to produce the same physiologic responses in the body as endogenous hormones (those made by the body).

Substances that are most similar to what our body produces naturally are thought to support human functioning without increased risk of allergic reactions and sensitivities. For example, studies have shown human-identical insulin to be more effective for diabetic patients. Moreover, an often overlooked aspect of biologically identical HRT is that it may vastly improve the quality of life for women suffering from a wide range of physical, mental, and emotional symptoms.

Although there have been a number of smaller studies on biologically identical hormones, there have been no large-scale efforts similar to the WHI research.

In the late 1800's, laws were passed in the United States that allowed medicines to be patented only if they were <u>not</u> natural substances. Because biologically identical hormones occur naturally in the female body, they cannot be patented and therefore large pharmaceutical companies have no financial incentive to fund research on these types of hormones.

Even the WHI authors acknowledged that results might have been different if biologically identical hormones had been used: "The results do not necessarily apply... to estrogens and progestins administered through the transdermal route. It remains possible that transdermal estradiol with progesterone, which more closely mimics the normal physiology and metabolism of endogenous sex hormones, may provide a different risk-benefit profile."

Today's women prefer natural hormones. In a survey of a nationally representative sample of 1009 women age 40 and older, 83% said they would prefer to use hormones that are similar to their own body's hormones. Bio-identical hormones include estrone (EI), estradiol (E2), estriol (E3), progesterone, testosterone, dehydroepiandrosterone (DHEA), and Pregnenolone.

To summarize:

SYNTHETIC = SUBSTITUTION
BIO-IDENTICAL = REPLACEMENT

Synthetic hormones are not found in humans, and are not identical in structure or function to the bio-identical hormones they are intended to replace.

Biologically identical hormones can be prepared by a compounding pharmacy in dosages and various administration forms to suit one's individual needs.

<u>What are the benefits of BHRT?</u>

1.   Fewer side effects versus synthetic derivatives.

2.   Protection against heart disease.

3.   Reduced risk of breast cancer.

4.   Improved cholesterol and lipid profile.

<u>What are the major Goals of BHRT?</u>

1.   **Alleviate the symptoms** *caused by* the natural decrease in production of hormones by the body.

2.   **Provide protective benefits**, which were *originally provided* by our naturally occurring hormones.

3.   Re-establish a **hormonal balance.**

<u>How does hormonal balance relate to weight loss?</u>

Well, many women gain weight prior to or during menopause, after a partial or complete hysterectomy or any other condition affecting hormones.

Even when these women (or men) eat semi-healthy, and exercise.... the body will not respond and weight loss does NOT occur! Why? The body is not in balance and is therefore unable to respond; or unable to heal itself!

It is advised to balance one's hormones naturally FIRST, and then incorporate a sensible weight loss program. Does that make sense? Sure, especially knowing that most weight loss candidates are women in their pre-menopause or menopause. To learn more about BHRT, read Suzanne Somers' books: The Sexy Years (2004) & Ageless (2006).

If you are on prescription hormones, I highly recommend you switch to bio-identical hormones. Your physician will most likely disagree with these recommendations, and this is why: he/she is NOT trained in bio-identical hormones and therefore can NOT recommend them; he/she is NOT trained in health, but only in disease; he/she is bombarded on a daily basis with prescription drug information from the medical repre-sentatives of drug companies. Regardless, YOU need to take control of your health. How? Keep reading!

BHRT Conclusion:

If you assume your hormones are out of balance, you are probably right. Before you spent money on a blood test and BHRT, take away the cause. You know what the cause of all disease and all symptoms is, right?

If money is not a concern, you can certainly accelerate and assist the restoration of your hormonal balance with BHRT.

I personally helped and witnessed many women and men restore their hormonal balance and reduce or abolish common related symptoms of hormonal imbalance (night sweats, hot flashes, mood swings, uncon-trolled emotions, low libido, fatigue, headaches, weight gain, insomnia etc.). Just note that BHRT alone will not cure anything. BHRT will assist in restoring hormonal balance. ONLY taking away the cause will deliver lasting results and optimal health.

9.6. Key Points

Daily stresses affect our health in a drastic way and contribute to the cause of all so called disease: toxemia. We need to learn how to minimize our daily stress by getting organized, manage our time and our finances, and prioritize our activities. We need to be proactive and prepare for unexpected emergencies.

We also need to combat the remaining stress by reposing our mind. Meditation, yoga, tai chi, or any type of mental relaxation will repair, renew and rejuvenate the mind.

Our mind doesn't cause disease nor cures disease. Our mind can influence health and disease. The only cure for so called mental disease is the same as the cure for physical so called disease: take away the cause. The cause of all disease is toxemia.

Emotions and feelings are normal responses of the body to external stimuli and do not cause disease. However, intense or abrupt or prolonged emotional stimuli contribute to toxemia.

To control our emotions we first need to know what emotions affect us and in what situations they do so. Next, we need to take ownership of our emotions and acquire the skills to control them.

Learn to choose your response to situations on the spot (don't react, relax, do the opposite or remove yourself from the situation), be proactive, change your perspective on life, develop a YES-attitude, eliminate false core beliefs and recognize thoughts and ideas that would worsen negative emotions.

Help others and pay-it-forward. Feel good about yourself without bragging about it.

Nature provided us with specific plants called 'adaptogens' which are highly effective in balancing bodily functions and adapting to stress.

Bio-identical hormones can assist in the restoration of hormonal balance.

Chapter 10 – Overstimulation & Overindulgences

Overstimulation and overindulgences rob our body and mind of energy. The occasional event of overstimulation or overindulgence can be overcome by our body, if we allow our body to recover and rebuild our energy reserve. However, intense and prolonged or regular overstimulation and overindulgences exceed the body's energy capacities. In the continuous attempt to preserve life, the body will be forced to put important, daily tasks and functions on hold. The body operates in a continuous emergency state of 'putting out the fires'.

As a result, normal metabolic functions including elimination of toxins are impaired, and toxemia takes place. Disease takes form and progresses silently until (maybe decades later) sickness suddenly rears its ugly head. And then we wondered what happened.

The only way to obtain and maintain optimal health is to recognize acts of overstimulation and overindulgence, and cease to expose the body and mind to these draining and toxic activities.

10.1 Perversions

Perversion comes from the Latin word 'perversus' which means 'turned the wrong way'. In health and disease, perversions are functions, actions and instincts that suffer inversion, meaning they have converted from their RIGHT use and purpose into a WRONG use and purpose.

Common rule is that every creature on this planet handles the laws and powers of nature with which it is endowed with a skill that is stunning and complete to meet the highest purpose of its being and to the fulfillment of its functions in unity with nature.

Man is the ONLY creature that has succeeded to be in constant antagonism with the harmony of nature. My explanation is that humans, unlike animals and other creatures, have the freedom to choose their response. This freedom and awareness has cost us our health and happiness, and has very much lowered the standards of our species.

Even though our mind and body, and nature around us TELL US EXACTLY what response to choose with any given stimulus or in any given situation, we tend to ignore that advice and choose the WRONG response.

Drinking beer for the first time results in a vomit party, accompanied with headaches, nausea, poor reaction time, loss of short term memory etc. What is our body trying to tell us? Of course: Don't drink beer! It's not natural, the body doesn't recognize it, it doesn't have any nutritional value, it doesn't serve the body, it only depletes energy and power, it contributes to toxemia. What do we do? We do it again and again and again. The body responds with no longer throwing a vomit party because that costs too much energy. It will preserve life differently: storing the sugars from alcohol, storing the toxins in adipose tissue, etc. But this comes with a huge price... to be paid later when the body no longer can compensate for the toxic overload.

Then this activity of drinking beers at regular intervals becomes a perversion, a wrong action, an action opposite of what nature intended, an action that promotes disease not health, an action that promotes depression not happiness.

Have you ever seen an animal in the wild overindulging on alcohol or anything else for that matter? No. Their instinct keeps them in harmony with nature and promotes optimal health.

The following is a limited list of some of our perversions:

Consumption of alcohol, use of tobacco, use of drugs, use of stimulants, use of medicines, drinking milk from other species, eating synthetic foods, anorexia, bulimia, eating and drinking for pleasure (feasting), cannibalism, cachexia (dirt eating), sadism, masochism, and many sexual perversions such as fetishism, exhibitionism, pedophilia, masturbation (that's right), sex for pleasure, prostitution, rape, pornography, polygamy, etc.

10.2 Overstimulation

Overstimulation starts upon conception. The pregnant mother who should rest and feed healthy instead continues to overwork, stress about everything, worries and fears the unknown, may become depressed before or after the delivery etc. She compensates by overeating and consuming more so called comfort food which is a nice term for poisonous food (sweets, sugars, deserts, ice cream or whatever she craves). The fetus is already mal-fed and overstimulated. Development requires proper nutrition and rest, not excitement and movement.

Babies need to sleep most of the time and should be kept quiet. Cuddling and pampering them, holding them in your arms, sleeping in the mother's arms, bright lights, too much noise, loud talking, family visiting all day, baby-buggies, cars, toys hanging over their heads, waking them up to unnecessarily feed them etc. are causing the baby to become sick. It's not the germ! All the overstimulation robs the baby from energy until it is depleted and weak.

A baby when born should be in perfect health. We succeed in making it sick immediately and often thereafter. You wonder how? Overstimulation is the only cause of all so called baby diseases. Take away all the unnecessary stimulation and put the baby in the right conditions to develop mind and body, and be healthy. It's that simple. But yet again it's not that simple because the parent is the problem and often selfishness is interpreted as love of children. Love is often a selfish ambition.

When one truly loves their child, one would do what's best for that child so it can develop a healthy mind and body and continue to be in perfect health. Smothering the child and holding it all the time, attending the child all the time and overstimulation bring on disease and innervation.

Children do not need entertainment. When children are left alone, they discover themselves and become acquainted with themselves... that's the entertainment they really need. Teaching a child to be content on its own, teaching poise and self-control should be started at birth.

Children that are coddled, entertained all the time, spoiled and attended to, develop discontent. Habits of irritability, temper, and overeating form. The reason children are irritable is because they are pampered and have not been allowed to learn self-control. This discontent brings on toxemia.

Last week I went for a 3 mile walk on the beach and to my delight I saw a 4 year old boy playing, all by himself, no toys, just himself and his imagination. He was making warrior sounds and his arms were slaying a dragon maybe... I didn't ask. He was content and happy. He was discovering himself. He didn't need to be entertained.

When children come to school age, things get worse. School work, homework, exercise, examinations, competition of all kinds, peer pressure etc. are just a few examples of all kinds of excitement and overstimulation. I'm not stating that kids shouldn't learn and be active, but our kids are just overburdened and it drains them from energy. They become irritated and frustrated, they worry unnecessarily, they fear, they are frightened to fail, they are anxious. These emotions, especially fear and worry, are destructive beyond your imagination. I'm dead serious, with the emphasis on 'dead'.

Children are subject to so many unnecessary fears: fear of the dark, fear of the bogy-man, fear of punishment by the parents and at school, just to name a few. This constant fear is health-altering and life-changing, no doubt.

If that's not enough, school lunches are atrocious. The government is responsible for ruining the health of millions of young men and women, and teaching them the sick habit, promoting the good, old S.A.D. (Standard American Diet). Not only are the school lunches the cheapest, filthiest, nutrient-depleted, toxic pile of man-made garbage, but they are also forced upon our kids at a certain time of the day. Our kids are forced to eat when not hungry, promoting the appetite habit. Furthermore, they are forced to drink with their toxic meal. It's beyond sad!

During the school years, it doesn't stop with unnecessary emotional stress, overstimulation and toxic food. Kids are pressured into straightening their teeth (if they were healthy that wouldn't be necessary), tonsils and appendices must be removed, and vaccines and serums must be injected to immunize from disease (more about vaccines later). I hope you can understand now that all these measures are senseless fads, in fact they are disease building not disease solving. The cause of disease is toxemia. Health only can return when the cause is taken away so nature can cure.

Our children are dissatisfied and overstimulated, promoting disease. An independent spirit and pride will save this world.

Older children may reach out to tobacco, coffee, excessive sweets (candy, pastries etc.), and alcohol. Self-abuse begins early in many (and causes stomach problems). Adolescence comes with excessive partying and dancing, smoking, drinking, insomnia, sex and venereal disease, and lots of fear springing from all the possible consequences.

And then there is our TECHNOLOGY: T.V., computer, game boy, play station, X-box, and most of all the cell-phone which allows us to call, text limitlessly, face-time, skype, instagram, facebook, tweet, google, take pictures, play games, and so much more. Talk about overstimulation. Just observe kids and adults getting lost for hours and hours in this technology excitement and entertainment, constantly updating profiles, posting pictures, texting friends etc. It's a crazy business overstimulating all of our senses constantly, robbing each one of us from vital energy and surely contributing to sickness. Use it when necessary ONLY, not for entertainment. What happened to family time, time with friends, outdoor activities, or plain and simple rest and relaxation?

When I was growing up my family and I would sit around the dinner table every evening and consume relatively healthy foods, freshly prepared and nutritious. We also had a conversation and enjoyed our time together at the dinner table. I assume that today, with a single parent environment or with both parents working (often a necessity), and the kids involved in many activities, traditional dinner has ceased to exist for the most part. Cheap fast foods, deprived from essential nutrients and loaded with sugars, hydrogenated oils, salt etc. are the common meal at dinner time... a recipe for disaster. No wonder more than one third of our children are overweight or obese and plagued with sickness. It's even predicted that this is the first generation of children in our history that is not expected to outlive their parents.

Just as explained in Chapter 1 that we are most likely guilty of nutritional homicide, it should be a crime to allow children to make poor choices when it comes to health. Children should be compelled to obey. Discipline must be taught by respected parents. This type of discipline brings love, not fear. No child can thrive while living in a state of fear and anxiety in the home or school. Fear and love are antidotal. For example, man has been taught to fear God and at the same time love Him. Where the fear is real, the love is not. Love is the basis on which ethics are build, thus love founded on fear builds a foundation of bad ethics and morals, including all conventional lies of our civilization.

Parents are ill-equipped to be parents. They lack knowledge on health and on how to place the body and mind in the RIGHT conditions to promote health and wellbeing of their child. They need a USER MANUAL and I hope this book can be that user manual.

Parents WORRY all the time. Worry comes from their lack of knowledge. If parents would know about healthy nutrition and emotions and overstimulation etc. one would be in control. Being in control promotes inner peace and happiness, not stress and fear and worry.

Parents need to know about proper nutrition, clean food, clean water, and clean air, the importance of sunshine, the effects of emotions on health, and the effects of overstimulation and overindulgences on health. Parents need to teach their children healthy eating habits (or how to break bad eating habits), and teach them how to repose their mind, avoid excess play, control emotions and feelings, and teach them about self-pollution and toxemia. That's their responsibility.

With the knowledge you acquire in this book, parents can raise their children properly so they can achieve health and happiness in life. Parents need the skills to teach discipline and self-control to their child. Most of us are not even aware of many facts such as overstimulation causing all so called baby diseases.

I agree that you may have been misled by your uneducated doctor and the media and the government, and that you trusted them with your health and the health of your child. Learn and move forward. Now you know and now you can do something about it! Remember that it's NEVER too late. As long as you are breathing, every cell in your body will try to return to perfect health. It cannot do otherwise. So take the one and only cause of disease away and REGAIN CONTROL of your health, and teach others.

If you ignore this information and you DO nothing about it, you are guilty of child abuse. If you love your child, you should set them up for success and happiness in life, not for failure, disease and depression. Even if you don't love your child, they're still your responsibility.

As adults, we have much fear and anxiety in our lives also. The constant fear of being able to provide for our families, having a secure job, making enough money to make ends meet, our children's behavior and their fears, etc.

Worries at work are very common. However, work doesn't cause worry. A job well done is a delight and is character building. Ineffective work, a job that doesn't satisfy, a job carried out for the purpose of money and without pleasure, a job without responsibilities brings on dissatisfaction and worry, and therefore promotes disease. So the cause of worry is lack of control. One must understand personal habits and occupation and gain control, be productive and be satisfied with a job well done.

Gossip, envy, jealousy, grief, shock, anger, egotism, hate, jealousy etc.

are all emotions that when intense or prolonged have severe damaging effects on the body and mind of the individual. As explained in the previous chapter, investigate which emotions you are guilty of and pinpoint the stimuli that bring them on. This self-knowledge is required so you may utilize the skills to start controlling these excess emotions. Once one achieves control over their emotions, inner peace and happiness can be obtained.

10.3 Overindulgences

Similar to overstimulation, overindulgences refer to activities in excess of normal. We could use the term perversion in this context also since anything in excess of normal would be contrary to what nature's purpose would be.

Self-indulgence is abnormal selfish indulgence. Self-pity, selfishness and being inconsiderate to others, the use of stimulants (coffee, tobacco, beer, drugs etc.), consuming comfort foods, overeating, feasting, partying, overstimulation (excess video gaming, watching TV, texting and cellphone use, social media participation etc.), excess sex, all are destructive to mind and body.

Overwork is mostly destructive because of the dissatisfaction of the work rather than the physical exhaustion, but both contribute to toxemia.

Physical activity is important for health, but excess activity without proper rest and sleep is extremely destructive. Besides a negative energy balance and poor elimination of toxins, free radicals run galore and start a cascade of damage to vital cells.

Dissatisfactions and overworked emotions are heavily contributing to toxemia, the cause of all disease. Worry, fear, anger, grief, passion, temper, irritability, overjoy, egotism, pride, depression, envy, jealousy, dishonesty and lying, gossip, failure to meet appointments and obligations, taking advantage of misunderstanding, abusing confidence of others in us, taking advantage of friends and taking things for granted, all build disease. The emotions and feelings are inherent to the individual. The individual participating in gossip is the individual who pays the price and will suffer for gossiping. Some call it karma, I simply see it as self-destructive behavior.These excess emotions translate to destructive behavior: alcohol abuse, drugs, overeating, robbery, prostitution, criminal activity, murder etc. Some of these behaviors are punished by our legal system (robbery, murder, prostitution) while others are not (alcohol, overeating) and as long as food-drunkenness retains its prestige with the professions (prescribed by doctors) it will take more than statutes to enforce law and order. Funny because most of our laws are made while the lawmakers are drunk on food and tobacco.

The doctor, the surgeon, the psychologist, the psychiatrist, the laws and the law-makers perhaps relieve some effects but cures are based on causes. Jails, rehabilitation programs, prescription drugs have been proven NOT to work. Of course not: our wants are based on our subconscious needs; sentiment and ethics have nothing to do with it. The cause has not been addressed. Legislatures are quack doctors. Self-control is the only cure. To develop self-control, the need must be understood.

When these self-destructive emotions accumulate and express themselves over a long period of time, disease pops up but often also expresses itself in an emotional breakdown. For example, a murder or a suicide ends the physiological storm of emotions. Murder and suicide are committed by people with less consideration for others. As opposed to murder, suicide involves less self-love. You may think these people are crazy, or there is something wrong with them when they commit these crimes...but this could happen to anyone, including you. The only way to prevent these events is to take away the cause: overindulgences and lack of control over one's emotions.

The simplest way to remove and abandon your overindulgences is to live for service. Help others help themselves is what we must do.

The first step is to realize the above information as a simple truth, and start controlling that truth. Learn to control your feelings and emotions, and remove overstimulation and overindulgences. Focus on helping

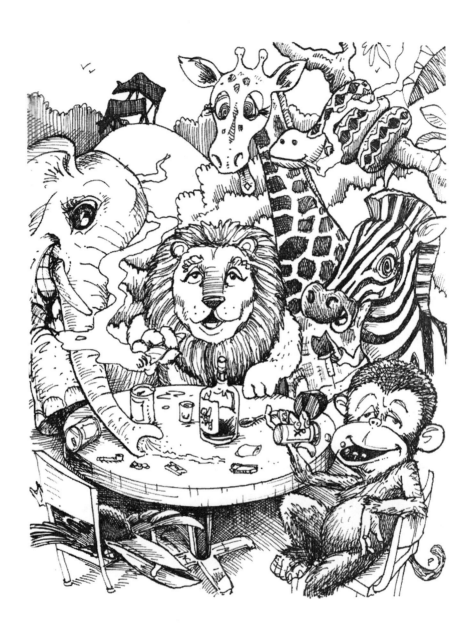

Illustration 17 – Party Animals

others and ban the self-destructive habits from your life. When (not if) you find inner peace and happiness, show others how to find it!

10.4 Key Points

Intense and prolonged overstimulation and overindulgences contribute to toxemia.

Perversions are functions or actions in antagonism with the harmony of nature. These actions have converted from their RIGHT use and purpose into a WRONG use and purpose. Man acquired a multitude of perversions due to his freedom to choose his response.

Overstimulation drains us of vital energy. Stimulants, overeating, competition, peer pressure, excess light, excess noise, excess play, excess sex, excess emotions contribute to sickness far more than one may assume.

Self-knowledge and skills are required to control emotions and control life. Health and happiness can only be achieved by taking away the cause of disease and dissatisfaction.

Overindulgences include acts of self-indulgence (self-pity, selfishness, use of stimulants, overeating, partying, overstimulation etc.) which are destructive to the individual. Overwork, excess exercise, excess emotions (as a result of self-indulgence) promote destructive behavior. This behavior cannot be cured by any so called doctor or psychiatrist or the law. Only taking away the cause of such behavior will cure. Self-control is the ONLY cure.

The simplest way to remove and abandon overindulgences is to live for service. Help others help themselves.

Chapter 11 – Exercise Controversy

Exercise and activity are vital to health. However, activity must follow rest and rest always must be followed by activity.

11.1 Exercise is Vital

Life is dependent on cell function and cell function is dependent on proper nutrition, assimilation, elimination, body temperature etc. This requires that all the cells of the body are in perpetual motion or movement. It's our circulation that stimulates and perfects all vital functions of our body. The blood carries all nutrients and oxygen and the lymphatic system carries fluids and wastes. Without activity, cell function is sluggish and impaired.

Exercise is the most important tonic of the body, strengthening and invigorating the entire bodily system. Exercise is far more than building muscle though; it is literally body-building. Every cell and fiber in the body is invigorated when exercising. The tone and quality of not only the muscles, but also the bones, the organs, the digestive system, elimination system and every single tissue in the body is invigorated.

Because exercise promotes circulation, it speeds up metabolism and therefore elimination. Activity assists in eliminating toxins and hastens the absorption of exudates and deposits.

Exercise thus promotes optimal health while lack of regular exercise promotes disease. Lack of exercise makes one weak and sluggish, metabolism slows down, cell functions are impaired, toxins build up, toxemia occurs and the disease process takes form.

While some people today have a sedentary job and lack exercise, others perform hard physical labor and are overworked. The sedentary ones are fat, bald, and fatigued while the overworked ones develop injuries. These injuries occur because the activities performed are repetitive and specialized, only exercising certain parts of the body while neglecting others. The sedentary person needs to incorporate regular whole body activities or exercise, while the manual laborer needs to incorporate exercises that counteract the one-sided tendencies.

It really doesn't need mentioning that animals in the wild and cavemen have plenty of activity hunting for their food and running away to avoid being another creature's meal. Everything is done by foot and hunger makes one hunt. Industrialization and commercialization made us sedentary. Even our pets are fed and they also became fat and lazy. The puppy is full of energy and wants to play around while the older dog is lazy, fat, and fatigued and can't be bothered.

Another concept that requires our understanding is the fact that well developed and formed muscles do not necessarily indicate strength. Bulk of muscle is by no means a reliable measure of strength, and far less one of health. Strength comes from within. Strength refers to one's vital, internal energy. This energy largely depends on clean food, clean air, clean water, plenty of sunshine, controlled emotions, balanced activity and rest, and absence of overstimulation and overindulgences. Without this vital energy, a well-formed and developed muscle lacks strength.

A simple analogy is that of a motor and fuel. One may have a bigger motor but without the fuel, not much will happen, the motor is useless. A smaller motor with fuel will accomplish much more. Keep in mind that a bigger motor has bigger potential, but also requires more fuel.

Without this vital energy, one cannot expect any type of development either. It's not exercise or activity that causes development, it's the internal vital energy that causes development. A newborn for example develops and grows much faster when sleeping more, since rest renews energy and activity uses energy. So exercise and activity only render occasion for development.

Overdevelopment is impossible because when exercise is in excess and carried beyond the point of usefulness, vital energy is depleted and exhaustion and atrophy ensue. Having said that, our organism always strives for perfection, so in order to obtain optimal health and strength, one must apply the rules and laws of nature.

In order to benefit from exercise (in regards to health) one must rest and sleep proportionately and live C.L.E.A.N. Fact remains that exercise is a destructive and exhaustive process, consuming vital energy and breaking down tissue. Repair and recuperation of energy take place during rest and sleep. Rest and sleep are constructive. Both activity and rest are vital to health and life.

Exercise, just like feeding, should not be in excess. In excess, exercise causes depletion of vital energy and consequently toxemia. Furthermore, exercise gives rise to more free radicals and therefore the consumption of even more antioxidants becomes crucial. We will talk more about top athletes later, but this explains why some of these top athletes suddenly drop dead or acquire cancer. The excess activity causes excess free radicals damaging the cells and promoting disease, including cancer. Toxemia is accelerated unless counteracted by high quantity, potent antioxidants. Top athletes only benefit from multiple workouts if these workouts are alternated with sufficient rest and sleep, and an adequate supply of antioxidants is consumed to neutralize the damaging effects of the free radicals. Top athletes need to live by the C.L.E.A.N. rules if they want to maintain good health and prevent disease.

We can conclude that we then must exercise daily if we desire health, strength, beauty and symmetry. These valuable commodities cannot be obtained without effort. Only useless stuff in life can be obtained without effort. That's why one should not be upset by the results one didn't get with the work one didn't do.

Exercise should address all body parts, thus involve the whole body. If asymmetries and injuries preexist, one should make efforts to counteract these with specific exercises.

Health thus includes an abundant amount of vital energy within the body combined with a well-formed, lean, muscular, symmetrical body on the outside, and a healthy mind of course.

Herbert M. Sheldon talks about 3 types of exercise:

Hygiene exercise is whole body activity to promote entire system circulation and therefore optimize cell function and health.

Educational exercise is the learning of new activities that involve coordination between the mind and body. When these activities are repeated enough, they become automatic, a habit. The mind is no longer involved and the muscles are trained to serve the mind. These activities increase efficiency and effectiveness, and consequently preserve energy.

Corrective exercises are exercises implemented to correct deformities, asymmetries and faulty postures.

11.2 The Controversy

Most physicians and health care professionals, including therapists, wrongly prescribe cardiovascular exercise to their patients/clients that are post-operative, obese or are suffering from fibromyalgia etc. The literature and exercise physiology books however tell them it's NOT the best choice!

Cardiovascular exercise such as walking, jogging, bicycling, swimming etc. at a low intensity for a longer period of time is a poor choice because this type of exercise has NO bearing with activities of daily living (ADL's). Cardiovascular exercise also demands too much energy from the client/patient. The post-operative patient, fibromyalgia patient or obese client has NO energy reserves and is unable to 'walk for 30 minutes' without depleting the body or without making the 'problem' worse or causing injury. On top of that, inflammation occurs with continuous exercise exceeding 20 minutes, caused by the constant friction between the muscles.

The type of exercise we need to prescribe is the type that most effectively increases energy production (ATP) in the tissues, thereby increasing oxygen levels and restoring full aerobic respiration of the cells. We are looking for the type of exercise that most effectively increases the number of mitochondria (oxygen factories) and nuclei in the muscles. That type of exercise is called: PRE or Progressive Resistive Exercise.

Yes, this type of strengthening exercise is far more effective than cardiovascular exercise for the post-operative patient or obese client. Don't believe it? Why don't you open that exercise physiology book again and learn that "for every increase in muscle tone there is a 40% increase in vascularization". This means that there's a substantial increase in the number of micro-circulation pathways and in the lumen of existing blood vessels. This vastly improves the circulation of oxygenated blood to the affected areas. In short, PRE is more effective in improving cardiovascular condition that cardiovascular exercise, there you have it!

Emphasis has always been in developing endurance in patients, but strength must ALWAYS precede endurance. If not, what's there to endure? A great example is the physical therapist dragging a patient with a cane or walker through the hallways of the hospital. What's the point? Should we not build strength first, and then when the patient has regained the strength and is able to actually walk, build endurance?

The 'Physiological law of Specificity of Exercise' states that "Performance of a task only builds limited strength in that task."

In Sports Medicine we always say: "Don't play to get into shape, get into shape to play". A football player does not just play football to get in shape for the new season. He does strength training, cardiovascular training, technical drills (throwing the ball, receiving the ball, tackling etc.), tactical training etc. Each facet or component of the game is trained.

What is PRE?

PRE is Progressive Resistive Exercise. PRE builds the largest number of mitochondria (energy production in your oxygen factories) and nuclei as a normal response to work.

PRE is a type of strengthening exercise with emphasis on strengthening muscles in short sets (anywhere from 7 to 10 repetitions per set) with a high resistance or intensity (70% of 1RM). 1RM is the weight with which we can execute 1 complete repetition, but are unable to complete the second one. We take large rest segments in between sets (2 to 5 minutes) to avoid draining energy reserves. The total duration is short to avoid inflammation. We only perform a few exercises (3 to 5 of them) but each one of them addresses multiple muscle groups.

In more depth:

The resistance or weight we use is pretty heavy, about 70% of 1RM. We will use our body weight and if necessary add some extra weight (dumb-bells or a gallon of water etc.). In short, we should be able to complete 7 to 10 repetitions, but not much more. If it's too easy to complete 10 repetitions or more, the weight or resistance needs to be increased. As muscles become stronger, resistance is gradually increased.

I recommend 3 sets for each of the 4 recommended exercises (we will discuss later which 4 exercises these are). Each set contains 7 to 10 repetitions. Start with 7 and gradually increase to 10 repetitions. If 10 repetitions become easy, increase the resistance. Make sure to take 2 to 5 minutes of rest in between EACH set. Deep (diaphragmatic) inhalation during the rest segments is recommended.

I suggest implementing 3 sessions per week initially, totaling about 120 minutes.

Now, what actual exercises do I suggest? The idea is to keep the total duration short while strengthening a maximal amount of muscles. So I personally looked into the exercises our astronauts perform while in space. NASA recognized that 70% of all leg and pelvic muscles PUSH, while 70% of all arm and torso muscles PULL, and came up with the following exercises for the astronauts:

Leg presses (such as a squat) address most of the muscles in the legs and pelvis, including gluteus muscles, hip flexors, hip abductors and hip adductors, quadriceps, hamstrings, calf muscles etc.

Pull-downs (or lat-pull) address most of the muscles in the arms, shoulder girdle and torso, including wrist flexors and extensors, biceps, triceps, latissimus dorsi, pectoral muscles, deltoid, trapezius, rhomboids etc.

Back extensions address the paraspinal muscles of the upper, mid and lower back.

Crunches address the abdominal muscles.

These 4 exercises address most muscles and muscle groups in the body and are highly effective.

11.3 Exercise Prescription

It's very simple... do what you like to do and incorporate activity in your daily schedule. It's not necessary to participate in an actual organized sport or go to the gym, but you can of course. You just need to move... that's all. You may play in the yard with the kids, go for a walk, or enjoy any outdoor activity... as long as you stimulate circulation. Ideally, you activate and use all body parts, not just the legs or the arms. This is your HYGIENE EXERCISE REGIMEN. That's all you need if you are in good health and want to stay in good health.

However, if you are in poor physical shape right now, you may need to select a more specific exercise program to regain normal physical condition. Most of us have poor form, poor strength and physical endurance so the above described PRE EXERCISE REGIMEN may be a great option to get started. Perform the PRE program 3 times per week and schedule a fun activity on the other days. Consider learning a new sport or fun activity (surf, paddle board, skate, spin etc.), or learn a dance and join some classes. This is EDUCATIONAL EXERCISE.

If you are obese you need to start losing weight (refer to chapter 12) and ease into an exercise regimen (PRE and non-weight bearing activities such as stationary biking or aquatic exercise) to prevent injury. If you suffer from any so called disease that supposedly causes your fatigue and muscle pains (chronic fatigue syndrome, fibromyalgia etc.), you need to start with corrective exercises and PRE, and prevent energy depletion and inflammation.

If you have poor posture, obvious asymmetries, strong and weak body parts, or other deformities you need to start with specific CORRECTIVE EXERCISES to regain balance and symmetry in the body. A knowledge-able Physical Therapist may be able to assist you in the right selection and execution of these specific corrective exercises.

You may employ any combination of hygiene, educational and correc-tive exercises. Of great benefit would be to incorporate diaphragmatic breathing as discussed in chapter 6.

As a general guideline, start with 120 – 200 minutes of exercise per week (about 20-30 minutes per day) and gradually increase up to 300 – 350 minutes per week (40-50 minutes per day). You may divide 40 minutes of exercise per day in two sessions of 20 minutes for example. Again, it's about movement and circulation. Remember that actively playing and running around in the yard with the kids or grand-kids or playing some ball counts as exercise, as well as a dance class.

The more you exercise or participate in physical activities, the better your circulation and the better cell function and health. However, the more exercise or activity the more rest and sleep one needs to repair and replenish energy reserves AND the more one needs to be aware of the extra free radical production.

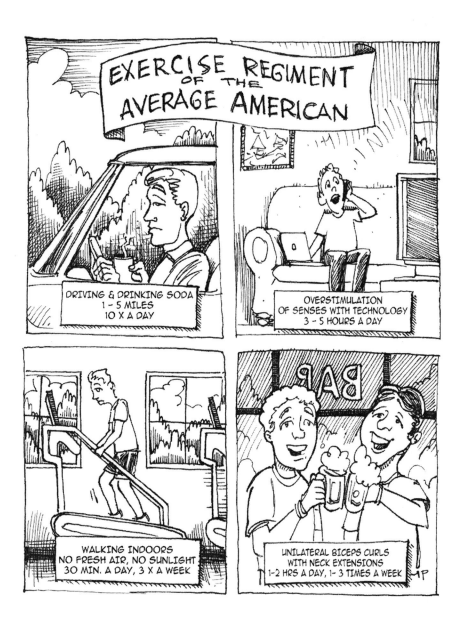

Illustration 18 – Exercise Regimen of the Average American

Make sure you alternate adequate exercise with adequate rest, and when you exercise regularly you should consume enough healthy foods and antioxidants to neutralize the extra free radicals and eliminate toxic by-products effectively.

11.4 Athletes Be Aware

Athletes train hard and workout in preparation for a competition. The high physical and mental demands of (usually) daily exercise expend huge amounts of energy and break down tissue, causing a cascade of free radicals and toxic by-products.

Athletes ONLY will benefit from this extreme type of exercise if adequate rest and sleep can repair the tissue and replenish vital energy. This constructive task can only be fulfilled if the RIGHT materials are available, meaning the right nutrients. Furthermore, excess amounts of antioxidants and phytonutrients are crucial to counteract the damaging effects of the excess amounts of free radicals produced as a result of intense exercise.

Every individual has his/her limits to how much energy he or she can spend. When one exercises too much and spends more energy that can be recuperated, exhaustion and injury occur.

Top athletes need to live C.L.E.A.N., if not they will pay a huge price at some point in their lives. Additionally, I recommend a potent anti-oxidant supplement such as liquid Vemma to 'supplement' their healthy, nutrient-rich, natural diet to assure neutralization of free radicals.

Top athletes: do not underestimate the importance of rest and sleep, especially for those of you who exercise much more than the average person. The more energy you spend, the more you need to repair and replenish... it's that simple.

How to improve your performance?

I'm not going to expand on training methodology and increasing VO2-max or increasing lactate tolerance etc. This knowledge is out there and the better coaches and trainers are able to apply these methodologies in their training sessions and maximize the performance of their athletes as a result.

However, there are a few things even top and Olympic coaches may not have considered or they just lack the knowledge or skill to implement them.

First of all, the individual has physical limits as to the development of body and muscles, and skills. I just assume that the capable coach knows how to maximize these. That's the motor. The coach optimizes the motor, the machine. A better and bigger motor will have more capabilities and possibly a better performance. But the fuel needs to be there to run that motor. Not just quantity of fuel, but quality. The fuel of the motor is like the vital energy of the body... the more the better, but the quality also will dictate the performance. It's not just good and clean food and nutrition that makes up vital energy, but also clean air, clean water, sunshine, rest and sleep, controlled emotions, healthy mind, absence of overstimulation and overindulgences etc. If you want to improve the quantity and quality of the fuel, teach the athlete on how to live C.L.E.A.N.

A great illustration of this effect would be the one of lactic acid production. For the laymen in sports physiology, I'll try to simplify things. As we exercise or compete at high intensity, our muscle tissue produces lactic acid. This lactic acid is removed from the muscle tissue and makes its way to the blood. The acid lowers the pH of the blood and in an attempt to maintain homeostasis (balanced pH of 7.35 – 7.45), the blood needs to buffer or neutralize this acidity by using alkalizing minerals (calcium, magnesium, potassium etc.).

As the intense activity continues, more lactic acid is produced and more needs to be buffered until the production exceeds the elimination of acid. That's when the body shuts down to protect the organism and preserve life. This is the moment the athlete slows down and can no longer continue to perform at the previous intensity.

Now, the coach and athlete can train both the aerobic capacity of the athlete in order to minimize acid production and simultaneously train lactate tolerance. In other words, athletes train to reduce acid production and increase acid elimination in an effort to optimize athletic performance. All coaches can do that with their athletes, but there is a limit. Assuming all top athletes reached this limit, what else can we do to prolong the time when acid production exceeds acid elimination?

The answer: start off with a higher pH to begin with! In other words, if the athlete is alkaline it will take more acid to reach the lactic acid threshold. Does that make sense?

It's like if we would clone Michael Phleps, and keep all variables the same, except one. Michael Phelps #1 continues his current nutritional regimen and the other Michael Phelps #2 starts to live C.L.E.A.N. and alkalizes his body. What will happen?

1. Michael Phelps #2 will have a higher, more alkaline starting pH and therefore the lactic acid threshold will be higher.

2. Michael Phelps #2 will have more alkalizing minerals in his body, due to his natural diet. More bio-available alkalizing minerals increase the effectiveness of the buffer capacity of the blood, resulting in faster and more effective elimination also resulting in a higher lactic acid threshold.

Michael Phelps #2 will kick Michael Phelps #1's butt pretty significantly!

So athletes: understand that more exercise may improve physical performance given enough rest so that physical adaptations are made (better and bigger motor), but without enough quality fuel that work would be in vain. Also note that there is a limit on how big and good your motor will be; however there is no limit on the amount and quality of fuel you drive that motor with.

11.5 Key Points

Exercise is vital for cell function and optimal health. Exercise doesn't necessarily mean one has to go to a gym or play organized sports. Exercise means movement and movement promotes circulation which in turn promotes cell function and vitality.

Hygiene Exercise refers to daily activities involving all body parts to stimulate whole system circulation. This type of activity is sufficient for the healthy person.

Educational Exercise is referred to as learning a new exercise or activity. Both the mind and body are involved in the learning process. Once mastered, the activity becomes effective and efficient and the mind no longer participates.

People in less than optimal health should start with specific exercises to restore normal physical condition. In most cases, I would suggest the PRE Exercise Regimen to improve strength, and learn a new, fun activity. Gradually progress and exercise 20-40 minutes per day.

If one exhibits a deformity, asymmetries, or a faulty posture then corrective exercises are indicated. These exercises are designed to counteract the imbalances and deformities in order to regain normal posture and symmetry.

Exercise expends energy and is destructive. Therefore exercise needs to be compensated for with adequate rest and sleep, which is constructive by repairing tissue and replenishing the body with vital energy.

Too much exercise with inadequate rest or less than optimal nutrition results in energy depletion, impaired elimination and toxemia.

Exercise results in extra production of free radicals that need to be neutralized with extra antioxidants.

Athletes often only focus on improving body physics (motor) while neglecting the quantity and quality of their vital energy which is the driving force of the body (fuel for the motor). Living C.L.E.A.N. will guarantee improved physical performance.

Chapter 12 – Sensible Weight Loss

Attention: This chapter is loaded with interesting info and insight, exposes the flaws of common popular diets and weight loss programs, and shares the keys to effective and lasting weight loss. However, the reader who is NOT overweight or obese can skip this 'obese' chapter if he or she wishes to.

Obesity is nothing NEW. The Venus of Willendorf, also known as the women of Willendorf, is a limestone statue of a female body estimated to have been carved around 23,000 B.C. The Venus represents an idealization of the female figure (refer to next page).

In Medicine, obesity was regarded as a disease since the 1700's. Yet, even now it is not fully recognized as a disease even by some members of the medical profession.

Currently, obesity is not just a disease anymore. We truly have an OBESITY **EPIDEMIC**, and that is NEW!

TODAY, it's a bitter irony that as developing countries continue their efforts to reduce hunger, some are also facing the opposing problem of obesity.

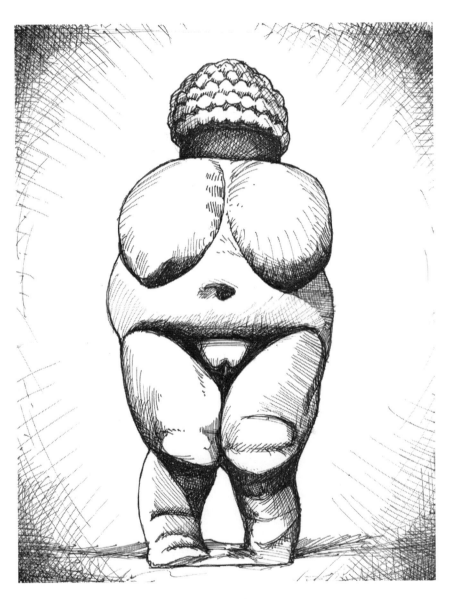

Illustration 19 – The Venus of Willendorf

Obesity carries a higher incidence of chronic illness including diabetes, heart disease and cancer. And while some of the poor are becoming plumper, they are not necessarily better fed. Obesity often masks underlying deficiencies in vitamins and minerals.

"We believe obesity is a significant problem that needs to be dealt with, along with the problem of the underfed," says Prakash Shetty, Chief of the Food & Agriculture Organization of the United Nations' (FAO) Nutrition Planning, Assessment and Evaluation service.

Just a few years ago, such a statement was rare. Experts hesitated to draw attention to obesity when so many lives were crippled by hunger; and out of a total of 815 million hungry people around the world almost 780 million are in developing countries. But startling data released a few years ago by the Worldwatch Institute challenged conventional wisdom. For the first time, the number of overweight individuals worldwide rivals those who are underweight. And sadly, developing nations have joined the ranks of countries encumbered by obesity.

A United Nations' study found obesity in all developing regions, and growing rapidly even in countries where hunger exists. In China, the number of overweight people jumped from less than 10 percent to 15 percent in just three years. In Brazil and Columbia, the figure hovers around 40 percent, a level comparable to a number of European countries. Even sub-Saharan Africa, where most of the world's hungry live, is seeing an increase in obesity, especially among urban women. In all regions, obesity seems to grow as income increases.

The existence of obesity in the developing world is not a surprise to FAO. "We already knew that the world produced enough food to feed everyone," remarks Barbara Burlingame, Senior Officer in FAO's Nutrition Impact Assessment and Evaluation Group. "Unfortunately, food doesn't always get to the people who need it most." Hunger is one result. Obesity is another."

In addition, practically all of the hungry and many of the overweight are weakened by a third type of malnutrition: a lack of vitamins and minerals referred to as micronutrient deficiency.

"The thinking used to be that if people get enough energy in their diets, the micronutrients will take care of themselves," says Dr. Burlingame. "But increasingly people are eating larger quantities of cheap food that fill the stomach but still leave the body without those micronutrients."

Though data on obesity in the developing world is limited, preliminary studies indicate that some of the same nutrient deficiencies in the underfed also afflict the overfed.

FAO maintains that a sound approach to nutrition must focus on quality as well as quantity. "One of our most important roles is to promote a diverse diet including traditional foods, which are generally balanced and high in nutrition," says Dr. Shetty.

The American society has become 'obesogenic,' characterized by an environment that promotes increased food intake, non-healthful foods, and physical inactivity. Obesity has become the 'disease of diseases' with far-reaching pathophysiology and co-morbidities. Even the AMA (American Medical Association) has now characterized obesity as a disease.

Even though the facts and statistics are conclusive, there continues to be a lack of understanding and education in medical schools.

Physical Attractiveness

A myriad of research also supports the importance of physical attractiveness. 'Looking good' is an indicator of the teacher's judgment of student intelligence and an indicator of the juror's judgment in simulated trials. Physical attractiveness also predicts job success and compensation levels. If you are overweight, the likelihood of being hired, getting a raise or a promotion is definitely lower.

Attractive people experience greater professional and personal success. Studies also indicate the existence of more negative attitudes towards the obese, even seen in young children, and that the obese are less likely to get help or favors.

12.1 Obesity: Terminology & Facts

Overweight is defined as the excess amount of <u>body weight</u>, including fat, muscle, bone and water. Someone is considered overweight if their Body Mass Index (BMI) exceeds 25.

Obesity is defined as an excess amount of <u>body fat</u> (BMI > 30). The terms overweight and obese are used interchangeably.

BMI (Body Mass Index) is a measure of an adult's weight in relation to his or her height, specifically the adult's weight in kilograms divided by the square of his or her height in meters. However, BMI is a very crude and inaccurate measurement tool. Athletes for example can have a high BMI but are usually not obese!

Another definition of obesity is the excessive accumulation of stored energy in the form of body fat. The reason for this excess storage is the fact that our survival instinct has become extinct. Our body has a stronger resistance against weight loss than defense against weight gain. Due to the constant food supply in western countries, we are limited today by our conscious cessation of eating, not by our food supply running out. Also, there's no need for physical activity since we don't have to go hunt down our food anymore. Food consumption exceeds resting energy expenditure, indicating the need for increased activity.

Waist-Hip Ratio (WHR)

The WHR is a predictor of abdominal fat. WHR is the waist circumference (in cm) divided by the hip circumference (in cm). Men are considered at risk when WHR > 1.0, and women when WHR > 0.85. The WHR correlates best with increased risk for cardiovascular disease.

How to measure WHR?

For accuracy and consistency always measure at the exact same level. You can achieve this by measuring the distance from the floor to the point of hip or waist measurement and record this distance as to assure accuracy with each consecutive measurement. The point of measurement for the waist is at the midpoint between the lower border of the ribcage and the upper border of the pelvis (hip-bone). The point of measurement for the hip is at the level of the hip-joint, palpable on the outer thigh.

Some more Obesity Facts

1. Excess weight is the #1 nutrition problem today.

2. Of the 10 leading causes of death in the U.S., being over-weight is a risk factor for half of them.

3. An estimated 40-55% of adult Americans and 20-30% of children are overweight.

4. Obesity is not just a cosmetic problem, but a serious health hazard.

5. Americans spend over $40 billion/year on weight loss treatments (that don't work).

6. The cost to society exceeds $100 billion/year.

Health Risks associated with obesity

Cancers & obesity: the association is unclear (not to me and the readers of this book though), but statistics show a definite link. There's an increased risk in post-menopausal women for breast and endome-trial cancers, and prostate cancer for men. Over 50% of breast cancer is diagnosed in obese women and the mortality rate is 1.5 times greater for some cancers in overweight women. Also, high-fat and low-fiber diets are indirectly related to colon cancers.

Diabetes: 80% of people with type 2 diabetes are obese. Losing as few as 10 pounds can reduce the risk of type 2 diabetes by 30%. Reducing body weight by 5% also significantly improves blood sugar levels and can improve insulin sensitivity.

Gallbladder disease: an increase in body weight drastically increases the incidence of symptomatic gallstones. Middle-aged women who are 40% overweight have a 33% greater chance of having gallstones.

Heart disease: The American Heart Association (AHA) classified obesity as a major risk factor for heart disease and stroke. Over 70% of diagnosed cases are related to obesity. A weight gain of 20 pounds or more doubles the risk of heart disease! A weight reduction of 5 to 10% increases HDL levels ('good' cholesterol) and reduces LDL ('bad' cholesterol) and triglycerides.

Hypertension: Obesity and being overweight are established risk factors for hypertension, and hypertension is approximately twice as prevalent in the obese versus the non-obese. Losing just a few pounds can lower your blood pressure.

Respiratory problems: Sleep apnea is linked to obesity and losing 10 to 15% of body weight can cure sleep apnea.

Psychological & social effects: Obesity can lead to emotional suffering, discrimination at work and social settings. Rejection, shame, and depression are common. As we discussed before, the American society equates thinness with attractiveness and therefore makes overweight people feel unattractive.

Death: according to the Framingham Heart Study there is a 1% increase in risk of death in the next 26 years for every pound of weight gain from age 30-42; and a 2% increase in each pound for ages 50-62. The study also indicated that weight loss reverses disease and the risk factors.

Note that the average American gained 1 to 5 pounds each year over the last 1-2 decades.

In light of this book, we can simply state that when one is overweight or obese (a symptom), toxemia has occurred. It then makes sense that this being overweight or obese shows up alongside a variety of other symptoms or so called diseases that are also caused by toxemia.

Western medicine tries to chase symptoms and study pathology, while there is NO pathology, just symptoms. Symptoms continue to evolve unless the cause is taken away. The above so called risk factors are yet again symptoms that occur as a result of the toxemia.

Note

Obesity has increased by over 50% over the last decade. Industrialization and commercialization have caused the mass production of processed, synthetic foods, loaded with colorings, preservatives, toxins and chemicals, hormones, antibiotics and carcinogens. Furthermore, these foods are deprived of essential nutrients and micronutrients!

Currently, there's virtually NO consumer education and prevention in place. The majority of insurance companies do NOT yet reimburse for the treatment of obesity itself (just for its related symptoms). The food industry spends billions of dollars yearly on advertising and almost nothing is spend on promoting healthy eating habits!

National consumption averages

The average American male consumes 2,800 cal/day and the average American female 1,800 cal/day. A study on dietary recall indicates that the average person estimates that they consume 30-40% less than they actually do!

Trends

Some of the trends below I shared already with you in chapter 1, but another quick review won't hurt anyone.

A decrease in consumption of foods high in fat is noted because people wrongly assume that fat makes you fat. BUT there has also been an increase in the consumption of foods with added fat such as fried foods and butter.

An increase in the consumption of fruit and vegetables is also noted.

WOW, you may think...but hold on: 18% of all vegetables are potatoes in French fries!

Cheese consumption increased by 250% due to the increase in pizza and cheeseburger consumption.

According to a UNC-study, the calorie content of food has increased also. For example, the calorie content in soft drinks increased by 49, fries by 68, salty snacks by 93, hamburgers by 97, and Mexican food by 133.

Visits to restaurants increased by 200%, resulting in higher fat and sugar consumption.

Standard American Diet: S.A.D.

We discussed the <u>S</u>tandard <u>A</u>merican <u>D</u>iet (SAD) earlier in this book, but it's beneficial to explain it again in another context. I state "American "diet because I live in America, but this holds true for almost the entire world.

Our genetics have not changed BUT more and more diseases currently exist (including obesity) and affect more and more people worldwide, including our children. Why is that? I will answer that question, but first you need to KNOW the following about OUR BODY:

1. Our body is the **MOST COMPLEX** piece of machinery on planet earth! We can build and control a nuclear plant, send a rocket ship into space and put a man on the moon; however we are far from figuring out the human body and its workings, and conventional medicine has no answers to any of our so called diseases.

2. Our body **CAN HEAL ITSELF**, but it needs to be in **BAL-ANCE** and **PUT IN THE RIGHT CONDITIONS** in order to do that. Our body is only in balance when all bodily systems and cells function optimally and in synergy.

3. Our body continuously **REBUILDS & RENEWS** itself. All cells in our body replace themselves, some daily, some monthly, some every 90 days etc. In other words, every few months we are a totally 'new' person and that – of course - is just physically speaking.

4. In order for our body to rebuild and renew itself, and be in perfect balance, we need to provide our body with the right tools or **ESSENTIAL NUTRIENTS** to do so. If you drive a BMW and continue to replace parts with second hand parts or parts from other brands such as Mercedes or Toyota, your BMW will eventually encounter some mechanical and functional problems, and will not be a 'real' BMW anymore. It will be a MUTATION! Translated to health, it will be a degenerative disease or CANCER. Another great analogy is the compatibility issues of different brands of technical devices such as computers.

5. The essential nutrients our body needs to rebuild, renew and balance itself are nutrients our body recognizes; these nutrients are the nutrients from **MOTHER NATURE** (natural foods, whole foods, plants, herbs, grasses, fruits and vegetables). Our body is able to assimilate and utilize these nutrients. Synthetic, processed foods are not recognized by our body and our body has major difficulties breaking these foods down in usable nutrients. It requires excessive amounts of calcium, potassium, enzymes, vitamins and minerals. In many cases, our body lacks these nutrients and is unable to break down these unnatural foods, and is consequently forced to store them.

6. Our body's health depends on the health of our cells. Every cell in our body (I believe there are about 70 trillion) has about 10,000 receptors on its outer membrane. The RNA or messenger of each cell 'tells' the receptors continuously what the cell needs to function optimally and rebuild or renew itself. The receptors will 'stick out their neck' and scan the environment (extracellular fluid) to

look for these necessary nutrients. Our S.A.D (Standard American Diet) does NOT provide our body with these essential nutrients and therefore the cells have to settle for less (synthetic, 2nd hand parts). As a result, cells lose their ability to function properly and optimally, organs are affected, disease takes over, and degeneration and mutation occur. We fall apart. Luckily we have prescription drugs to provide a band aid and keep things together... ha-ha!

7. Conclusion: We have to provide our body with the ESSENTIAL NUTRIENTS it needs to function optimally and stay in balance.

So, let's answer this question: How come we have to cope with more and more so called disease, including obesity?

First, the world population has grown out of proportion and there is not enough food from nature (whole foods) available to feed every mouth. Industrialization and commercialization have caused the mass production of synthetic and processed foods.

These man-made foods contain harmful preservatives, colorings and toxins which are foreign to the body and may cause disease, including but certainly not limited to allergies, immune-diseases, degenerative disease, cancers and more.

At the same time, these synthetic, processed foods do NOT contain adequate nutritional value. In other words, our body does NOT get the nutrients it needs to function properly and renew itself. Our body has to continuously utilize useful nutrients like vitamins, minerals and enzymes to neutralize the harmful toxins we ingest.

Next, as we lack essential nutrients and elimination suffers, toxemia starts and metabolism slows down. Every cell function becomes slow and sluggish, and ineffective. The body stores fat instead of breaking it down. It puts less vital tasks to the side, hopefully to be dealt with later.

12.2 Obesity: Causes & Treatment

Nature or nurture?

Studies show that 80% of children born to two obese parents will become obese; only 14% of children born to normal-weight parents become obese. Studies on adopted children show that genetics account for only 33% of a child's weight. So, we can use our GENETICS as a lame excuse of being overweight or being unable to lose weight. BUT the above numbers also indicate that we can CONTROL our weight at least 66%, right? That seems more than enough control if we just want to lose 5, 10, 20 or even 40% of our body weight.

What is it that we CAN CONTROL then? Lifestyle factors such as physical activity and eating habits. A slow metabolism can be partially controlled by our genetics, but you will learn later how we easily can speed-up our metabolism through some healthy practices!

So is the statement: "You are what you eat" true? Well, basically it is, but remember that other factors such as clean water, clean air, adequate sunshine, rest and sleep etc. also play a role in correcting toxemia and obtaining an optimal body composition.

"Move it or lose it"

According the Centers of Disease Control (CDC), 37% of obese people don't exercise. A sedentary individual may begin to gain weight on as few as 1800 calories. Regular exercise burns calories and builds lean muscle mass, which in turn burns more calories. Some top athletes may even burn up to 5,000 calories/day. Lack of activity can certainly contribute to obesity.

Fast Food

Fast food contains more calories and fat, and people consume more than needed. Usually, lower calorie items are available at these fast-food places, but most people don't order them. The typical fast food meal averages 700-1200 calories. "Supersizing" with fries and soda seems like a bargain but comes with a huge caloric price. For example, a small order of fries contains 210 calories and 10 grams of fat while a supersized order has an astonishing 540 calories and 26 grams of fat. A small soda has 150 calories versus the whopping 310 calories in a 32-ounce one!

Fast food is also consumed... too fast. Researchers have shown that the best way to moderate how much you eat is to eat slower, relax, enjoy your food and focus on your meal. We will expand on this topic in our Behavior Modification section of this book.

Smokers

Smokers gain up to 10 pounds after quitting. However, most return to normal weight after 1 year. The reason for the initial weight gain is the intake of extra calories within the first months after quitting, with a peak at 6 months. After people quit smoking they commonly 'substitute' their cigarette for food.

Also, nicotine may increase metabolic rate. So, when people stop smoking their metabolism slows down a little bit, possibly contributing to the initial weight gain.

Women

According to the American Journal of Clinical Nutrition, the earlier a girl reaches puberty and has her first menses, the heavier she's apt to be as an adult. In a study, 26% of girls who matured early were obese by age 30, compared to only 15% of girls who started their periods later in life.

After pregnancy, most women gain 5 pounds or more, and many of them never lose that extra weight, especially if they gained more than 35 pounds during pregnancy. Many women lose 10 pounds immediately following delivery, and another 5 pounds in the first month or two after delivery. The rest of the weight usually continues to drop slowly over the next 6 to 12 months, depending on caloric intake, activity level and whether or not the mother is breastfeeding.

Sleep & weight

Less sleep equals more weight! An extensive study showed that people who sleep less than 7 hours are significantly more obese. Those of us who sleep less than 6 hours per day have a 27% increased rate of obesity and those who sleep only 5 hours have a 73% increased rate.

Children who sleep less than 10 hours per day have a 3.5 times greater incidence of obesity compared to children who sleep 12 hours per day. Sleep deprivation at 30 months can predict obesity at the age of 6.

People who work night shifts average 42 minutes less sleep per 24-hour period.

How does that work then?

Well, less sleep results in less growth hormone activity. Growth hormone is responsible for recuperation, regeneration, renewing and rebuilding processes within our body during sleep.

Less sleep also increases cortisol, insulin and ghrelin levels, while decreasing leptin. Ghrelin is a hormone, produced by the stomach and pancreas, which stimulates hunger. Leptin is a protein hormone, mainly produced by white adipose tissue (fat), which controls appetite and satiety (feeling of being full).

Less sleep also causes increased daytime fatigue, resulting in less physical activity or exercise.

It's generally accepted for adults to sleep 8 hours per day, with a minimum of 7 hours. An extra 30 minutes per day can reduce body weight. I recommend to rest and sleep enough as to restore expended energy and assure a positive energy balance.

From our newly acquired knowledge we can state that lack of rest and sleep causes an energy deficit which then slows down metabolism and elimination processes. Toxemia starts and obesity and other symptoms may appear.

Hormone imbalances

Other common causes are hormone imbalances, in both men and women. In women, this can be caused by menopause and/or by surgical interventions such as a hysterectomy.

The most obvious and common cause of obesity

Most people consume excess calories. Calorie intake exceeds energy expenditure. Often, people are unable to control portion size. People eat larger portions because our processed foods do NOT contain the essential nutrients our body needs, and therefore our body continues to ask for more food by increasing the 'hungry feeling'.

Most people consume mostly acid-forming foods. Acid-forming foods deplete our body from alkalizing minerals such as calcium and potassium, and slow down metabolism. A slow metabolism results in the storage of fat and toxins.

Most people lack physical activity and many people are taking prescription drugs that make one gain weight.

Treatment of Obesity

Surgical treatment options

The ultimate biological basis of severe obesity is still unknown according to Western medicine (but we already know it's toxemia) and therefore specific therapy for the severe obese is not yet available. Severe obesity is accompanied by a reduction in life expectancy (duh).

In 1978, the National Institutes of Health (NIH) formed a consensus on surgery for severe obesity and considered primarily intestinal (jejunoileal) bypass, which exerts its weight loss effects through poor absorption, decreased food intake, and possible other mechanisms. This surgery seemed effective, but came with serious complications! During the next 2 decades, other surgical procedures developed.

Bariatric surgery provides substantial weight loss and ameliorates co-morbid conditions, including sleep apnea, hypoventilation, glucose intolerance, diabetes, hypertension, and serum lipid abnormalities. It possibly prevents end-stage organ damage as seen in renal disease, stroke, heart attack and heart failure; and may improve mood and other aspects of psychosocial functioning.

Major types of surgery for the severely obese include vertical-band gastroplasty, Roux-en-Y gastric bypass and biliopancreatic bypass. However, it's not the intention of this book to expand on the surgical interventions for the severely obese.

What I like to point out is the many risks involved with these type of surgeries. Why? Well, many people who are obese (but not severe enough to have surgery), will opt for surgery because they ASSUME it's the easy way out!

The immediate mortality rate is very low; however morbidity in the early postoperative period is as high as 10%. WOW, 1 out of 10 people die? Almost unbelievable! This high morbidity rate is due to wound infections, dehiscence (a previously closed wound that reopens), leaks from the staple line breakdown, stomal stenosis (narrowing of the stomach), marginal ulcers, various pulmonary problems, and DVT (deep venous thrombosis, or simply a blood clot).

In the later post-operative period other problems may arise such as pouch and distal esophageal dilation, persistent vomiting, cholecystitis (infection of the gallbladder), and failure to lose weight or keep the weight off.

Long-term complications such as micronutrient deficiencies are also common, especially B12, folate and iron.

"Gastric dumping syndrome" is another possible complication. This happens when the lower end of the small intestine expands too quickly due to the presence of hyper-osmolar food from the stomach. Symptoms include nausea, vomiting, bloating, cramping, diarrhea, dizziness, fatigue, weakness, sweating, and dizziness.

Mortality and morbidity rates are higher with reoperation. In other words, it's key to keep the weight off after the first surgery (if you survive).

And then there are some quality of life considerations. Not only will there be reorientation and adjustment to the side-effects of the surgery, but one has to also consider the effects of a changed body image. Euphoria can be seen in the early postoperative period; and some patients experience significant late postoperative depression.

Surgery is ONLY recommended if the body weight is in excess of over 100 pounds (BMI: 35-40+), if co-morbidities threaten the patient's life, AND ONLY if ALL OTHER conservative measures failed!

Common Non-surgical treatment options

Very Low Calorie Diets (VLCD) have great success with significant weight reduction (for example 40 pounds in 12 weeks), but if not combined with behavior modification participants regain their weight within 1 year. Many of these VLCD's are liquid diets and calories are restricted to 800 cal/day, which is very unhealthy! These diets are unsafe and unnecessary since they show no better results than low calorie diets (LCD).

Behavior Modification is a therapeutic approach based on the assumption that habitual eating and physical activity behaviors must be relearned to promote long-term weight change. We will discuss behavior modification techniques later in this book.

Exercise and physical activity have limited effect on initial weight loss, but are vital to lasting results and maintaining an optimal body composition. We learned about the exercise controversy and effective exercise prescription earlier in this book.

Drug therapy – Remember to check the prescription and Over-The-Counter (OTC) medications you are taking, and have your doctor substitute the drugs that cause weight gain. Even better, flush them all down the drain and learn how to regain your health and resolve your medical problems. In other words, it would be better if you just discontinued your medications and replaced them with more effective, natural alternatives that don't have a side-effect profile...

Back to drug therapy for weight loss. The common goal of drug therapy is to promote a negative energy balance. The pharmacological mechanisms' focus is on:

1. Reducing energy intake: reduce hunger, increase satiety, reduce absorption, and reduce fat or carbohydrate preference,

2. Increasing energy expenditure by increasing metabolic rate, increasing thermogenesis and stimulate activity (fidgeting, exercise),

3. Increasing fat oxidation.

Contraindications to drug therapy include pregnancy and breastfeeding (of course), unstable cardiac disease, valve disease and pulmonary disease, uncontrolled hypertension, severe systemic illness (rheumatoid arthritis, lupus, congestive heart failure, uncontrolled diabetes, kidney or liver disease etc.), unstable psychiatric history (anorexia), and incompatible medications (MAO's, migraine drugs and adrenergic agents).

The following is a brief history of weight loss agents:

1890: Thyroid extract
Problem: catabolic effect on heart and bones.
1930: Dinitrophenol.
Problem: neuropathy and cataracts.
1937: Amphetamines
Problem: addiction.

1967: 'rainbow' pills (amphetamine, digitalis, diuretics)
Problem: deaths.
1971: Aminorex
Problem: pulmonary hypertension.
1978: VLCD (collagen based)
Problem: deaths.
1997: Fenflramine/phentermine ('Fen-Phen')
Problem: primary pulmonary hypertension (PPH) and vascular insufficiency.

Current weight loss agents:

Adrenergic agents:

Adrenergic agents increase the neurotransmitter concentration in the hypothalamus (Norepinephrine).

Brand names:

DEA schedule III:
Bontril (benzphetamine, phendimetrazine).
DEA schedule IV:
Fastin, Adipex-P, Tenuate
(diethylpropion, phentermine).

Phentermine is the most commonly prescribed appetite suppressant and the HCl-form was FDA-approved in 1973. According to the literature, Phentermine is the most effective agent BUT was NEVER tested against other agents. Weight loss with Phentermine continues for 20 weeks, but the FDA limits the use of Phentermine to 12 weeks.

Serotonin agents:

These agents alter energy intake, energy expenditure, adipose stores and substrate utilization.

Brand names:
DEA schedule IV: D-fenfluramine – withdrawn in 1997.

Fluoxetine, Sertraline.

Anti-absorption agents:

Orlistat (Xenical) was FDA-approved in 1998, but is NOT very effective (<5%) and has many GI side-effects!

Off-label pharmaceuticals:

Metformin (Glucophage) is approved for Type 2 diabetes and reduces insulin resistance. Some studies report an 8kg weight loss in 6 months.

SSRI's only have shown short-term weight loss results. Participants regain weight within 1 year.

Meridia (Sibutramine) is a combined serotonin and adrenergic reuptake inhibitor. Meridia has been FDA-approved since 1997 for long-term use. Several studies show effectiveness up to 16 weeks with 6 to 10% weight loss in 1 year. However, results are very dose dependant.

Phen-pro (by Michael Anchors, MD) is a combination of Phentermine and Prozac. Phen-pro increases the activity of Norepinephrine and serotonin with a complex interaction in the hypothalamus to help reduce hunger and increase satiety (the feeling of being full). Phen-pro is proven better than SSRI's or Phentermine alone. BUT NO long-term benefits were ever reported and Dr. Anchors recommended plenty of water, food pyramid guidelines, and aerobic exercise along with his Phen-pro prescription. Is that maybe why participants achieved short-term weight loss? Of course!

Bottom-line: drugs are poisons and ALWAYS cause adverse reactions and impaired health, plus the results as shown above are very poor to state the least.

Supplement Ingredients:

Ephedra (MaHuang) has been proven effective as a weight loss agent for thousands of years. Ephedra has also been proven to be very effective in combination with caffeine. But again, the FDA showed an unprecedented abuse of power. Ridiculous reports by the FDA on the adverse effects and deaths by the use of ephedra surfaced from 1997 – 1999. I'm not in the mood to state AGAIN that the FDA is corrupt, but if you need proof, read "Ephedra – Challenging a 5,000 year legacy" by Dr. Jim Morris.

<u>Caffeine</u> is the world's most popular psychoactive substance. It's an energy booster (read depressant) and fat burner. Caffeine is a central nervous system and metabolic stimulant, and is used both recreationally and medically to reduce physical fatigue and restore mental alertness (short term effect only). Caffeine works for weight loss by speeding up metabolism, but it also binds to fat cells increasing their removal and inhibiting their storage. They recommend you take only minimal doses (100-200mg/day) depending on body weight and caffeine sensitivity. Although most people get their caffeine fix from coffee and sodas, the best way to ingest caffeine for fat-burning purposes is in the form of a natural caffeine supplement. Caffeine from natural sources does not cause the stereotypical caffeine high-followed-by-the-crash effect. The energy is long-lasting, so replace these chemical drinks with natural caffeine! My recommendation: NO caffeine.

<u>Panex Ginseng</u> has been proven to improve glucose tolerance but no studies show an effect on weight loss.

<u>Chromium & Chromium Picolinate</u> also improve glucose tolerance and aid in absorption but studies reveal mixed results. These supplements seem to work better in type 2 diabetes patients.

Clinical trials with <u>Cinnamon</u> show that it improves blood sugar levels and lipid levels in diabetics. Weight loss trials in vitro (rats) look promising and also the USDA is currently conducting studies.

In vitro studies on mice with <u>Conjugated Linoleic Acid (CLA)</u> show decreased fat deposition: a decrease in triglyceride absorption, increased fatty acid oxidation and increased fat cell death. However, no improvement in BMI is seen over a 12-week period in humans.

Pyruvate is the end-product of glucose metabolism. There is lack of research supporting the use of pyruvate as a weight loss agent, and it's very expensive.

Phenethylamine (PEA), also referred to as the "body's endogenous amphetamine", acts as a releasing agent of norepinephrine and dopamine. In the early 1980's, researcher Michael Liebowitz, author of the popular 1983 book 'The Chemistry of Love', remarked to reporters that "chocolate is loaded with PEA" and this evolved into the now eponymous "chocolate theory of love". The PEA in chocolate is believed to be a great mood enhancer and the chemical that mimics the brain chemistry of a person in love. For weight loss purposes, PEA elevates mood and suppresses appetite simultaneously. Some studies however point out that PEA is rapidly metabolized, preventing significant concentrations from reaching the brain and thus causing a psychoactive effect.

Cocoa extract provides all the benefits of chocolate without the added calories from sugar and fat. Active ingredients include PEA, caffeine, theobromine and tyramine which work synergistically to suppress appetite and stimulate fat-burning, while providing energy. While no research has been done yet, anecdotal evidence is extremely positive.

1,3- Dimethylamylamine (DMAA) is a derivative of geranium oil which resembles the body's own chemical messenger, epinephrine (adrenaline). Like adrenaline, DMAA is a powerful central nervous system (CNS) stimulant, increasing one's energy, clarity, brain function, and physical performance. For fat loss, DMAA works through a similar pathway as ephedrine, causing a rise in cAMP, the chemical messenger that triggers fat release. Because this natural supplement seems to work very well is small doses, the FDA may make DMAA illegal in the future. Like other stimulants, overdosing may cause damage to the internal organs. In reality, all stimulants are depressants.

Dietary fibers:

Psyllium husk (Plantago Psyllium) promotes satiety and cleanses the colon. There is an improvement in glucose and lipid levels, but no weight loss benefits have been shown.

Glucomannan (Radix Amorphophallus Konjac) inhibits glucose absorption in the gut and reduces fat absorption. Be aware of the incidence of GI obstruction.

Guar gum (Cyamopsis tetragonolobus) helps with satiety, but NO benefits were shown for weight loss versus placebo.

Hydroxycitric Acid (garcinia Cambogia) is a tropical fruit from India. This fruit inhibits mitochondrial citrate lyase, thereby decreasing fatty acid synthesis and Acetyl Co-A production. Clinical trials show mixed results.

7-keto DHEA is the type of DHEA that can't be converted into androgens or estrogens. It stimulates metabolism and thermogenesis, increases thyroid hormone production and lean body mass in women. I found no studies related to the benefits for weight loss.

5-HTP & L-tryptophan increase serotonin levels in the central nervous system (CNS). 5-HTP, an intermediary between serotonin and L-tryptophan, at a dose of 600mg/day decreases overall caloric intake while a dose of 900mg/day promotes satiety and reduces carbohydrate cravings. L-tryptophan was withdrawn in 1990 because of some concerns about Eosinophilia Myalgia (EMS) due to possible contamination. It's still used in infant formulas and OTC-drugs in Europe.

Yerba Mate (Ilex Paraguariensis) grows in the forests of South America, and is a traditional tonic and stimulant ('Mate' tea). Yerba mate consists of over 250 natural compounds including flavonoids (rutin, quercetin etc.) and alkaloids such as caffeine, theophylline, and theobromine which stimulate the CNS, act as diuretics, boost metabolism and suppress appetite. Yerba Mate is a good supplement to assist in weight loss and probably one of the most potent energy boosters (without the well-known crash effect afterwards).

Hoodia or Hoodia Gordonii is a plant that originally grows in the desert of South Africa. The plant takes 5 to 7 years to mature, at which age it contains the P57-molecule. P57 has strong appetite curbing properties. The research available shows no safety issues with the use of Hoodia. The Pfizer company pulled out an exclusive agreement to market Hoodia in 2003, and Phytopharm has now the rights to P57 in partnership with Unilever (Slim Fast). Just know that this patented and isolated P57-molecule is far less effective than the whole plant. Just make sure that the supplement you take contains authenticated South African Hoodia. In other words, the Hoodia is only effective if it comes from Africa and when the plant is picked at maturity!

hCG-injections

hCG stands for Human Choriogonadotropin, the hormone produced by pregnant women in the early stages of pregnancy. hCG is also used to treat infertility.

Research suggests that a small, daily injection (approximately 125 – 200 IU) results in a weight loss of 1 to 2 pounds per day, and often more, when accompanied by a VLCD (very low calorie diet) of approximately 500 calories.

That's a joke, isn't it? THAT'S THE ONLY REASON WHY THIS WORKS! It's NOT the hCG injection, it's the forced starvation that makes you lose weight. You can do that without an hCG injection. Oh, and men... be aware! If you take hCG injections and follow-up with a pregnancy test, your results may be positive. For those of you who test positive: CONGRATULATIONS!

I could explain Dr. Simeons' original hCG diet, but it would be useless! For those who want to know more about hCG injections, look it up online or read Kevin Trudeau's book; "The Weight Loss Cure They Don't Want You To Know About". Mr. Trudeau is right: You really don't want to know about hCG injections. Stupid and NOT SENSIBLE!

What is Metabolic Syndrome?

It's a term used to describe a combination of medical problems that increase the risk of heart disease and diabetes. People with metabolic syndrome have some or all of the following: high blood glucose, high blood pressure, abdominal obesity, low HDL, elevated cholesterol and high triglycerides. The root causes of metabolic syndrome are being obese or overweight, lack of physical activity, and possibly some genetic factors.

Common primary targets for risk reduction are smoking cessation, lowering LDL and blood pressure, and drug therapy to target individual risk factors. But if excess weight is the cause, wouldn't it be more SENSIBLE to just lose weight? I thought so! Along with some lifestyle changes, weight loss in the ANSWER. In the weight loss treatment of patients with metabolic syndrome, most health care professionals use the glycemic index (GI) as their guideline.

What is the Glycemic Index (GI)?

In 1981, Dr. David Jenkins - at the University of Toronto – developed dietary guidelines for diabetics based on an intrinsic system of 'exchanges'. Dr. Jenkins and his team charted how quickly various foods affect blood sugar levels, and assigned each of these foods a 'GI-number'. The GI-numbers are derived by comparing the rate of a given food's digestion to that of a reference food known to digest rapidly, such as pure glucose or white bread. The reference food is assigned a GI of 100 and the tested food is charted against this standard. Foods with a high GI (70 and above) are foods that break down quickly and cause a spike in blood sugar levels. Foods with a low GI (55 and below) break down more slowly and steadily, providing a sustained supply of energy.

Many popular diets and weight loss programs wrongly assume that foods which rapidly raise blood sugar levels are responsible for weight gain, and base their entire program on this misconception. They ignore the substantial amount of research that runs counter to their 'theory', and have taken a controversial nutritional concept out of context.

Diets composed of low GI-foods slow down the conversion into blood sugar and lower glucose levels and peaks. These diets also reduce the progression of type 2 diabetes by lowering insulin levels, and satisfy appetite without consuming extra calories. These diets are the new standard for managing diabetes in Canada, UK, France, Australia and New Zealand.

However, the American Diabetic Association (ADA) has not yet endorsed GI. The ADA raises questions about its practical importance since differences in rates of digestion do not warrant changing the diet for diabetics, and "what if different foods are eaten together at meals"? Good point! Furthermore, the ADA points out that fats have a low GI, including peanuts and chocolate; and that therefore a diet exclusively based on low GI puts the individual at risk for heart attack and stroke. Atkins is a good example of this.

Contrary to what most people and health care professionals believe, white bread and baked potatoes (low fiber, high milled content) raise blood sugar levels with both speed and magnitude, even worse than table sugar. Oats, rye and barley have a lower GI. Amylose and compact sugars such as vegetables, pasta, and oatmeal digest slower. Fructose (simple sugars in fruit) digests slow too since they are processed by the liver prior to entering the blood.

There are not enough clinical trials on GI yet to make a conclusion, but the diets and weight loss programs featuring low GI (low carbo-hydrate, high protein) plans took the GI out of context. GI is meant to identify the rate of digestion of different foods and possibly incorporate that knowledge to optimize the dietary guidelines for diabetics.

BUT also note that most foods with a low GI are fruits, vegetables, grains and beans...NOT meat, milk and cheese! So, all these diets such as Atkins, The Zone and others promoting a high protein intake through the consumption of meat, and restricting the intake of carbo-hydrates (considered high GI-food) are NOT only totally UN-Healthy, but also ignore the fact that our healthy foods (fruits, vegetables, grains) have an even lower GI than the meats and fats!

Conclusion: Our Sensible weight loss program can be considered a low GI-diet, but is not meant to be! What I mean is, the sensible weight loss program promotes the consumption of healthy foods, including grasses, grains, fruits, vegetables and beans...which all have a low GI, even lower that meats! Even diabetics would benefit much more from our SENSIBLE weight loss program than from any other low GI diet.

WHY? Popular low GI-diets advocate the consumption of meat which increases the risk of heart disease and stroke due to its high fat content. Our SENSIBLE weight loss program promotes foods with a lower GI than meats (in other words, less spikes in blood sugar levels and a more sustained energy) AND does NOT result in major health risks. In fact, it reduces the risk profile for all diseases. PERIOD.

12.3 Popular Diets & Weight Loss Programs Exposed

This whole business of losing weight can be a frustrating, constant struggle. Many diets are so unnatural and so unrealistic that it's virtually impossible to incorporate them long-term and be a part of your lifestyle; they are impossible to live with...let alone enjoy! Most programs don't even deal with our cravings and our desires, or with our feelings of hunger and fullness. Eventually, we become 'just plain tired' of the hunger, lack of flavor, lack of flexibility, the lack of energy and THE FEELING OF DEPRIVATION.

We quit our diets and then GAIN BACK THE WEIGHT WE HAVE LOST... AND SOMETIMES WE GAIN EVEN MORE!!!

A tragic statistic – Only 3% of diets and weight loss programs on the market are successful. Why is that? What are the common denominators? What are the common flaws of these diets? And more importantly, what is the SOLUTION to this obesity problem with epidemic proportions? First piece of advice: STOP listening to UNQUALIFIED mass-marketers and START taking the advice in this book.

What are the common flaws of these 'FAD' diets and popular weight loss programs? Well, there are many! For one, they are all 'One-Size-Fits-All' approaches. That means that these diets are NOT individualized or customized. If 1000 people sign up for Nutrisystem (or any other diet for that matter) today, all 1000 people will be put on the exact same diet with the exact same guidelines. Does that make sense? Of course not! Should someone who is 150 pounds be put on the same diet as someone who is 270 pounds? I don't think so! What about people's medical history and specific dietary needs? What about their individual goals, body composition, eating behaviors, physical activity level etc.? Also, there's NO supervision of a knowledgeable health care professional and therefore these diets can be potentially dangerous.

Next, most of these popular diets and weight loss programs are low calorie diets (LCD), and that's usually the ONLY reason why people lose weight on these diets. What is a LCD and what are calories, you may ask? Well, calories are basically energy. And all of us need a certain amount of energy or calories to sustain life on a daily basis (also referred to as BMR or Basic Metabolic Rate). People who are mostly sedentary and inactive may only require 1200 to 1500 calories per day, while Michael Phleps (so I've heard) burns over 5000 calories per day. Now, these LCD's restrict your caloric intake. You are taking in less calories than your body needs on a daily basis, and you end-up with a calorie deficit. Your body officially is in a 'starvation mode' and is forced to get the energy it needs from somewhere else. Eventually, the body will break down your own valuable muscle tissue to retrieve energy from its proteins.

And yes, you do lose weight on these diets, BUT it is mostly muscle weight and water weight due to dehydration, NOT FAT! That's why you will REGAIN weight after you stop these diets. Your body comes out of starvation and immediately starts storing fat in preparation for a possible next starvation period (your body has a memory and adapts to external conditions). That's also why they call these diets "yo-yo" diets: when you are on these diets you will lose some weight, when you're off them you will regain the weight, and many times you will regain more than you initially lost! ALL these diets and programs only obtain SHORT-TERM results.

Even more importantly, most of these diets and weight loss programs are unbalanced and therefore unhealthy. With unbalanced I mean that most of these diets promote the consumption of one food group and restrict the consumption of another...which is all BOGUS! Take Atkins for example (I often use Atkins as an example because most people know or heard about it): It promotes the consumption of meat and restricts the consumption of carbohydrates. In the long-term this drastically increases the risk for cardiovascular diseases, causes ketosis, and results in many, severe micronutrient deficiencies. NO GOOD!

Each time we go on another diet of deprivation, the weight becomes more difficult to lose and we become even more frustrated and discouraged. Then, we eat more and exercise less, causing ourselves more frustration, discouragement and depression. Soon we find ourselves in this **'vicious cycle'**. **No one can realistically live in the "diet" mode for the rest of their life, depriving themselves of the true pleasures of healthy eating and activity!**

Then we think to ourselves...Oh, why bother?? We start to blame ourselves for having no will power when what we really need is a <u>clear, common sense, realistic program that we can follow and get results that are quick and permanent!</u>

Are you with me so far? Keep reading...

The SENSIBLE weight loss program explained in this book will also put emphasis on a lower caloric intake BUT without putting your body in a starvation mode.

HOW? Well, we make sure that your body receives ALL the essential nutrients it needs on a daily basis during your weight loss program, including vitamins, minerals, digestive enzymes, essential amino-acids, omega fatty acids, fruits, vegetables, grasses, grains, and powerful antioxidants. You will reduce calories (and therefore lose weight) while providing your body with all it needs. The body does NOT need to break down valuable muscle tissue and the weight that is lost will be FAT! The results will be LASTING.

Furthermore, the nutrition plan is balanced and healthy, and focuses on detoxification and elimination, optimization, and supplementation. To assure maintenance of weight loss we incorporated behavior modification techniques, a simple – short – yet effective personal exercise regimen, and an easy compliance and support system. Keep on reading, it gets much better…

How to recognize or identify a 'FAD' diet?

1. Promises quick weight loss, often more than 3 pounds per week.

2. Promotes methods too good to be true.

3. Implies that weight can be lost without exercise or lifestyle changes.

4. Uses scare tactics to promote the diet plan.

5. Restricts or eliminates certain foods or food groups and prescribes an unbalanced, unhealthy diet plan resulting in major nutrient deficiencies such as vitamins, minerals, dietary fiber and protective phytonutrients.

6. Rarely addresses portion size.

7. Insists on consuming specific foods or combinations of foods that don't comply with the laws of nature.

8. Offers rigid menu plans that do not comply with the laws of nature.

9. Encourages the dieter to eat as much as he/she wants of a particular food while prescribing a daily caloric intake well below average requirements for a healthy adult.

Despite the poor success rate of all these popular diets and weight loss programs, they continue to grow in popularity among overweight Americans. More than 50% of the best-selling diet books have been published since 1999.

Why? People try a diet, it doesn't work or only gives them short-term results, or it's too hard to follow, and they give up. BUT they still want to lose that weight AND they jump on the next diet hitting the market (and promoted by celebrities).

Silly? Maybe, but there's no other option...until NOW!

A USDA review of popular diets

In 2004, the Feinberg School of Medicine at Northwestern University, conducted an evidence based evaluation of the most popular diets and weight loss programs on the market. Their quest was to find the 'magic bullet' for successful weight loss.

Here's the evaluation:

Calories:

A total caloric intake averaging 1400-1500 calories daily results in weight loss, regardless the macronutrient composition. Physical activity can enhance weight loss, but when on low-calorie diets without exercise, weight loss is still achieved.

Dieters who adhered to low-fat, high carbohydrate diets rich in fruit, vegetables and grains consumed less calories than those on other types of diets. This reinforces again that there is an inverse relationship between carbohydrate intake and body weight and that the statement "carbohydrates are fattening" is a myth!

Moderate-fat weight loss diets also result in loss of body weight and body fat even when food is consumed ad libidum. The mean caloric intake of individuals following general diets (the USDA food group pyramid with a diet composition of 55% carbohydrates, 25% fat and 20% protein) is 1895 daily; and the mean caloric intake of those on a high-fat, low carbohydrate regimen is 2166 calories daily.

This makes absolute sense when we know that 1 gram of protein or carbohydrate gives us 4 calories, while 1 gram of fat consumption results in 9 calories.

In the table on the next page we can see that no matter what diet is prescribed, the average total caloric intake (1400-1450) is far less than the total calories consumed during the typical American diet (2200), and therefore people will lose weight on these diets. However, we already established that the results will only be short-term.

We can conclude that it's therefore MUCH HEALTHIER to take part in a balanced diet that does NOT promote one food or food group and restricts another one. The restrictive, popular diets do NOT obtain any better weight loss results, but can be health hazards!

Nutrition Adequacy:

High fat, low carbohydrate diets cause deficiencies in vitamins A, B6, D, E, thiamin, folate, calcium, magnesium, iron, potassium, and dietary fiber. WOW, NO GOOD!

Moderate fat, low carbohydrate diets, which usually follow the USDA food pyramid guidelines, promote a balance of the 6 food groups: grains, fruits, vegetables, meats, dairy and fats/sugars. If 1 or more food groups are eliminated, inadequate intake of nutrients occurs. Even though I don't fully agree with the USDA's pyramid model (especially the dairy part), it's a more balanced approach which does not cause any immediate health hazards.

Low fat, high carbohydrate regimens cause deficiencies in vitamin E, B12 and zinc. Individuals following these diets need to fortify with supplements also.

Weight reducing diet & body composition:

Weight loss can indicate loss of body weight, body fat or lean muscle mass, or a combination. A total daily calorie restriction (approximately 1500 calories daily) sustained over a longer period of time promotes

Type of diet	Total calories	Fat grams (% calories)	Carbohydrate grams (% of calories)	Protein grams (% calories)
S.A.D. Typical American Diet	2200	85 (35%)	275 (50%)	82.5 (15%)
High fat, low carb (Atkins, Zone Diet, Sugar Busters, Protein Power)	1414	96 (60%) Fat level range 35-60%	35 (10%)	105 (30%)
Moderate fat diet (USDA food pyramid, DASH diet, ADA, Weight Watchers, Jenny Craig)	1450	40 (25%) Fat level range 21-34%	218 (60%)	54 (15%)
Low- and very low fat diet (volumetrics, Dean Ornish's, Eet more – weigh less, New Pritkin program)	1450	20 (13%) Fat level range 10-20%	235-271 (70%)	54-72 (17%)

Illustration 20 – Popular Diets

loss of body fat, regardless the macronutrient composition of the diet. Physical activity is recommended because it facilitates loss of body fat by increasing energy expenditure, increasing lean muscle mass and increasing metabolism.

Physiological changes during weight loss:

Weight loss is directly correlated with a decrease in total blood cholesterol, LDL-cholesterol (especially with low-saturated fat intake), and plasma triglycerides. Caloric restriction improves glycemic control by lowering blood sugar levels and insulin levels regardless the macronutrient content of the diet. Weight loss also decreases blood pressure.

Hunger, satiety and adherence to diets:

Long-term weight loss is regulated as follows:

1. Insulin stimulates the uptake of glucose and proteins into the cells and possibly increases appetite.

2. Leptin is a hormone released from fat cells. It increases our metabolism and assists in suppressing appetite.

3. The secretion of insulin and leptin is influenced by macronutrient composition, but the mechanism is unclear.

4. During weight loss, blood insulin and leptin levels drop.

Fat restricted diets (with low-caloric intake of course) offer satiety due to the high-fiber, high water content of low-fat foods, which give the enhanced feeling of fullness. Low-fat regimens develop an aversion to fatty foods over time, contributing to the long-term success. High dietary fiber intake lowers insulin levels and is correlated with long-term maintenance of weight loss.

Neurochemical factors, gastric signals, emotional factors, individual taste preference and other contributing factors account for differences in appetite, food intake and body weight.

An American Cancer Institute Review

The American Cancer Institute's quest was to find out whether the advice given by popular diets and weight loss programs, about nutrition and weight loss, is based on scientific science. The Institute also wanted to evaluate the potential effectiveness and possible health risks associated with these diets. The Institute evaluated 4 books:

1.   Dr. Atkins' New Diet Revolution by Dr. Robert Atkins.

2.   The New Beverly Hills Diet by Judy Mazel & Michael Wyatt.

3.   Protein Power by Michael Eades, MD.

4.   Suzanne Somers' Get Skinny on Fabulous Food.

The American Cancer Institute concluded that ALL 4 plans are essentially low calorie diets, even though they were NOT advertised as such. Each one encourages the dieter to eat as much as he/she wants of a particular food while still prescribing a daily caloric intake well below average requirements. All the diets also recommended omitting certain foods or even entire food groups resulting in major nutrient deficiencies. Dr. Atkins recommends supplementing his diet and conveniently offers his own line of products.

The diets lack a balance of protein, carbohydrates and fat; and prescribe a daily intake high in protein and low in fat and carbohydrates. This is a far cry from the recommendations by AICR, AHA, ADA, USDA and the Surgeon General.

Unbalanced diets also can lead to ketosis. Maintaining these diets causes a fasting state of the body, and the body starts metabolizing muscle tissue (after fat tissue). Symptoms include muscle breakdown, nausea, dehydration, headaches, light-headedness, irritability, bad breath and kidney problems. Long-term adherence to these diets can be fatal to the fetus of pregnant women and individuals with diabetes.

All 4 diets promote loss of water weight. The diuretic effect of high protein, high fat, low carbohydrate diets give a false sense of accomplishment. The water weight also returns quickly.

The American Cancer Institute also pointed out some significant other health risks while on these diets:

1. Long-term restriction of carbohydrates leads to lack of fiber causing constipation and GI-problems.

2. High amounts of cholesterol and saturated fat increase the risk of heart disease and some cancers.

3. Higher risk of osteoporosis because excess protein leaches calcium from the bones.

4. Increased risk of Gout because of the increased intake of foods rich in purines (meat, poultry, nuts, seeds, eggs, seafood) which cause an increase in uric acid levels in the body.

5. Uric acid and calcium oxalate stones formed by high protein diets can cause kidney stones.

6. High protein diets cause a significant loss of fluids and electrolytes, which may cause a rapid drop in blood pressure and fainting.

7. Bad breath can also occur as a result of an incomplete breakdown of fatty acids, also called 'keto-breath'.

Conclusions by the American Cancer Institute:

The Atkins diet follows NO logic. Other cultures follow high-carbohydrate, low-fat diets. The diet is also unsafe and most of the weight loss is due to its diuretic effect. The diet also has POOR real-world results in keeping the weight off.

Popular notions are based on studying the chemistry of foods, and wrongly assume that sugary foods (candy, ice cream) that are composed of simple carbohydrates are absorbed immediately while starchier foods (bread, potatoes) provide long-term energy. We already established earlier that the exact opposite holds true.

All the above are some important subtleties and contradictions ignored by authors of popular diets.

Other Popular Diets

Weight Watchers:

Established in the 1960's, Weight Watchers promotes weight loss of 5 to 10% of one's body weight. Their strictly dictated meals are based on points. Exercise allows for more point consumption, and the latest program has a zero-point food list. Weight Watchers conducts weekly support meetings and has online support.

The ADVANTAGES are that it's the #1 rated weight loss program by Consumer Reports. It educates the participants on food and has been proven more successful than do-it-yourself plans in the long-term. Peer pressure seems to work. It's a better choice than most other diets that lack balance in their nutritional recommendations.

The DISADVANTAGES are that some people are embarrassed during the public weight measurements and meetings, that the program is rather expensive, and that Weight Watchers has NOT been proven better than any other diets or programs.

South Beach Diet:

Developed by a cardiologist in Miami, this diet puts emphasis on a low-carbohydrate phase followed by increasing amounts of low glycemic carbohydrates. The diet also restricts high glycemic foods and foods high in saturated and hydrogenated fats.

The ADVANTAGES are that the South Beach diet allows for healthy fats and carbohydrates, reduces insulin, improves lipids and lowers appetite.

The DISADVANTAGE is that it is based on glycemic index (GI), which is not approved by the ADA.

Nutrisystem:

Toxic, nutrient depleted meals are mailed to your doorstep. The system works with 'military rations' of 1200-1500 calories/day, and is based on low GI-foods with a total intake of 55% carbohydrates, 25% protein and 20% fat. The cost is about $280/month and they offer some phone support. BAD, BAD, BAD!

High Fiber diets:

High fiber diets include soluble fibers (fruit, beans, oats) and insoluble fibers (vegetables, grains), with a recommended daily dose of 25-40 grams (the average person consumes about 10 grams per day).

The ADVANTAGES are reduced appetite, reduced GI-problems, improved lipid profile (protects against heart disease), and reduced risk for most cancers.

The DISADVANTAGES are a reduced absorption of minerals and the fact that many people are allergic to wheat products.

Meal Replacements:

Usually meal replacements are high protein shakes or snacks that replace a meal. In general, there's an improved compliance versus diets alone because participants feel like they have to sacrifice less: "fast food that's good for you", and also feel a greater satisfaction.

The ADVANTAGE is that studies show greater weight loss (25-60%) with meal replacements at 3 months and 1 year compared to regular diets.

I personally think that it's a GREAT STRATEGY to implement a GOOD meal replacement in a weight loss program.

Ornish diet:

This is a vegetarian diet that gets 10% of the calories from fat. It allows NO cooking oils, nuts or advocados, and excludes fish. There are NO calorie restrictions.

The ADVANTAGES are improvements in blood pressure and lipid profiles. The diet also reverses angina and artherosclerosis.

The DISADVANTAGES are that the diet is very difficult to follow, and that there's a potential for deficiency of essential fatty acids.

The Ornish diet is a prevention diet for people at risk for heart disease, and a reversal diet for people with a known heart disease.

Some other considerations:

The average protein consumption should be 15% of the caloric intake. This is the absolute minimum when on a diet. So make sure you consume at least 1 to 1.5 grams of high-quality protein per kilogram of body weight when on a low calorie diet (LCD).

When consuming less than 50-100 grams of carbohydrates per day, the body becomes ketogenic. This leads to excessive protein breakdown and dehydration. Note that for every 1 gram of glycogen or protein broken down, 3 grams of water is released!

12.4 Keys to a Successful & Sensible Weight Loss Program

The 7 Keys to success:

1. A correct ASSESSMENT

2. OBJECTIVITY

3. CUSTOMIZATION – Individualized approach

4. A Balanced and HEALTHY nutrition program

5. LIFESTYLE changes – Behavior Modification

6. SUPPORT system

7. COMPLIANCE system – Facilitators

Key 1 - Making a correct assessment

What caused the obesity? We know there's ONLY ONE CAUSE of ALL so called disease: toxemia. Treating obesity then means taking away that cause. So the action plan will be the same as the action plan to regain optimal health. However, we can add a few specific recommendations to facilitate weight loss.

There are other questions that need to be answered to assist you in your quest to obtain and regain an optimal body composition:

Why are you overweight? It's important to get an answer to that question and identify the *causative factor* or factors. We know the answer is toxemia, but now we need to identify why there's toxemia; what are the habits that led to toxemia? When we know what caused the toxemia, we can address these causes and also make sure we control them while trying to maintain a healthy and optimal weight.

WHEN did the weight gain start?

This weight gain could have started during pregnancy and/or post-partum (after delivery of the baby), during the pre-menopausal period or during menopause because of hormonal imbalances.

Weight gain also can be a result of a medical condition in which the ambulatory status or activity level is affected.

One can also gain weight as a result of a trauma. This can be a physical trauma such as a car accident, or an emotional trauma such as the loss of a spouse or family member. These traumas cause significant amounts of stress which in turn slow down metabolism. Also, many people dealing with a lot of stress cope by finding comfort in food.

Next, what does the current diet consist of? How much do you currently consume? This is called the *'current diet assessment'*. What are your current eating habits? What is your current diet composition? Are you on the "Standard American diet" (SAD)? How much fast food do you consume? What macro - and micronutrients are you lacking? Do you use supplementation? In what circumstances do you crave food? Are there any important environmental factors?

We also need to inquire about one's *current physical activity level* or exercise regimen.

We need to look at one's *previous attempts to lose weight*. What diets and weight loss programs have you tried? What were the results? What was your experience? Why did you quit?

When we suspect *hormonal imbalances* (weight gain started during menopause or after a hysterectomy for example), we need to prescribe a complete hormone panel and also screen for cancer (we don't want to administer hormones when there's a cancer present).

Even a great weight loss program will produce limited results if one's hormones are out of balance. The test results will indicate deficiencies and/or excesses of specific hormones, and with the prescription of bio-identical hormones we can safely replace these 'missing' hormones and re-establish a healthy hormonal balance.

Key 2 – Objectivity

With most popular diets and weight loss programs, the scale indicates whether you lost weight or not. However, the scale does NOT indicate WHAT was lost: body fat, lean muscle mass or water? Therefore, the scale is really not an objective way of measuring the effectiveness of a weight loss program. People on a diet or weight loss program usually need to lose excess body fat and maybe even gain some muscle mass, but certainly can't afford to lose valuable muscle tissue or water. There is NO way to really measure 'true' progress with a scale to evaluate the effectiveness of the program.

A wonderful body shape or a healthy body is not defined as 125lbs., but as a % of body fat. It is the lean body mass that forms the body shape, so having a lighter weight does not necessarily define a beautiful body. Factors that guarantee a beautiful body are based upon the balanced ratio of lean body mass to fat mass.

Having The Same Weight does NOT always mean having the Same Body Shape.

While trying to shed weight, the amount of each component and its proportion in our body change. Since muscle is heavier than the same volume of fat, a person with more muscle looks slimmer. Although it could be important, weight alone does not tell us anything about body composition. Therefore, what is important is our body composition, not our weight, and the well-balanced ratio of its components is a critical health indicator. Body weight alone is not a clear indicator of good health because it does not distinguish how many pounds of fat you have and how many pounds of lean body mass you have.

A healthy person maintains a balanced body composition. However, if this balance gets disturbed, a proportion of each component changes; excessive fat causes obesity; insufficient proteins cause malnutrition; excessive water causes edema or swelling; insufficient minerals cause osteoporosis. The purpose of body composition analysis is to evaluate the body function and improve your health condition. Therefore, it is crucial to pursue personal health and fitness by understanding body composition such as muscle development, nutrition and possible obesity through regular body composition check-ups.

We should measure our body composition with a body composition analyzer, such as the InBody520. This accurate piece of equipment measures your percentage of body fat, water balance and segmental lean muscle mass. Now, we will be able to set specific goals (for example: lose 40 pounds of fat and gain 10 pounds of lean muscle mass), monitor progress and revise the plan of action if indicated.

With the results of the body composition analysis we also will be able to design a personal exercise regimen based on the segmental muscle mass measurements.

Does this make sense? We just want to make sure you are losing fat, not muscle or water AND with a body composition analysis we can accurately monitor this. That's what I call OBJECTIVITY. It also motivates the participants when they see objective progress is being made.

You may want to investigate if a physician office, weight loss clinic, gym or wellness center in your area has such a BCA available. If not, don't worry about it, our SWL (Sensible Weight Loss) works great even without a BCA.

Key 3 – Customize & Individualize

We need to get away from these 'One-Size-Fits-All' approaches and customize the client's weight loss program, including nutrition, exercise, BCA results, and lifestyle changes.

Based on your symptoms and if indicated, we also may prescribe a complete hormone panel. If your hormones are out of balance, BHRT (Bio-identical Hormone Replacement Therapy) is recommended.

An LRA-test to identify the foods that should be eliminated form your diet (due to their delayed allergic response) may also be conducted. For more information on the LRA-test, refer to Chapter 15 (Allergies).

Key 4 – A balanced & healthy nutrition program

We also have to make sure that this customized diet or nutrition program is balanced and healthy, and provides the body with all the essential nutrients it needs on a daily basis. Through nutrition and supplementation, we will try to RESTORE normal health and balance in the body, including pH levels and metabolism.

An acidic pH slows down metabolism, and by introducing more alkaline foods into someone's diet or nutrition program, we will help speed up metabolism and restore normal functioning of the body, therefore assisting in effective elimination and weight loss.

Fasting and an effective detoxification regimen are also crucial in effective weight loss, as well as some unique supplements that may facilitate initial efforts.

The nutrition program of our SENSIBLE weight loss program is easy to follow, does NOT dictate to participants WHAT they should eat which in turn increases compliance, and makes sure the participant is NOT starving or has to sacrifice all the time.

Key 5 – Lifestyle changes

A diet or weight loss program that does not address lifestyle changes will ONLY produce short-term results. It's absolutely necessary to address eating habits, emotional eating, and portion size and break some bad habits while relearning new ones. We will provide what we call 'behavior modification' techniques to assist you in making these crucial lifestyle changes.

Key 6 – Support system

It's hard to do things by yourself, especially when we want you to make some lifestyle changes. General website support, phone support or online support, chat rooms etc. may be of valuable assistance. However, peer support or support from a health care practitioner who is educated in the Hygiene system is even better. He or she understands your personal medical conditions and history, and can communicate with you on a personal level, monitor your progress and modify your plan of action if indicated; and most importantly makes your weight loss experience SAFE!

If you don't have a personal doctor or health care professional available to assist you in weight loss, find some outside support (online, weekly conference calls with Q&A, a knowledgeable physician that can assist you personally through email or by phone etc.).

A great tip is that when you decide to enroll in a SENSIBLE weight loss program, try to involve all the members of your household; or find a friend to do it with you! How difficult would it be to try and eat healthier and lose some weight while everyone else at home continues to eat fast food and junk all the time? It would benefit everyone you love to participate so that you can support each other, and end-up a healthier and happier family.

Key 7 – Compliance system

Compliance is one of the major reasons why people quit diets and weight loss programs. Fad diets are too difficult to follow; you feel like you are starving and/or you have to sacrifice too much...you try, but it won't last and eventually you will quit.

Overcoming compliance issues is therefore of utmost importance in establishing a successful weight loss program. Our SENSIBLE weight loss program is designed specifically to increase compliance and make it easier for the participant to follow.

The prescribed nutrition program is simple, yet very effective and ONLY incorporates foods that are palatable to the individual's taste.

The personal exercise regimen is short, simple and effective and can conveniently fit in everyone's daily schedule without interrupting that schedule.

Because the nutrition plan is balanced and healthy, participants do NOT encounter the well-known 'plateau'. For those who may not know what a 'plateau' is....it means that you suddenly stop losing weight on a particular diet after you lost some weight initially. This usually discourages the participant and he/she quits.

The reason why people on most popular diets and weight loss programs hit the plateau is because the diet is unbalanced and tricks the body in losing weight. The body will eventually protect itself from health hazards, or is unable to retrieve the necessary energy from its own resources such as muscle tissue. Due to our body's inherent defense mechanism no further weight loss occurs and the so called 'plateau' is reached.

Personal support and guidance, with the ability to customize, monitor progress and modify the plan of action increases compliance.

Long-term results are maintained by simply continuing to implement the nutrition program, new habits, and exercise regimen. It's a lifestyle change and it has become part of you. You feel great, you have obtained an optimal body composition, a metabolic and hormonal balance, and you are taking the road to optimal health.

Nothing will stop you!

Popular diets & weight loss programs	SENSIBLE Weight Loss
One-Size-Fits-ALL	Individualized
General guidelines	Skilled supervision
No medical history	Health history
Unhealthy	Healthy
Subjective	Objective
Subjective progress	Monitor progress
General support (if any)	Individual support
Plateau	No plateau
Poor compliance	Excellent compliance
Short-term results	Long-term results

Illustration 21 – Sensible Weight Loss

Secrets to Effective Weight Loss

As you already discovered, it's very easy to get discouraged in your quest to lose weight and more importantly to keep the weight off. People who were able to successfully lose weight and obtain and maintain their optimal body composition usually have the following in common:

1. They participated in a common sense program that emphasized a balanced and healthy nutrition program.

2. They participated in a weight loss program that overcame feelings of hunger and/or sacrifice, and offered a solid support and compliance system.

3. They were willing to learn about proper nutrition and implemented new habits and lifestyle changes.

4. They believed they could do it and used their past failures as empowerment to take control over their weight and health.

5. They lost the weight because they wanted to for themselves, not for someone else.

6. They had a plan of action to cope with temporary weight gain and implemented that plan immediately. For some people this plan was to exercise more, for others is was to cut back on sweets or to cut portion size.

7. They gave positive feedback and reinforcement to themselves even when they made a 'mistake'.

8. They learned to face and confront their feelings and implemented the behavior modification techniques they learned.

9. They asked for support from friends and family.

12.5 Exercise & Weight Loss

Our **Basic Metabolic Rate (BMR)** is the energy our body uses to sustain life on a daily basis; the energy necessary to sustain all biomechanical reactions and bodily systems. The BMR consumes about 60 to 70% of the total energy at a rate of 1kcal/kg/hour.

The thermal effect of our digestive process demands another 10% of that total energy. We have limited control over our BMR and thermal digestive effect; however we can control the energy we spend through activity and exercise. Exercise can demand anywhere from 10-40% of the total available energy.

Example of energy expenditure: A 75kg person burns 100kcal when walking 1 mile, and 1 pound of fat equals 3500 kcal. So this person would have to walk 35 miles to burn 1 pound of fat.

Research & Benefits of Regular Exercise:

Regular exercise results in a decrease in the loss of fat-free mass (muscle) associated with weight loss. Exercise also increases muscle mass and results in more effective fat oxidation (more fat is burned per unit of exercise).

A quick increase in fat metabolism is observed within 3 weeks of exercise at a frequency of 3x/week and within 10 days of 1-hour of exercise/day.

Exercise improves maintenance of weight loss; exercise helps sustain weight loss results. Exercise is more beneficial for maintenance than for initial weight loss and does not have a major impact on short-term weight loss results.

As an overweight or obese person loses weight, it takes more and more exercise just to maintain the weight loss.

As we all know, exercise also improves cardiovascular and metabolic health (independent of weight loss).

In studies, NO advantage is shown with supervised versus non-supervised activity in the long-term. In other words, going to the gym and/or having a personal trainer does not benefit you; however initially it may be advised that a knowledgeable person assists you in the proper execution of your exercise program to assure optimal effectiveness and prevent injury.

Compliance is shown to be higher when exercises are performed home based vs. group based. I assume that is true because group based exercise interrupts people's daily schedule (they have to be at a certain place at a certain time) and when people's personal schedule changes (kids off school during summer, different job, spouse out of town etc.) they are inclined to 'give up'.

A single bout of exercise can increase BMR by 5-15% for up to 48 hours (due to an increased systemic nor-epinephrine). Example: if a 70kg person burns an extra 160 kcal/day, he/she loses an extra pound of fat every 20 days.

Ideally you need to exercise 120 – 200 minutes/week for weight loss. In our Sensible Weight Loss program (SWL) we suggest you incorporate exercise within the first month of the program, even though we established earlier that exercise does not have much of an effect in initial weight loss. Why? The client has to learn the appropriate exercises, and gradually increase the frequency and duration BECAUSE when the client reaches his/her optimal body composition, exercise will be crucial to keep the weight off. I recommend you start with 120min/week and gradually increase to 200min/week. We already discussed the type of exercise, intensity, frequency and duration of our PRE exercise regimen.

Exercise decreases appetite short-term due to reduction in visceral blood flow and catecholamine elevations. Exercise does not increase food intake in the long-term in normal individuals.

So, the key is to combine diet with exercise. You will lose more weight than diet alone and the body composition changes: increased fat loss, less lean muscle tissue loss and decrease in visceral fat. Exercise is key factor in maintenance of weight loss.

Conclusion so far:

Diet = key factor for initial weight loss.
Exercise = key factor for sustained weight loss!

Many dieters will 'plateau' (unable to lose more weight at a certain stage within a popular weight loss program) UNTIL they increase exercise.

Final conclusion on Exercise

Develop, personalize and customize the exercise program based on the results of the Body Composition Analysis (if available), current activity level and limitations, and the client's medical, physical and psychological readiness.

Keep a record of the exercises on an exercise log.

Initially, perform maximum 4 exercises in PRE-mode for a total of 120 minutes/week; for example: 4 times 30 minutes/week. As we gradually increase our exercise regimen to 200 minutes/week, I suggest we incorporate cardiovascular exercise. At this point, you have the energy reserves to successfully complete a cardiovascular workout (or a fun activity) without draining the body or causing injury. This will also provide some variety in the person's exercise regimen. Make sure you choose an activity you like to do.

To increase compliance, we suggest performing the exercises from home unless you prefer to join a gym. At home, you can fit in your short exercise session into your daily schedule, even if that schedule is prone to change all the time.

A great example is a client of mine, his name is Steve. Steve came to me about 5 years ago for weight loss. He is a construction worker and lives in an apartment by himself. He usually gets up around 5:30am in the morning and comes home after 6pm, exhausted. Steve eats fast food and rarely cooks a healthy meal. When he comes home, Steve often snacks in front of the TV and watches 2 to 3 hours of crime scene investigation episodes. Steve has no time to go to a gym and cannot

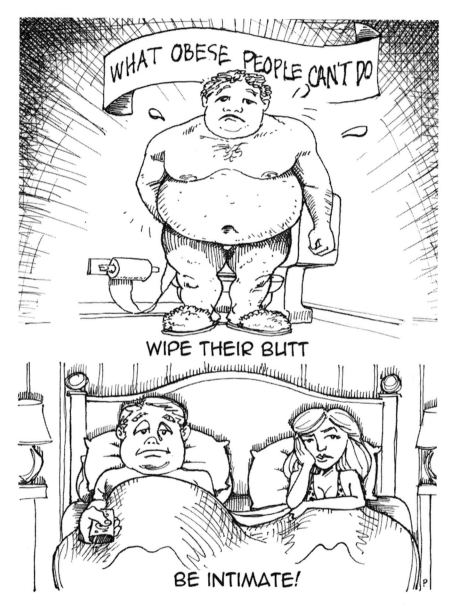

Illustration 22 – What Obese People Can't Do

afford it either, but even more importantly he doesn't want to miss his CSI. We HAVE TO make sure we FIT Steve's exercise regimen into his daily schedule without interrupting that schedule in order to guarantee long-term compliance. In Steve's case, the InBody520 results showed that his segmental muscle mass in the arms and core (trunk) was above average, but his muscle mass in his legs could benefit from an increase. Steve has no exercise equipment at home, and he doesn't want to invest in equipment anyway. We decided to prescribe Steve some simple squats from a chair. We instructed Steve to squat during every single commercial while watching the crime scenes. Yes, he was sore the first weeks because as you know…those commercials can be pretty long! Steve's lean muscle mass in his legs improved quickly and continues to improve. Steve is still doing his PRE exercises from home! The regimen does not interfere with his daily schedule. Steve does not feel he has to sacrifice and most of all he experiences the benefits.

12.6 Here's YOUR Action Plan.

In order to regain and maintain an optimal body composition, a sensible approach is recommended.

The Sensible Weight Loss program (SWL) is a common sense approach with emphasis on improving WHAT you eat while consuming less calories. All ESSENTIAL nutrients are provided on a daily basis so that the body is NEVER put in a starvation mode. Participants gradually lose more and more weight, feel healthier and more energetic, and most of all KEEP THE WEIGHT OFF!

The SWL will be the LAST diet or weight loss program you will EVER do! OH, and it's very easy, simple, and you will never feel like you have to sacrifice. It's simply AWESOME. Many already lost their target weight and never regained it. NOW, It's your turn!

In essence the SWL program or action plan is exactly the same as the ACTION PLAN to regain control of your health in the back of this book. By living C.L.E.A.N. you automatically address toxemia, the cause of all so called disease including obesity and being overweight. That's it.

However, if losing weight is a primary emphasis we can recommend a few things that may assist you further and facilitate you weight loss efforts.

The SWL program is a **6-week, step-by-step, EDUCATIONAL** approach. After the 6 weeks, participants continue the program on their own until they reach their target weight.

For your convenience, you can find all the instructions, accompanied by reading materials and youtube videos on my website www.health4life.info.

Before you start, ask yourself the following questions and write down the answers on a piece of paper. Display a copy and read aloud twice daily.

1. Are you willing to learn about proper nutrition and implement new habits and lifestyle changes?

2. Do you believe you can do this? Why?

3. Are you ready to lose some weight? Are you doing this for yourself or for someone else?

4. Do you have a plan of action to cope with temporary weight gain and will you implement that plan immediately? For some people this plan will be to exercise more, for others it will be to cut on sweets or to cut portion size. For other options, please review the chapter on behavior modification.

5. Will you maintain a yes-attitude, a positive attitude and give yourself positive feedback and reinforcement, even when you make a 'mistake'?

6. Are you ready to face and acknowledge your emotions and feelings, and implement the behavior modification techniques you learned (chapter 13)?

7. Did you ask for support from friends and family?

WEEK 1 – SWL SET-UP

Below you will find your TO-DO LIST:

- ✓ Print your 'My SWL record' document online. Complete all your initial measurements: weight, waist circumference, hip circumference, salivary and urine pH, and 'Subjective Feelings' section. Also, take some standard 'before' pictures (front view and side view, minimal clothing) with plain background.

  For instructions on how to obtain correct hip and waist measurements, refer to the beginning of this chapter.

- ✓ Purchase the pH-strips for urinary and salivary testing. Read the package instructions and test the pH of your urine AND saliva prior to starting the SWL-program, and follow my personal protocol:

Day 1: take 3 urine measurements and 3 salivary measurements, totaling 6 pH measurements. The first urine and salivary measurements are in the morning, prior to breakfast; the other ones are respectively after lunch and after dinner.

Day 2: same as day 1. Now, total the 6 urine measurements (3 from day 1 and 3 from day 2) and divide by 6 to get an average urine pH measurement. Do the same for your salivary measurements. Record the average urine measurement and the average salivary measurement on your SWL-record. Initially, repeat this entire procedure bi-weekly; after 3 months repeat monthly.

Your urine pH measurement will be approximately 0.5 lower (more acidic) than your salivary measurement. If your urine pH reading is below 6.5 (even below 7.0) you are advised to alkalize your diet. Note that occasionally one's initial pH readings are always highly alkaline (greater than 7.5), which is due to catabolism (the process of breaking down). In this process, nitrogen (in the form of ammonia and alkaline amino acids such as arginine, asparagines, glutamine and lysine) is lost and the urine becomes excessively alkaline. If constant 7.5 to 8.0 readings should occur in your case, you should stimulate your anabolic (repair) mechanisms, thus reversing the catabolic cycle.

Generally speaking, the exact reading is not that important. What is important is that you will see a gradual rise in pH, in other words your pH has to become more alkaline (meaning that you are cleaning up your 'internal fish tank').

WEEK 2 – The Alkaline Way

✓ Download and print the 'Acid-Alkaline Forming Food List' on-line and follow these instructions:

1. Take a yellow high-liter (marker) and high-lite ONLY the foods you like to eat.

2. Buy and eat more of the high-lited foods in the ALKA-LINE FORMING categories.

3. Eat less of the high-lited foods in the ACID FORMING categories or eliminate them if you can.

✓ Incorporate FOOD COMBINING Rules.

✓ Incorporate the Back To Basics rules (Chapter 5; 5.2.).

✓ Facilitate initial weight loss with effective, safe supplements (B LEAN or BODE BURN and PEA PROTREIN). Refer to our chapter on supplements for more info.

WEEK 3 – BEHAVIOR MODIFICATION

✓ Acquire the following HABITS:

1. Only eat when you are hungry! Anytime you grab for food,

ask yourself if you are hungry; if not don't eat and do something else.

2. Prolong your meals by: eating slowly, putting down your eating utensil between each bite, and do not pick up your eating utensil until you have swallowed the bite, hesitating between bites, even if you're eating finger foods.

3. Choose a specific place in your home or office to eat all of your meals. This will become your 'designated eating place' and should not be changed. Try not to eat at your desk at work. This would make you prone to eat all day long and not just at meal time.

4. Do not do anything except eat when you sit down for a meal. Do not read, watch TV, talk on the phone, work, etc. Make yourself aware of the food you are eating. Focus on the conversation and enjoy your meal.

5. Do not keep food in any room in your house except the kitchen. Do not keep food such as cookies out on the counters. Do not store items in 'see-through' containers.

6. Do not buy junk food. Neither your mate nor your children need it.

7. If possible, serve individual plates from the stove and do not serve family style on the table. If this is not possible, put the serving dishes on the opposite end of the table.

8. When preparing a meal, freeze in the excess immediately so there's just enough food for today's meal.

9. Serve yourself on a smaller plate.

10. Develop a habit of leaving at least one bite of each item on your plate. If you can master this, it becomes easier to stop eating when you feel full. You will be used to leaving

food on your plate.

11. Plan your meals for the week, make a list and go shopping only once for the whole week. Make sure you have a balanced plan. I also recommend you go shopping after you had a meal so that you are less likely to load up your shopping cart with junk, which is another reason to make a list.

12. Replace 'bad' eating habits with other activities. For more information, read Chapter 13 on Behavior Modification techniques.

13. Record habits that are successfully implemented on 'MY SWL Record'.

All of the above are eating techniques that aid in behavior modification.

WEEK 4 – DO I REALLY HAVE TO EXERCISE?

We established that activity and exercise are vital to cell function and health in the previous chapter.

You can lose weight without exercise, BUT you will lose weight FASTER with exercise. Lean muscles speed up metabolism and in turn BURN FAT! The best way to lose weight is NOT cardiovascular exercise but PRE (Progressive Resistive Exercise). Also, in order to keep the weight off...EXERCISE is crucial.

✓ Print the SWL Home Exercise Program and Exercise Log, from week 4 online. You can exercise from home OR gym (your choice). The exercise sessions are relatively short. Make sure to fit them in your daily activities.

✓ Start recording the number of exercise sessions bi-weekly in 'MY SWL Record'.

PRE - Rules:

1. Pick 1 exercise out of each category, for a total of 4 exercises.

2. Execute 3 sets of each exercise; with 7 – 10 repetitions/set.

3. Use a high resistance (70-80% of 1RM) or use your body weight. You should be pretty exhausted after your 7-10 repetitions; if not you need to increase your resistance. For example, when doing squats and using your body weight as resistance, you can add some weight by holding a gallon of water in each hand, or some dumbbells.

4. Rest 2-4 minutes in between sets.

5. Exercise every other day or 4 times per week.

6. Gradually increase your exercise duration from 120 minutes/week PRE to a total of 200 minutes/week PRE and cardiovascular exercise or a fun activity.

7. Keep your exercise log up-to-date.

WEEK 5 – BODY DETOXIFICATION

✓ Start drinking at least the number of ounces of pure water/day equaling your body weight in pounds divided by 2. For example: if you weigh 160 pounds, you need to drink at least 80 ounces of pure water/day. I strongly recommend CLEAN water obtained from a home purification system. Tip: additionally you may squeeze some lemon or lime in your pure water to improve taste and help alkalize your body even more.

✓ Start buying organic foods and whole foods, try to avoid all processed and canned fruits and vegetables. Visit your nearby farmer's market!

✓ Make sure to incorporate our Detoxification program in your regimen (if you didn't already).

✓ Make sure to add the Vemma (refer to chapter on supplements) to your program (if you didn't already). This supplement will provide the essential nutrients for your body, and the grasses and grains help detoxify your body naturally.

✓ Discontinue soda and soft drinks, and also beverages containing high fructose corn syrup. ELIMINATE them NOW.

✓ Tighten up 'The Alkaline Way' program and try to eliminate more acidic foods, especially fried foods, processed meats, white flour products and white sugar.

✓ Replace sugar with raw honey, stevia or blue agave.

✓ Discontinue milk at all cost. If you use milk with cornflakes or cereals in the morning, try to use almond milk. It's sweeter and you will get used to it after a few days!

✓ Record successfully integrated detoxification practices on 'MY SWL Record' under the Behavior Modification section.

WEEK 6 – LASTING RESULTS

✓ Continue to implement the 5 steps above, and continue to improve upon them. Soon, old habits will be broken and healthy new habits acquired!

✓ Increase your exercise regimen from 120 minutes of PRE per week to 200 minutes per week by adding approximately 80 minutes of cardiovascular exercise per week (walking, jogging, running, swimming, cycling).

✓ Take a picture (front and side view) every 4 weeks.

✓ Continue until your reach your desired, optimal weight.

✓ Take your FINAL 'after' picture and submit 'before' and 'after' pictures along with your SWL record and testimonial to Dr. Mike (not required).

✓ You can opt to discontinue the meal replacements, but ONLY if you commit to staying healthy. However, most participants fall in love with the PEA PROTEIN meal replacement and continue...forever. It's convenient.

✓ Continue to eat alkaline forming foods and use the R3 Essentials or liquid Vemma.

✓ Due to the continuous onslaught of toxins on our body, you need to continue the detoxification practices outlined in week 5.

✓ Become a LIVE testimonial and encourage other people to enroll in the SWL. IT WORKS!

So, that's THE ACTION PLAN!

Take it step-by-step and START with week 1. Do NOT try to look ahead and absorb too much information at once. Simply follow the directions week by week and make yourself accountable. Once you start shedding some extra pounds, feel the health benefits of healing and balancing your body with essential nutrients, and rid your body of toxins, you will get EXCITED because YOU NOW KNOW that it REALLY works. This process usually takes anywhere from 3 weeks to 3 months, depending on your current health condition.

What is it exactly that you may feel? The list can be lengthy and varies from person to person; but most commonly people will feel more energetic and less fatigued, and will experience less digestive problems.

Optional, but beneficial

You may opt to do a LRA test. You will receive a test kit and someone local (your physician, a nurse or a phlebotomist) will have to draw some blood. The blood samples are mailed to a laboratory where your blood is introduced to 100-400+ food items, molds and colorings.

Your report will list the highly reactive food items and discuss in detail their origin, possible source of exposure, and plan of action. Many of these highly reactive food items are wreaking havoc in your body and are therefore slowing down your metabolism. By avoiding these specific food items, you give your body a huge break and reestablish a healthy metabolism, which in turn will facilitate your weight loss efforts.

Also, if possible, I advise you to find out if someone in your local area has an InBody520 to conduct a Body Composition Analysis (BCA). Call around since some gyms or doctor's offices may have one OR contact www.biospaceamerica.com and they may be able to locate the nearest provider for you.

The BCA will give you accurate measurements of percentage of body fat and segmental lean muscle mass. You will be able to follow your progress and make sure you lose body fat, NOT valuable muscle tissue or water.

Good luck! Actually, you don't need any luck, you just need to follow all of the above instructions step-by-step and accurately. The better you follow the plan, the better your results...it's that simple!

Good to know... Health Freedom, LLC donates net income from supplements to CHILDREN INCORPORATED, INC. Every single time you or someone else purchases a supplement online, you are HELPING KIDS in need. Is that AWESOME or what? I thought you may want to know...

12.7 Key Points

Obesity has become an EPIDEMIC. It's a bitter irony that as developing countries continue their efforts to reduce hunger, some are also facing the opposing problem of obesity.

Both the hungry and the obese are weakened by a lack of vitamins, minerals and many essential micronutrients.

The mass produced, synthetic foods we consume today are loaded with preservatives, colorings, chemical toxins, carcinogens, hormones and antibiotics AND are also deprived of essential nutrients. Our body does NOT get the essential nutrients we need from the food we consume, resulting in obesity and disease.

Obesity is associated with many health risks, including heart disease, diabetes, cancer and death. Our society equates thinness with physical attractiveness and therefore people who are overweight tend to feel unattractive.

Genetics play a role in obesity BUT are a lame excuse for being obese or overweight since we can CONTROL our weight by modifying eating habits and physical activity.

Common causes of obesity are bad eating habits, lack of activity, lack of sleep, hormone imbalances and prescription drugs. We already know the cause of any so called disease, including obesity: toxemia.

Surgical treatment options are ONLY recommended if one's body weight is in excess of over 100 pounds, if co-morbidities threaten the client's life, and only if all other more conservative measures failed.

Many non-surgical treatment options including very low calorie diets (VLCD), drug therapy, hCG-injections and many supplements are NOT proven effective at all OR are detrimental to your health.

Metabolic Syndrome is best treated with a sensible weight loss program and the Glycemic Index (GI) of fruits, vegetables and grains is lower than the GI of meats and dairy.

Only 3% of popular diets and weight loss programs on the market are successful. The USDA and American Cancer Institute agree that these popular diets and weight loss programs are ALL low calorie diets and pose a health hazard to the consumer because of the unbalanced food-intake approach.

Most popular diets and weight loss programs recommend a daily caloric intake well below average intake, resulting in short-term weight loss. 97% of participants regain the weight after discontinuing these diets. The actual weight that is lost with most popular diets is water weight and lean muscle tissue, NOT fat!

Another contributing factor to the very poor success rate of these popular diets is the fact that they all are 'One-Size-Fits-All' approaches, lacking individualization.

Our SWL (Sensible Weight Loss) plan is exactly the same as the ACTION PLAN to regain control of your health in the back of this book. By living C.L.E.A.N. you automatically address toxemia, the cause of all so called disease including obesity and being overweight. That's it.

However, if losing weight is a primary emphasis we recommended a few things in this chapter that may assist you further and facilitate your weight loss efforts.

Chapter 13 – Behavior Modification

All of us exhibit many bad lifestyle habits or perversions, including but not limited to poor food choices, consuming unnatural foods and drinks, drinking unclean water and breathing unclear air, lack of sunshine, uncontrolled emotions, stress of various types, lack of rest and sleep, overstimulation and overwork, overindulgences of all kinds, lack of activity and exercise, use of stimulants and so on.

Many of these bad habits are actually addictions, even when many of them are not recognized as such in the current medical world. One of the addictions we all are guilty of is FOOD.

In order to REGAIN CONTROL OF OUR HEALTH, we need to break these bad habits and incorporate good, healthy lifestyle changes.

To guarantee long lasting success in obtaining and maintaining optimal health, it's paramount that we understand more about what HABITS are and HOW we can change them.

13.1 About Habits & Behavior

In behavior modification theory, all behavior is defined as being externally controlled by aspects of the environment. In this sense, both the inside and outside of our body constitutes an environment. For example, behaviorists believe that if a person sees a lion and runs away, he is not running because he is 'scared'. Instead, he is running because those that did not run in the past died, and therefore the urge to run is a result of the survival of those that ran and lived to pass on their genes.

In addition, the subjective feeling of being 'scared' is considered a flight or fight reflex, not an emotion. The heart races and adrenaline increases as the central nervous system reacts to the 'environment' of the body. Therefore, anything a person does, from snoring to talking, can be target for behavior modification.

Feedback

Like the definition of behavior, the concept of positive and negative feedback is used differently in behavior modification than in everyday language. Anything that increases a behavior is considered positive feedback or reinforcement and anything that decreases behavior is considered negative feedback or punishment. Positive feedback refers to something added to the environment and negative feedback refers to something that is taken away.

An example of positive feedback might be giving a child a hug when he or she does a good job or turning off an annoying sound when the child does a good job. An example of negative feedback is making a child do extra chores after he or she does something bad or taking away the child's favorite toy when he or she is bad.

Conditioning

To modify behavior, good behavior must receive positive feedback and poor behavior must receive negative feedback. It's a simple system of bonuses and consequences. Bonuses alone are not effective, and con-sequences without bonuses aren't result promoting either.

Behaviors themselves are typically broken down into components so that the individual gets reinforced for every action that more closely approximates the desired behavior.

For example, if one overeats we can define the different components of overeating for that individual. Let's assume this individual eats 3 meals per day, one of them fast food, eats too fast, eats when worrying, eats when seeing food in the kitchen, and indulges on a second plate when food tastes good. In order to change this behavior of overeating we need to reinforce every component, with either negative and/or positive feedback. If the individual skips breakfast we may add $2 to his account for a new pair of running shoes or if he or she skipped breakfast for the entire week, a deserved relaxing day at the beach or a free yoga class may be considered positive feedback. If the individual drives by McDonalds and orders a supersized Big Mac meal, T.V. or computer time is taken away for the day or an extra 30 minutes of exercise is due. Don't reinforce good behavior with bad behavior and vice versa. For example, don't reward good behavior with a Big Mac Meal or with not having to exercise.

As each component changes from bad to good, the bad behavior or habit will gradually evolve from bad to good.

Although the concept of behavior modification may seem theoretically complicated, its real life application is actually quite simple. If a person is reinforced every single time he or she does something good, eventually the reinforcement loses its power. When using behavior modification with the general population, such as your coworkers or family, initially reinforce what you want with consistency, then as they start to respond, change your schedule of reinforcement to every third time they do what you want. After a while, change it again to every fifth time. For example, if you want your husband to open the car door for you then first arrange a situation where he has to open the door, such as holding a huge bag of groceries. Once he opens the door the first time, look at him in the eye and tell him what an amazing person he is. Don't explicitly connect the comment to the door opening, but do make sure that the comment directly follows the desired behavior. It might take some time but eventually he will open the car door on a fairly consistent basis. Once that happens do not compliment him every time. Instead, change from a modification stage to a 'maintenance' stage and compliment on average every third to seventh time he opens the door.

Habits

Habits, good or bad, are formed by repetition. We will address common habits in this chapter, but let's use eating habits as an easy example. Eating habits are no exception: they are formed by repetition as any other habit. If you are in the habit of snacking when you watch TV, you were reinforcing that habit until finally it became a part of you. Other habits are formed in the same way. Some of these habits are: eating while reading, eating when coming home from work or your office, eating while cooking dinner, etc.

We also find that a certain mood or emotion, and circumstances can cause us to eat ...even if we are not hungry. For example: anxiety, anger, boredom, fatigue, happiness, loneliness, and nervousness all may trigger an eating response. The list is endless. Habits are hard to break. We must not only break old habits, but we must make it our goal to form new ones in the same manner...which is through REPETITION. We must then make some daily commitments. We must work to meet these commitments each day whether you feel like it or not, until the habit is changed. Your daily commitments will help you form good habits.

Resisting temptation is difficult. However, if you succeed in resisting the first time, it becomes easier to resist the next time. Before long, you will have formed the good habit of resisting temptation every time it confronts you.

Because of the human weaknesses mentioned, we must use what has become known as behavior modification techniques.

13.2 Behavior Modification Plan

Behavior modification simply means changing your behavior. The behavior modification techniques work only if you commit to them and consistently repeat them, so that they become a new habit and part of a new you.

In order to be successful, we need design an individual PLAN.

Here's your 3 step ACTION PLAN to succeed in breaking those poor habits and acquiring some good new habits:

Knowledge: you need to identify these poor habits and acknowledge you possess them. You need to pinpoint each cause or situation that elicits a bad habit, and record them.

Skill: you need the skill to transform these poor habits into healthy new habits. We will provide you with some sample behavior modification techniques in the next few pages.

Willpower: that's the only component of success we can NOT help you with. That's something you need to bring to the table! You need to decide that whether regaining optimal health and being happy is important enough or not.

For each and every one of the poor or bad habits you recorded for yourself, you need to design a behavior modification technique. If the technique doesn't work, you need to design another one.

Once you stick with the technique and the commitment it takes, you will surprised how fast a bad habit actually can turn into a good habit. It's silly to put a number on things like this, but if you deny a bad habit 12 times on average, it will have turned into a good habit and then you are 'stuck' with that good habit. You no longer feel you have to commit or sacrifice because it's a habit now, a part of you, and you feel good doing it.

A good behavior modification plan has the following characteristics:

Sets reasonable goals which are challenging but attainable. These need to be written down in a diary.

Includes frequent contact with peers or a knowledgeable health care provider.

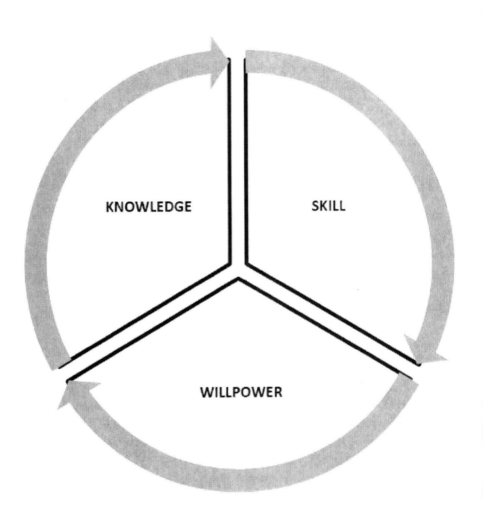

Illustration 23 – Habits

Includes record keeping and self-monitoring. You must write down your victories and failures on a daily basis and set new short-term goals if indicated to overcome those failures. These failures are just road blocks we have to overcome.

Includes rewards for achieving goals. Rewards can be set individually or decided by children and parents together, and should revolve around something that encourages positive behavior. For example, giving sporting equipment as a reward may encourage more physically active behavior. Avoid using food or bad stuff as a reward.

Encourages verbal praise.

Educates about health and body image, overcomes misconceptions and myths and false schools of thought, and therefore facilitates turning bad habits into realistic and positive ones.

Develops a social support network (family, friends and neighbors) that can encourage healthy eating and exercise habits.

13.3 Behavior Modification Techniques

Below are more sample techniques that you may use to convert bad into good habits and lifestyle changes. Often, you may have to tweak them to customize them, to make them workable for you.

Stimulus Control:

Remove cues for inappropriate behaviors and increase cues for appropriate behavior, e.g. remove cues to refrain from bringing ice cream into the house and increase cues to exercise more such as putting the exercise bike where it can be more easily seen and used.

Cognitive restructuring:

Learn to counter negative self-statements with positive ones. For example, instead of "I ate that candy so now I might as well eat the whole box," learn to say to yourself, "Eating candy is not a big deal. I'll just make sure I follow my meal plan closely for the rest of the day."

A sample list:

1. Eat when you are truly hungry, don't eat when you are not hungry. Therefore, plan your meals (just one good meal a day is recommended) and have two or three planned snacks (fruit, health bar, veggie juice) available daily. When tempted to grab for food because you smell it or see it, just ask yourself: "Am I hungry"? If not, don't eat. Don't confuse appetite for hunger.

2. Prolong your meals by eating slowly. Putting down your eating utensil between each bite and not picking up your eating utensil until you have swallowed the bite; hesitating between bites, even if you're eating finger foods. This technique prevents overeating since your body now has the time to signal you when you are full.

3. Choose a specific place in your home or office to eat all of your meals. This will become your 'designated eating place' and should not be changed. Try not to eat at your desk at work. This would make you prone to eat all day long (even when you are not hungry) and not just at meal time.

4. Do not do anything except eat when you sit down for a meal. Do not eat while you read, watch TV, talk on the phone, work, etc. Make yourself aware of the food you are eating. Focus on the conversation and enjoy your meal.

5. Do not keep food in any room in your house except the kitchen. Do not keep food such as cookies out on the counters. Do not store these items in 'see-through' containers.

6. Do not buy junk food. NOBODY needs it! Replace refined

snacks that lack vitamins, fiber, minerals, and phytochemicals with fruits and vegetables. Drink plenty of WATER to keep yourself hydrated, and remember that water fills you up and is calorie free!

7. If possible, serve individual plates from the stove and do not serve family style on the table. If you finish your plate, ask yourself if you are still hungry...if not, don't get seconds (I know it's difficult when the food smells good). Serve your meals on a smaller plate; you may not need that larger portion in order to feel 'really' full.

8. Develop a habit of leaving at least one bite of each item on your plate. If you can master this, it becomes easier to stop eating when you feel full. You will be used to leaving food on your plate... and that's just fine!

9. Plan your meals for the week, make a list and go shopping only once for the whole week. Make sure you have a balanced plan (for example: fish on Monday, pasta on Tuesday, soup and salad on Wednesday, chicken or meat on Thursday etc.). I also recommend to go shopping after you had a meal so that you are less likely to load up your shopping cart with junk, which is another reason to make a list. Do yourself a favor and SAVE some significant money this way! You will need this money later for some high quality supplements and for the – unfortunately - more expensive, organic whole foods. However, you will probably be eating far less.

10. Also, make sure you work on reducing stress and try to RELAX! Overeating is often caused by stress and over-scheduling. We also recommend you keep a record of your food intake and exercise.

All of the above are eating techniques that aid in behavior modification. Other behavior modification techniques not related to eating are to substitute activity for eating, which means exactly what it says: substitute another activity for between meal snacking. If you are in the habit of going straight to the kitchen and eating every time you walk in the house, try to change this habit by going to another room of the house when you come home. Delay going into the kitchen until the desire to eat is gone. When you are tempted to eat, try to substitute that temptation with activities such as walking, checking your e-mail, drinking water, playing with the kids or dog, calling a friend, writing a letter, reading a book, taking a bath, gardening, painting or any other activity or hobby.

I had a client who was always stressed at work when the boss was around (a few times per week). After their usual confrontation, my client would get up from her desk and walk over to the vending machines. She would buy a soda and snickers bar ...and vent. She consumed this JUNK not because she was hungry (she just had breakfast at home, which she shouldn't), but because it was her way of coping with the stresses at work (other people may go outside and smoke a cigarette).

In order to change this 'bad' habit and form a new habit, we had to identify the problem and acknowledge that the junk food consumption was a mood-related impulse. We decided to substitute the walk to the vending machine with a walk around the office building. When my client would go to the vending machine and stand in front of it, she would have to ask herself: "Am I REALLY hungry or do I just want something to deal with the stress?". If she wasn't hungry, she should save her money! Also, we decided that my client had to bring some pure water to work and drink it whenever stressed and unable to go for a walk. Water fills you up, detoxifies the body and has no calories.

My client has had no soda or snicker bar for over 6 months now, and saved lots of money too ($360 so far).

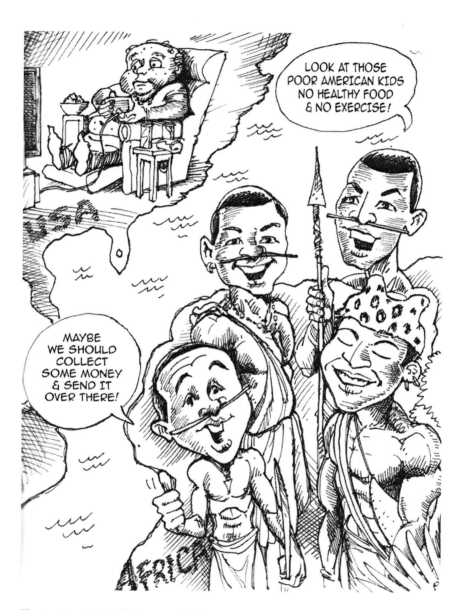

Illustration 24 – USA versus Africa

11. Limiting television/computer/video game time (including cell phone use, texting, social media) to only 30 minutes or an hour or so per day. The strategy of reducing your or your child's sedentary behavior can be more effective than a strategy of promoting physical activity.

12. Observe weekend eating. People tend to eat more on the weekends.

13. Limit (or avoid, if possible) take out, fast foods, high-sugar snacks, commercial packaged snacks, soda, and sugar-sweetened beverages (including too much juice).

14. Let children choose their own food portions. One study indicated that children naturally ate 25% less when they chose their own portion size. When they were given larger portions their bite sizes were larger and they ate more.

15. Do not criticize a child for being overweight. It does not help, and such attitudes could put children at risk for eating disorders, which are equal or even greater dangers to their health.

16. For young children, try the traffic-light diet. Food is designated with stoplight colors depending on their high caloric content: Green for go (low calories); yellow for "eat with caution" (medium calories); red for "stop" (high calories).

17. Never eat during, immediately before or after physical or mental activity.

18. Never eat when sick, in pain or mental discomfort.

19. Another way of slowing down your eating process is to properly masticate and insalivate. Actively count the number of times you chew on a bite of food (20-30 times is ideal).

20. Do not drink with meals. Only drink water 20 minutes before a meal or 3-4 hours after a meal.

21. Only drink when thirsty. Do not confuse appetite for thirst. When you think you are thirsty just ask yourself if you are really thirsty or just have a desire for a drink.

22. Start combining your foods the right way. Only combine protein with green, non-starchy veggies AND combine carbohydrates with starchy veggies.

23. Eat fruit by itself, never with or after a meal. Don't combine sweet fruits with acid fruits and eat melons alone.

24. Limit your consumption of sweet fruits to one piece a day.

25. Make a plan (and write it down) and gradually incorporate more alkaline foods into your diet, while avoiding more and more acid foods and drinks.

26. Buy pH-strips and monitor your alkalinity.

27. Avoid the consumption of yeast products such as breads, pastries, bakery goods, and beer.

28. Avoid the consumption of fungus and molds, which are abundant in algae (seaweed), cheese (dairy products) and mushrooms. Mushrooms are carcinogenic.

29. It's time to ban coffee, vinegar, soy sauce and sodas entirely from your diet.

30. Consuming dead meat with denatured protein and injected with colorings only overloads the digestive system. Limit meat and derive your protein from more natural sources such as beans and peas.

31. Always opt for raw, fresh, organic, and local food and

avoid overcooking food.

32. Duck-tape the door of your microwave or throw it out (don't donate it or you are committing nutritional homicide). A microwave nukes your food and kills the good and the bad, leaving even healthy foods empty in essential nutrients.

33. Replace your plastic ware in the kitchen with metal or glass.

34. Vacuum often, ban smoking indoors (you shouldn't be around smokers anyway), minimize the use of candles and wood fires, and use the exhaust fans in the kitchen, bath, and laundry areas.

35. Test your home for radon gas, which can cause lung cancer (test kits cost about $15). This is usually only necessary when you live in an older construction home.

36. Minimize the risk of deadly carbon monoxide gas by properly maintaining heating equipment, wood stoves, fireplaces, chimneys, and vents. Install carbon-monoxide alarms on all levels of your home.

37. Don't idle your car, run fuel-burning power equipment, or light a barbecue grill in your garage, basement, or in confined spaces near your home.

38. Don't store chemicals, solvents, glues, or pesticides in your house.

39. Use natural household products versus chemical ones, including detergents, soaps, cosmetic products etc. Many of these products release toxic gasses, e.g. hairsprays.

40. Consider a commercially available air filter designed to improve the quality of air indoors. It may be a great investment since your health (and that one of others) is priceless.

41. Most of us are air-conditioning junkies. Air conditioning in the house or office, or the car is yet another bad and (most of the time) unnecessary habit. Lifeless, reused air - cold or hot - doesn't serve any good purpose. But save some money and only use your A/C when extremely cold or hot. Open those windows in your house or office, and when driving a car open the roof, sunroof or windows and have the fresh air circulate.

42. Keep some green plants indoors. As you know plants and trees exchange CO_2 (Carbon Dioxide) for O_2 (Oxygen). Therefore, a few green plants in your home or office provide you with some fresh oxygen.

43. Open windows if you can, as much as possible, and let fresh air circulate. If you open a few you really get some circulation of fresh air (unless you live right by a busy highway or next to an industrial plant of course).

44. Spend more time outdoors. Go and eat your lunch (if you have any) outdoors, go for a short walk during a break or lunch time. Don't stay indoors.

45. If you exercise, maybe consider outdoor activities or suggest to your yoga instructor to do some outdoor classes.

46. On your days off or in the evenings, go sit outside to read a book or to relax or to have dinner with your family. The kids will love it also. Make some trips to parks and springs (lots of fresh air from trees and plants), or go to the beach if you are close (fresh ocean air).

47. Learn to breathe properly and maximize oxygenation through diaphragmatic breathing at least 3 times/day and whenever indicated.

48. Reduce and recycle. Avoid bagging your groceries in plastic bags, use actual towels versus paper towel rolls.

49. Plant an extra tree in your yard.

50. Walk or use the bicycle whenever you can. You will be more active and simultaneously reduce pollution.

51. Use air filters and replace them regularly.

52. Learn about signs of dehydration and restore the proper feeling of thirst.

53. Avoid buying and drinking bottled water and install a home purification system which will save you lots of money.

54. Incorporate the many ways to conserve water in the home. Make a check-list and get it done.

55. Only drink clean, pure, alkaline water. Squeeze some lemon in your water if you like.

56. Assure adequate rest and sleep in your life. Record your current habits and change them if needed. Rest and sleep are vital for repair and energy.

57. Learn about fasting and incorporate fasting in your new, healthy lifestyle.

58. No enemas.

59. Learn our detoxification program and make it an active part of your healthy life. Incorporate more detoxifying herbs and plants into your diet.

60. Learn about your emotions and feelings and how they affect your body and mind. Record the situations that elicit these emotions.

61. Take ownership of your emotions.

62. Acquire the skills to control your feelings and emotions.

63. Learn HOW to be proactive, change your perspectives, be optimistic, not worry, and acquire a YES-attitude.

64. Start helping others and pay-it-forward.

65. Use adaptogens to facilitate managing your stress.

66. Consider bio-identical hormones to restore hormonal imbalances.

67. Record your perversions (and don't be shy about it, we all possess them) and make a specific plan to abolish them.

68. Make a list of items and situations that contribute to overstimulation and overindulgences, including but not limited to excess food and drinks, light, sound, technology (cell phone, TV, computer etc.), emotions, activity and overwork, play, party, self-pity, jealousy, drugs, stimulants, and destructive behavior.

69. Live for service.

70. Practice hygiene exercise daily.

71. Learn new, fun activities.

72. Correct deformities and asymmetries with corrective exercises.

73. Learn the right type of exercise to obtain your goal.

74. Too little or too much activity or exercise is detrimental to health.

75. Athletes should be aware of the ramifications of their excess exercise and counteract with adequate rest and

sleep, and a huge amount of antioxidants.

76. If you are obese or overweight, incorporate the Sensible Weight Loss program which is the same, exact action plan as to regain control of your health. Learn the extra things you can do to facilitate your efforts to re-establish an optimal body composition.

77. Learn how to successfully incorporate behavior modification techniques.

78. Realize that supplements don't replace C.L.E.A.N. living, they just 'supplement' or assist in optimal health.

79. Learn the criteria to select the right supplements and don't waste your money and health on the 'bad' ones.

80. Avoid milk and dairy products at all cost. Dairy is poison and doesn't have any health benefits.

81. Don't worry about big pharmaceutical hoaxes such as cholesterol. Cholesterol is a vital substance. Learn more about cholesterol later in this book. The advice your doctor gives you and the statistics he throws at you in regards to an increased risk for stroke and heart attack are unsubstantiated.

82. NO soy or soy products, NO GMO.

83. Realize that doctors, drugs, surgeries and diagnostic tests are contributing to the disease process and need to be avoided (except in emergencies). Make a list of all the situations you or loved-ones have been in that worsened the condition (make sure you have enough paper).

84. Understand that ONLY the body heals and that any interference is ignorance. We just need to place the body in the RIGHT conditions to heal.

85. As humans we have the freedom to choose our response. Choose the RIGHT response from now on.

86. If you are not sure about the right response, ask what Mother Nature would have us do or what animals in the wild would do.

87. Know the C.L.E.A.N. principles and incorporate them; continue to improve upon them.

88. Read this book over and over, and fine-tune your behavior modification plan and techniques.

89. Incorporate the Action Plan in this book entirely and find inner peace, health and happiness. It's the normal way of living.

90. Share this user manual with others.

Your task is to set-up an individualized behavior modification plan with challenging but attainable goals, and design your own behavior modification techniques, including the deadlines, positive and negative feedback (which bonuses or rewards and consequences, and when), and record them.

You will then record daily progress (victories and failures) into a diary and revise techniques if applicable.

It may take several hours of mental work, but it certainly will be worth it. A NEW YOU is waiting!

13.4 Key Points

Behavior Modification is an essential part of regaining control of your health and obtaining happiness, and assures that the results are lasting.

Behavior Modification techniques are tools to assist you in transforming some 'bad' habits into some 'good' habits.

Knowledge, skill and willpower are the 3 components that one needs to address in order to successfully acquire new habits.

You will need to design and customize your own Behavior Modification Plan. Make sure to incorporate the characteristics of a SUCCESSFUL Behavior Modification Plan.

Chapter 14 – The Truth about Supplements

There are so *many* products (miracle cures, secret potions, elixirs, silver bullets) that *hit* the marketplace daily. Everyone has 'the' product that will cure all ills. ALL have good 'stories', but are NOT backed up by FACTS.

Furthermore, supplements are exactly what's in their name: they supplement. Without a solid base of C.L.E.A.N. living and healthy eating habits including fresh wholesome foods, supplements are virtually useless.

Nutrients NEVER work alone. Nutrients work as a team such as a cascade of antioxidants is needed to neutralize a cascade of free radicals. Nutrients in our body work in synergy. A single nutrient supplement won't benefit our body or our health. Kobe Bryant or LeBron James may be the absolute best basketball players but they wouldn't have a chance without their team mates against any team whatsoever. Agreed? As such will a single nutrient, even if proven highly effective in a laboratory, not render any positive effect in a real life situation without the support of a wide variety of other natural nutrients and wholefoods.

What are supplements?

Supplements are fragmented foods that have been isolated and separated from other nutrients, and never will work well on their own. All nutrients in wholefoods work synergistically for maximum absorption. Supplements are therefore incomplete foods that offer

343

incomplete nutrients.

Ideally, we do eat wholesome foods and these should provide us with enough potent and essential nutrients. I personally believe that in a perfect world that would be true, but in today's environment it's almost impossible to get all the nutrients, even from organic wholefoods. Why is that you may ask? First of all, our soils are depleted from nutrients and therefore the fresh vegetables and fruits grown on these soils will lack some essential nutrients. Next, many nutrients are lost during the time between harvesting the crops and consuming them.

Therefore I believe that adding high quality, proven supplements to a wholesome food diet is beneficial. However, the thought that supplements replace healthy living or the consumption of healthy foods is absurd. Supplements ONLY will be beneficial while LIVING C.L.E.A.N.

14.1 Do We Need Supplements?

Yes, we do! And anyone who disagrees is totally NUTS, or is living in another time (before industrialization). We know that there's too many of us on this small – so called blue – planet that loses all its green. Mass production of food for the masses has depleted the nutrients we need. Commercial foods are not only high in calories but are severely short in vital nutrients. Proper supplementation is a life insurance policy. However, we need to carefully select the RIGHT insurance policy, since many of them are just scams.

Sure, whole foods can give us all we need, but their availability is limited and even these whole foods lost much of their valuable nutrients before we ingest them. Did you know that when you pick an apple from a tree,

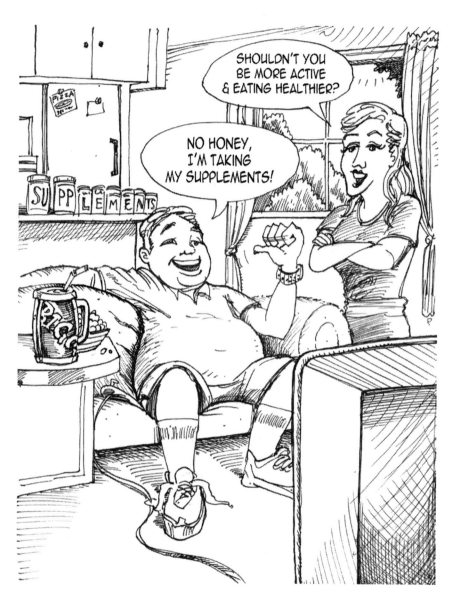

Illustration 25 – Supplements

50% of all the enzymes are DEAD within 30 minutes? Did you know that when you store asparagus for just 1 week, 90% of its vitamin C is gone? So, how many LIVE nutrients remain in your whole foods and organic foods? Hard to say, but I'm sure you don't get all the nutrients you need; it's just impossible TODAY (unless you move your family to an untouched pristine area... good luck).

Furthermore, most of our soil lacks essential nutrients so the plants and foods sprouting and growing from the soil are missing some essential nutrients. How come our soil is depleted you may ask? Well, commercial farms have been relying largely on chemical fertilizers to grow their crops. During the late 40's, farmers found that 3 minerals left over from the post-war armaments industry produced fine-looking crops. These 3 minerals are nitrogen (N), phosphorus (P) and potassium (K). The subsequent use of these minerals quickly replaced traditional mulching and the use of manure (feces). Over time, the NPK-fertilizers caused depletion of many micro-nutrients in our soils.

I'm not telling you not to buy whole foods and organic foods though...I buy them almost exclusively. Why? They are still a lot more nutritious than processed, synthetic foods AND our body recognizes these 'whole foods' from nature and therefore is able to absorb them. They are FREE of pesticides, harmful chemicals, toxins, colorings and preservatives. That alone is a GREAT reason to buy whole foods and organic foods!

As we learned we are also exposed to an onslaught of daily toxins as never before. Therefore we need to neutralize and eliminate more toxins than someone who would live in a pristine area.

It's obvious that besides living C.L.E.A.N. we DO need SUPPLEMENTS to obtain all necessary nutrients our body and mind need to regain and maintain optimal health.

14.2 Criteria to Select the Right Supplements

Let's learn what supplements you should avoid because they are unsafe, don't get absorbed, don't have any proven health benefits and are guaranteed to impair your health and waste your money, and which ones you should select.

The most important criteria when selecting a nutritional supplement:

1. Is The Supplement Safe To Take?

Supplements are simply an encapsulated group of ingredients taken from plants, or created in a laboratory. Inside the capsule can be many harmful substances – both immediate hazards and accumulative ones.

For years, the FDA (who else) advanced the argument that vitamin supplements and herbal products are unsafe but facts and statistics show clearly that fewer deaths are caused by dietary supplements than by air fresheners (LMAO). It pays to further state that NOT a single death has been reported of an adverse reaction or unintended cause from the consumption of dietary supplements. Reports show that every decade an average of 14 UNINTENTIONAL deaths occur due to the use of supplements (accidental infant poisonings) versus the annual (not decade) + 110,000 deaths caused by simply taking pharmaceutical drugs. Yes, they kill with a vengeance.

Considering that almost 50% of Americans consume one or more supplements on a daily basis, for an annual consumption of over 50 billion USD, this is a safety record without equal. However, as I'll explain later, most of these supplements are scams and do rob essential nutrients from our body while they should add them.

There are few regulations in regards to this whole business of supplements, but the better and more responsible companies and manufacturers voluntarily acquire the necessary licenses and accreditations to prove their commitment and show us they have superior products.

In the U.S. the manufacturer is responsible for determining that the supplements it produces are safe and that any claims made about the product are substantiated. However, the burden of proof for unsafe products and false or misleading labeling lies entirely with the FDA.

Of course, this corrupt agency has chosen so far NOT to invoke this authority. Consequently, there are no current U.S. regulations that enforce minimum standards of practice, no requirements for pre-market approval, no post-market surveillance, no product licensing, and no site licensing for the manufacturing of supplements.

Current reference standards are completely VOLUNTARY. This lack of regulatory oversight has created a market open to abuse, false and misleading marketing and labeling, misinterpretation, unsafe products, and less than optimal products. Thanks again FDA for protecting public health. BRAVO!

So, buyer be aware. That's why I have to educate you and make sure that you consume the RIGHT supplements that facilitate achieving and maintaining optimal health versus robbing you of essential nutrients and money.

The real issue with supplements becomes the manner in which the final product is manufactured. Purity, potency, identity, safety, and quality control are of utmost importance if you plan to take a supplement on a daily basis.

Check the source of the ingredients since many herbs from China and other regions in the world may be contaminated. In commercial cultivation, organo-chlorine pesticides and other toxins are often used. Make sure the supplements or products you consume are TESTED for contamination.

It's also a fact that with the majority of supplements the label does not match the content. That's a scary fact. If what's on the label is not in the bottle, what is then?

The best way to assure a safe product is to verify in what type of laboratory the product is manufactured and what licenses and accreditations that laboratory has. Look for GMP (Good Manufacturing Practices) standards, manufacturing regulatory compliance and uncompromising operational practices.

I personally look for the following, among other:

- cGMP's (certified GMP) for nutritional supplements in accordance with USP.

- Registration with NSF International as a GMP manufacturing facility.

- ISO certification and ISO/IEC accreditation of in-house laboratories.

- Veri-Match electronic label match to ensure content accuracy or a Certificate of Analysis which verifies that a third party takes a sample of the product and compares it to the original.

- VCP (Vendor Certification Program) to ensure raw material quality.

- FDA audit compliant (yes, the FDA contributes somehow in this situation while ignoring its primary purpose: protect the public).

- Approved facility to produce Certified Organic products.

2. Is The Supplement Absorbed?

Supplements (as well as food) travel from the stomach, to the intestines, to the blood stream and to their final destination – if everything goes right. There is a lot that can go wrong. Evaluate your supplements, their delivery 'vehicle' or technology, and make sure you're not wasting your money on supplements that have a poor absorption.

The ingredients in your supplement need to be organic whole foods or natural ingredients. Synthetically derived vitamins, minerals and other nutrients have a very poor absorption rate because our body does NOT recognize them. When our body doesn't recognize man-made substances it needs to utilize its own resources such as vitamins, minerals and other essential nutrients to break those man-made ones down.

THAT'S WHY THE CONSUMPTION OF THE MAJORITY OF SUPPLEMENTS ON THE MARKET RESULTS IN A NEGATIVE NUTRIENT BALANCE.

It's a sad fact. People are trying to be healthier and recognize the importance of supplements, and when they purchase these supplements they don't realize they rob the body from essential nutrients. Most of these supplements impair health, not promote health.

Most manufacturers use man-made, synthetic ingredients in their supplements. For example, many manufacturers use metallic minerals in their supplements because they are cheaper than their natural counterparts. These metallic minerals have an absorption rate of ONLY 8%. What a waste. Not only do we have a very poor absorption, our body utilized more nutrients in the digestive efforts of these metallic minerals than they produce. We end-up with a negative nutrient balance. It's more healthful to flush these supplements versus swallowing them.

Minerals derived from plants on the other hand are absorbed by our body for almost 100%.

Disintegration is another aspect we need to pay close attention to and is one of the most basic quality control parameters in the supplement market today. If a tablet, pill, or capsule cannot disintegrate, the individual nutrients within it are unable to dissolve into the intestinal fluids and thus unable to be absorbed by the body. Hence nurses often call supplements 'bed pan bullets'.

The 'vehicle' of a supplement or product refers to the medium in which the ingredients or nutrients are carried. Good 'vehicles' have health benefits themselves, optimize and synergize the nutrients, and facilitate the absorption of these nutrients. A 'good' vehicle is crucial since it is responsible for bringing the nutrients to their final destination: the cells.

Aloe vera (the inner gel and not the outer rind) for example is commonly used as a 'vehicle' in natural supplements. Aloe vera contains over 75 nutrients and 200 active compounds, including 20 minerals, 18 amino-acids, and 12 vitamins. Aloe itself has multiple health benefits and optimizes the absorption of other natural nutrients.

3. Are There Proven Health Benefits? This is a matter of potency and identity.

Companies will promote superior ingredients, liquid vitamins being better than capsules, capsules being better than tablets, etc. Don't be distracted by the hype! Bottom line – Are there proven health benefits from taking the supplements? Be aware that there is a difference between proven ingredients and a proven product and isolate a good nutrition company as a consumer.

Many companies will brag about the ingredients of their product and use reports, research and claims made regarding these ingredients. BE AWARE though! Often, their product contains a cheap rip-off of that original, natural, beneficial ingredient OR their ingredients are not plant-derived or not authenticated. In other words: they don't work.

Make sure the ingredients are all natural and organic, and come from parts all over the world where they are originally grown.

The organic foods or ingredients have to come directly from the pristine areas where these plants and foods ORIGINALLY grow. Many natural foods, plants and herbs are cultivated in areas other than the original one. The soil and climate are usually different and this alters the properties of the food, plant or herb.

Furthermore, it's important to know that certain constituents of foods and plants, which carry the beneficial health properties are ONLY found in certain parts of that food or plant. For example, the beneficial properties of Aloe vera are found in the nutritious inner gel of this cactus-like species and not in the outer rind of the leaf which is commonly used to scam the public.

And there is more to know. The maturation stage of each food, plant or herb also dictates its properties. A great example is South African

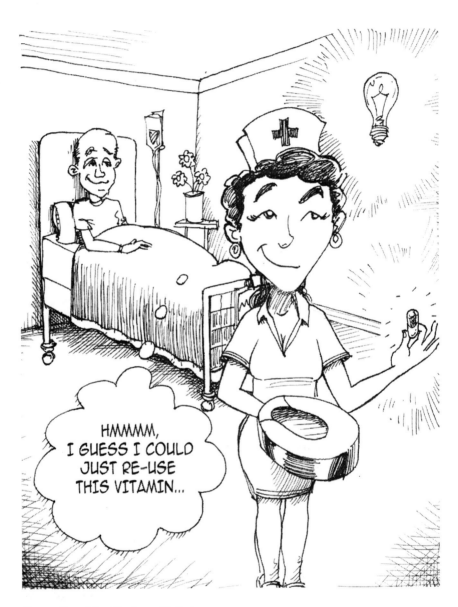

Illustration 26 – Bedpan Bullets

Hoodia which is known to be a potent, all natural appetite suppressant. This plant grows in the South African desert, and matures in 5 to 7 years at which age it contains the P57 molecule that carries the appetite curbing properties. In short, for the Hoodia to be effective, origin and maturity need to be authenticated. Unfortunately, most Hoodia sold on the market today is not from the South African desert and is prematurely picked.

4. Optimal Dosage

The Food and Nutrition Board of the Institute of Medicine, US National Academy of Sciences, has been setting national standards for nutrient intake for over 70 years. These standards are collectively known as Recommended Dietary Allowances (RDA's). The RDA's were developed during WWII to establish baselines for nutrient intake. These baselines were to provide guidance for the development of wartime rationing measures among the armed forces and civilians.

Therefore, these RDA's represent the absolute minimum requirements to avoid sickness and disease associated with acute nutritional deficiencies. The RDA's were NOT designed to address the levels of nutrient intake required for OPTIMAL health. These standards represent the dietary and lifestyle choices of the sick, unhealthy, bald, fatigued, fat couch potatoes.

Pressure from government and pharmaceutical lobbyists has kept these dangerously low levels of nutrient intake current.

Advances in nutritional science have led to the attempt to determine optimal levels of nutrient intake as a means of preventing degenerative disease. The Dietary Reference Intakes (DRI's) are a step in the right direction but still fall short from optimal levels.

As far as I'm concerned, one can never have enough essential nutrients. Vitamins, minerals, enzymes and other nutrients derived from nature are the fuel for our body and mind. Each and every one of our trillions of cells uses these essential nutrients and coverts them into energy. As established multiple times in this book already, we need lots of energy to maintain normal metabolism and continue to effectively eliminate toxins from our body in order to avoid toxemia, the cause of all so called disease.

It certainly would be recommended to have an energy reserve also, in times when extra expenditure may be necessary, e.g. to fight a pathogen or cold, or to overcome extra physical or mental work, or to compensate for lack of rest and sleep, or to deal with an episode of overstimulation and overindulgences.

In short, besides living C.L.E.A.N. and consuming whole foods, one should supplement with optimal doses of essential nutrients. Be aware that these optimal doses are much higher than any RDA's or DRI's.

A good friend of mine called me up not too long ago and asked if it's dangerous to have too much vitamin B12 because her blood test showed that her levels were far above the range. Conventional doctors would recommend discontinuing supplementation because of such test results. Again, they do not know much about health and only pursue a useless understanding of pathology, which doesn't even exist.

I informed my friend that there can't be enough of a good thing, and even if the body wouldn't have any use for it, no harm is done. Now, I believe the body has use for it and if not immediate, the body will convert the nutrients into energy and build an energy reserve.

All the standards designed to interpret lab results are man-made and are not scientifically valid. They are based on bare minimums to survive, not on achieving health. I never get a test done, and I never will... they are just useless and harmful for the healthy. However, they may save the life of someone who was almost dead anyway.

High-dose or better 'optimal' dose supplementing is very beneficial, but only if implemented long-term and consistently. It's not about trying to 'cure' symptoms, but about preventing toxemia.

5. Completeness

A huge flaw of the pharmaceutical companies is that the objective of their clinical trials is to evaluate a single biochemical nutrient for its therapeutic effect on a particular disease or symptom. Once that measurable effect has been established, the drug can be patented and sold to the misinformed public. Billions of dollars are made at the expense of the health of our children, ourselves and our pets.

The fact simply remains that isolating and testing a single nutrient or compound may make for good science in a test tube, but is not valid and realistic when dealing with a complex biological system such as the human body and mind. Our body simply doesn't rely on a single nutrient to prevent or treat disease.

First, there is no disease, only symptoms and symptoms are attempts of the body to regain optimal health. The body does NOT need any interference. Instead, our body uses the synergistic powers that exist between a wide variety of ONLY natural, essential nutrients.

Humans (and animals) require a full range of essential, natural nutrients in a properly balanced and optimal amount in order to support optimal health.

6. Rating Criteria

Besides the criteria to ensure a safe supplement, we have to look at other criteria such as:

completeness, potency, mineral forms, bioactivity of the ingredients, the type of ingredients (natural versus synthetic), the identity of the ingredients, the source of the ingredients, the antioxidant support, the degree in which the supplement supports bone health, cardiovascular health, liver health, metabolic health, ocular health, elimination of toxins, inflammation control, anti-aging, bioflavonoid profile, phenolic profile; and the absence of potential toxicities (vitamin A and iron).

14.3 Top Rated Supplements

A U.S. based company, NutriSearch, has been conducting an independent study in this field for over a decade and has compared over 1600 U.S. and Canadian supplements.

Only 1% of all 1600 supplements received a maximum score. Most supplements score very low, indicating yet again that they are a waste of money and most likely impair health versus improve health.

The companies and products that received a perfect score are the following (listed in the NUTRISEARCH Comparative Guide to Nutritional Supplements, 2011 edition by Lyle MacWilliam, MSc, FP):

USANA Health Sciences (Essentials and HealthPak 100)
TrueStar Health (TrueBASIC Solo and TrueBASIC Plus)
Douglas Laboratories (Ultra Preventative X)
Country Life (Superior)
Creating Wellness Alliance (Vitalize)
Life Extension Foundation (Life Extension Mix)
Rejuvenation Science (Maximum Vitality)
Source Naturals (Elan Vital and Life Force Multiple)
Swanson Lee (Swanson Signature Line Longevital)
Vitamin Research products (Extend Plus)

Please note that these products are all combination packs or multi-component supplements. Single nutrient supplements don't work without a solid base of synergistic nutrients.

Single nutrient supplements may be beneficial in addition to a potent multi-nutrient supplement or combination product.

Once I share with my clients or friends the companies that successfully produce health enhancing supplements, I'm often asked: "so what supplements do you take?".

Well, I don't conduct the research on the 1600 supplements myself (that would take up all my time and cost me) but I have put my confidence in

NutriSearch and I'm well aware on HOW they conduct their studies and what criteria they use to rate the supplements. So what I do is only look at those companies and products that received a perfect score (less than 1% or less than 20 in total).

I private-labeled the Douglas laboratories' supplements (they only sell to health care professionals) so that my patients and clients could use them in their efforts to resolve their medical issues (refer to chapter 16), and I personally use them when indicated. However, my family and I use the LIQUID VEMMA nutritional supplements.

Vemma is a unique, clinically studied, liquid antioxidant formula which contains a full spectrum of vitamins and essential minerals, mangosteen (the "queen of fruits"), organic aloe vera and green tea leaf extract (decaffeinated). I highly recommend these Vemma products to RESTORE your health (Chapter 16) and jump-start your C.L.E.A.N. Living efforts.

The Vemma supplements are tasty and are absorbed much faster and much better than any tablet or capsule (because they are liquid). The Vemma products are manufactured in an FDA-approved laboratory and comply with my personal criteria to select the RIGHT supplement (page 346-355).

The clinical studies conducted on the Vemma products showed an ORAC score of 4800+ which indicates a very high level of antioxidant potency. This scoring system (ORAC or Oxygen Radical Absorbance Capacity) was developed by scientists at the NIH (National Institutes of Health) to measure the antioxidant potency of a food or supplement. Studies also indicate a significant decrease in C-reactive protein after 30 days of use compared to a placebo. C-reactive protein is the number one marker for systemic inflammation in our body.

In short, LIQUID VEMMA effectively addresses the 2 major contributors to TOXEMIA: Systemic inflammation and Free radicals. I strongly suggest you start consuming this very potent liquid antioxidant formula NOW and keep using it DAILY.

14.4 Health 4 Life Supplements

Let's expand some more on the supplements we recommend to regain and maintain optimal health. Remember that supplements alone will NOT obtain optimal health. The action plan in this book, living C.L.E.A.N, is the key to success and happiness. The recommended supplements will not only facilitate your efforts but are a vital key to your success.

Please note that these supplements received a maximum score based on the criteria we discussed earlier in this chapter. They are tested and graded for MAXIMUM POTENCY, COMPLETENESS & ABSORPTION. That's pretty impressive! Again, I didn't put these supplements together, nor did I manufacture them. I just put my label on the best of the best so you could benefit from them also.

The Health 4 Life Supplements are professional grade which means that our products are formulated based on the very latest, most credible science to deliver optimal health benefits.

ALL of the ingredients in our supplements are SAFE & 100% NATURAL. Our products contain NO yeast, wheat, gluten, soy, milk, dairy, corn, sodium, sugar, starch, artificial coloring, preservatives or flavoring. Talk about PURE!

Our supplements are manufactured at Douglas Laboratories. Their facilities meet the highest industry standards (superior GMP and ISO certification and accreditation) and are audited by the FDA.

Here are some of the Health 4 Life supplements:

R3 ESSENTIALS

The R3 ESSENTIALS are Douglas Laboratories' Ultra Preventative X, rated in the top 1% among over 1600 supplements and receiving a Gold Medal of Achievement from NutriSearch. R3 stands for: 'RESTORE – RESOLVE – REJUVENATE' as in my wellness model which will be discussed later in this book.

Studies show that a high percentage of adults in North America and other developed areas eat less than the minimum daily allowance of 10 or more essential nutrients. Adequate amounts and proper balance of these nutrients are needed not only for maintaining good health, but also for the dietary management of the body's structure as well as the optimum functioning of its various systems, including the immune and gastrointestinal systems.

We know that we need to provide our body with all the ESSENTIAL nutrients so it can obtain and maintain optimal health. You could try to figure out yourself all the nutrients you may need and purchase 10's or even 100's of individual supplements...but that would be too costly and too time consuming. This job is already done for you. R3 ESSENTIALS provides all the ESSENTIAL nutrients you need, in the optimal dosages and combinations.

R3 ESSENTIALS has been carefully developed to contain the right proportions of vitamins, minerals, trace minerals, antioxidants, bioflavonoids, grasses and greens, and other essential nutrients in their natural form, without danger of toxic build-up or other side effects. Each ingredient is selected in consideration of its absorbability, competitive relationship with other nutrients, allergenic potential, and long-term safety.

R3 ESSENTIALS also contains Metafolin®, a patented, natural form of (6S) 5-methyltetrahydrofolate (5-MTHF) as well as 1,000 IU of vitamin D3 per serving. For more information, the label and a complete list of ingredients, visit our website.

Certain nutrients such as beta-carotene, vitamin C, vitamin E, and B-complex vitamins are included in high-potency amounts because of the vital roles they play in antioxidant protection, energy production, the maintenance of healthy blood cells, the nervous system, hormonal balance, and more.

Minerals and trace elements are provided in their safest and most bio-available forms.

R3 ESSENTIALS' herbal green food base also includes very important phytonutrients. Gluten-free grasses and several varieties of microalgae supply chlorophyll, carotenes, B-vitamins, and trace elements. Cruciferous vegetables, broccoli and cauliflower, offer protective sulforophane compounds known for their ability to induce protective phase 2 detoxifying enzymes.

PURE OMEGA 3

The only nutrients that are missing in the R3 ESSENTIALS are some potent omega 3 oils. We discussed the importance of these anti-inflammatory nutrients earlier in this book and their daily intake will allow for great health benefits.

PURE OMEGA 3 consists of Supercritical CO2 extracted oils in triglyceride form, manufactured in Germany exclusively for Douglas Laboratories and Health Freedom, LLC. PURE OMEGA 3 is unique among other fish oils for its' critical extraction, purity, bioavailability and concentrations.

'Critical Extraction Supercritical CO2' advanced technology is the superior protection against oxidation. The extraction method of fish oil uses less heat and no chemical solvents when compared to molecular distillation, resulting in fewer unwanted isomer formations and 'cleaner' oil. 'Critical Purity Supercritical fluid extraction' uses CO2 (carbon dioxide) instead of oxygen to gently extract the fatty acids, which also protects them from microorganisms that can't survive without oxygen.

No chemical preservatives, solvents, or undesirable compounds are found in PURE OMEGA 3. Heavy metal and contaminant levels measure significantly lower than the standard. Critical Bioavailability Recent scientific data shows the triglyceride form of fish oil is better absorbed when compared to ethyl esters.

Recent data have demonstrated that omega-3 fatty acids delivered in a triglyceride form may result in greater plasma levels and a higher omega-3 index compared with omega-3 fatty acids delivered in the form of ethyl esters.

Critical Concentration:

Many fish oils contain only about 30% omega-3 fatty acids, of which roughly 18% is EPA and 12% DHA. The remaining 70% is a varying mixture of other components. In other words, regular fish oil contains less than a third of the desired active ingredients and more than two thirds of 'other' components. These other components may include cholesterol, omega-6 fatty acids, saturated fatty acids, oxidation products and other contaminants. Highly concentrated fish oil, like PURE OMEGA 3, provide at least 75% active ingredients, leaving less room for nonessential compounds.

The benefits of omega-3 fatty acids continue to emerge and numerous health organizations around the world recommend adequate daily intake of EPA and DHA. More and more data support the crucial roles of EPA and DHA in cardiovascular health as well as many other areas, including neurological health, vision health, and joint health. The omega-3 fatty acid EPA is the direct precursor for the prostaglandins, which are involved in helping to maintain the body's normal inflammatory processes.

IMPORTANT MESSAGE:

I personally ONLY take 2 supplements on a DAILY basis: The R3 ESSENTIALS and the PURE OMEGA 3. This combination provides you with the absolute best essential nutrients your body needs on a daily basis to allow for optimal cell function and metabolism. Furthermore, any other supplement or single nutrient will work MUCH BETTER in synergy with the R3 ESSENTIALS and PURE OMEGA 3. Look at these two supplements as the base or structure necessary for all other supplements to work optimally. Remember that the nutrients in your body work as a team and the synergy between them has no limits.

I do use the other supplements also, but only when needed or when situations or conditions call for them. I'll clarify later.

PEA PROTEIN

I know there are hundreds of protein shakes and bars on the market, also referred to as meal replacements. Most of them are soy-based (you will learn later that soy is carcinogenic and best omitted all together) or whey-based (you will learn later in more depth that milk and dairy are not only useless to our body but dangerous instead).

That's why I suggest PEA PROTEIN for those who want to lose weight or for those who want to replace a meal and make it easy on themselves, or for those who need extra protein (athletes for example).

PEA PROTEIN is a nutritionally fortified protein drink that is a rich source of all the indispensable amino acids essential to health, as well as 25% of the nutrition provided by R3 ESSENTIALS, a multi-vitamin/mineral dietary supplement.

PEA PROTEIN's source of protein is from yellow peas, a low allergenic source that contains no genetically modified plant tissue and is pesticide, lactose and gluten free. PEA PROTEIN beverage powder also provides a significant amount of the prebiotic fructooligosaccharide (FOS).

The dietary protein provided by PEA PROTEIN supplies essential amino acids that participate in all of the body's metabolic and physiologic systems including the intestine, skeletal muscle, and the cardiovascular, nervous, and immune systems. Protein turnover in these systems is continuous and can be substantial. The dynamics of this constant degradation and resynthesis demand a daily supply of dietary protein and their constituent amino acids. Essential or indispensable dietary amino acids must be supplied by the diet as they are not made by the body.

Recent analyses of the dietary protein needs of people suggest that age and activity level may influence protein requirement for optimum health. For example, elderly adults may have a significantly higher protein requirement than young adults. This requirement may be as high as 1.0 g of protein per kg of body weight per day, or 25% more than that suggested for a young adult. This higher requirement may derive from a lower efficiency of protein utilization in advancing age, despite the associated decrease in muscle mass. Failure to meet these increased protein needs may negatively affect an individual's immuno-competence and recovery from medical complications.

Increased protein synthesis follows prolonged exercise. Athletes competing in body building or endurance sports may require significantly more protein that the normal requirement.

PEA PROTEIN contains BeFlora Plus™, a prebiotic soluble dietary fiber fructooligosaccharide (FOS). This dietary fiber passes through the small intestine into the colon without being digested or absorbed. Once in the colon, FOS selectively supports healthy levels of beneficial bacteria such as Lactobacillus acidophilus and Bifidobacteria, and other gramposi-tive bacteria.

PEA PROTEIN can help satisfy the body's need for not only the indis-pensable amino acids, but also for the essential nutrients needed for optimum structure and function of all the body's systems.

I personally use PEA PROTEIN regularly as an easy meal replacement (when I'm home alone and not in the mood to cook a meal) or after a swim or a workout at the gym.

C-MAX

This formula gives you a blast of antioxidant power (real power, unlike that from coffee, red bull and other stimulants). C-MAX contains Ester-C®, a non-acidic, calcium ascorbate form of vitamin C combined with potent antioxidants to support the healthy functioning of the entire body.

Vitamin C (ascorbic acid) has numerous biological functions. It is essen-tial for the synthesis of collagen and glycosaminoglycans, which are the building materials of all connective tissues, such as skin, blood vessels, tendons, joint cartilage and bone.

Vitamin C is essential for normal wound healing and capillary health, and participates in the biosynthesis of serotonin and certain neurotrans-mitters, including norepinephrine.

Vitamin C is among the most powerful antioxidants in humans and animals. In addition, vitamin C interacts with glutathione and alpha-lipoic acid, and regenerates vitamin E.

The antioxidant functions of vitamin C appear to have clinical significance in providing protection from free radical damage to the eyes, lungs, blood and the immune system.

Bioflavonoids (also called flavonoids) are a class of phytochemicals that are potent antioxidants, which scavenge many potentially damaging free radicals. Another aspect of the antioxidant properties of bioflavonoids is their synergy with vitamin C. The bitter tasting flavanones hesperidin and naringin, from the white albedo layer of citrus peels, have been shown to extend the nutritional functions of vitamin C. Bioflavonoids are also capable of binding to metal ions, which prevents these metals from acting as catalysts in the body to enhance free radical production. Many bioflavonoids, especially rutin and quercetin, support the health of the body's circulatory system by helping maintain capillary blood flow and proper vascular permeability, integrity, and resiliency.

Pycnogenol® is made exclusively from the bark of the European coastal pine, Pinus maritima, which grows along the Atlantic coast of southern France. Pycnogenol is one of the most powerful natural free radical scavengers yet discovered. As such, it reduces oxidative damage to vital tissues and helps maintain a healthy capillary system.

I personally supplement with C-MAX when I feel fatigued, when I feel I could use a boost, every time I travel, and when I feel I may get sick.

B12 MAX

Methylcobalamin Liquid High Potency Vitamin B12 (in a convenient dropper for use under the tongue) provides 1,000 mcg of highly bio-available vitamin B12 in a tasty and convenient liquid.

Vitamin B12 is essential for normal metabolism of carbohydrates, fat and protein; and is also required for nucleic acid (DNA) synthesis and normal myelin synthesis in the nervous system amongst other vital functions.

Along with vitamin B6 and folic acid, adequate levels of vitamin B12 are required to maintain normal plasma homocysteine levels. Certain populations, including the elderly, those with HIV/AIDS, and strict veg-etarians are often at risk for vitamin B12 deficiency, either due to low dietary intake or impaired absorption.

Most of the vitamin B12 found in supplements is in the form of cyanoco-balamin. While cyanocobalamin is an excellent source of vitamin B12, studies indicate that methylcobalamin, a coenzyme form of B12, may be better utilized and better retained in the body. Other studies indicate that methylcobalamin itself may play important roles in supporting neurologi-cal and immune health.

I personally don't take this supplement as I consider myself in good health (and closing in on optimal health). My R3 Essentials contain sufficient amounts of B12 to maintain good health. However, if you are deficient in B12 or in the process of regaining normal health, this B12 liquid is more potent than your average supplement and replaces B12 injections at the doctor's office.

OSTEO MAX

OSTEO MAX provides 1,500 mg of elemental calcium from calcium carbonate, citrate, and caseinate, together with significant amounts of vitamin D (1,000 IU) and magnesium oxide and citrate (420mg). Other nutrients are also included to assist the body in maintaining healthy bone structure.

The adult human body contains approximately 1,200 g of calcium, about 99% of which is present in the skeleton, and 20-30g of magnesium with about 60% located in bone. Bone is constantly turning over, a continu-ous process of formation and resorption. In children and adolescents, the rate of formation of bone mineral predominates over the rate of resorption. In later life, resorption predominates over formation.

Therefore, in normal aging, there is a gradual loss of bone. Intestinal calcium absorption ranges from 15 to 75% of ingested calcium. Vitamin D is a key regulatory hormone for calcium and bone metabolism. Adequate vitamin D status is essential for ensuring normal calcium absorption and maintenance of healthy calcium plasma levels.

Magnesium absorption is independent of vitamin D status and ranges from 30 to 60% of ingested magnesium. Osteoporosis, a condition of reduced bone mineral density that can increase the risk of fractures, affects a large proportion of the elderly in developed countries. Caucasian and Asian women typically have low peak bone densities, and therefore, are at the greatest risk of developing osteoporosis. It is generally accepted that obtaining enough dietary calcium throughout life can significantly decrease the risk of developing osteoporosis. Among other factors, such as regular exercise, gender and race, calcium supplementation during childhood and adolescence appears to be a prerequisite for maintaining adequate bone density later in life. But even elderly osteoporotic patients can benefit significantly from supplementation with dietary calcium.

OSTEO MAX provides a highly beneficial source of dietary calcium together with other nutrients that assist in the maintenance of healthy bone structure and function. For example, boron affects the composition, structure, and strength of bone. It appears to be necessary for calcium and magnesium absorption, their adequate renal reabsorption, and their incorporation into the bone matrix. Boron is absorbed at about 90% efficiency and is rapidly distributed among the tissues.

I personally don't take OSTEO MAX. This supplement is indicated for people with osteopenia and osteoporosis. R3 ESSENTIALS contains sufficient amounts of calcium, magnesium and vitamin D3 to maintain good bone health.

FIBER MAX

FIBER MAX is a convenient dietary supplement designed to provide a unique combination of all major classes of naturally occurring dietary fiber. FIBER MAX capsules supply a balance of soluble and insoluble, as well as fermentable and non-fermentable dietary fiber.

Dietary fiber is defined as "complex carbohydrates that are resistant to the action of digestive enzymes". They pass through the intestinal tract, unabsorbed. Dietary fiber includes substances such as cellulose, hemicellulose (xylans, galactans and mannans), pectins, gums, and lignin.

Dietary fiber has many nutritional benefits for the health of the gastrointestinal tract. Insoluble dietary fiber, such as cellulose and many hemicelluloses, are not efficiently fermented in the colon. As a result, they provide fecal bulk, bind water, and help soften stools. Soluble dietary fiber, such as pectin, many gums, and some hemicelluloses, are fermented in the colon to varying degrees. This results in lower colonic pH (acidity) and the production of short chain fatty acids, which are important for the intestinal microflora and the health of the mucosal cells. Short chain fatty acids also have a role in facilitating colonic water absorption.

Many insoluble and soluble fiber types bind dietary cholesterol and bile acids in the intestine, and therefore play an important nutritional role in the enterohepatic circulation of cholesterol and cholesterol metabolism in general. Most types of dietary fiber, when hydrated, contribute substantially to the volume of stomach contents and help provide a feeling of fullness.

FIBER MAX was formulated to take advantage of all of the physiological benefits of fiber by combining a wide variety of insoluble, non-fermentable and soluble, fermentable natural fiber sources. Glucomannan is a partially fermentable, soluble fiber extracted from the konjac root (yam family). This hemicellulose fiber is noted for its high water-binding capacity, and may have a beneficial role in cholesterol metabolism. Carrot and celery powders provide a rich array of soluble and insoluble dietary fibers, including cellulose, hemicellulose, pectin and lignin. Sodium alginate is a soluble partially fermentable fiber derived from seaweed. Pectin is a soluble dietary fiber noted for its ability to provide beneficial short chain fatty acids for the colon.

FIBER MAX provides both types of naturally occurring pectins: high- and low-methoxyl pectins. Slippery elm powder supplies a number of gums and mucilages that are important for the mucous lining of the gastrointestinal tract.

I take FIBER MAX as part of my 30-day detox program and whenever digestion and elimination are not optimal.

B LEAN

B LEAN is a novel weight management formula that includes three branded and clinically studied ingredients-- Meratrim™ plant extract, Capsimax™ capsicum extract, and Zychrome® chromium complex. This special combination of ingredients may improve lipolysis, thermogenic activity, and insulin function. The ingredients in B LEAN also help to increase adiponectin levels which facilitate proper fat metabolism and glucose regulation.

Meratrim™ is a proprietary plant extract blend for weight management derived from two plants, *Sphaeranthus indicus* and *Garcinia mangostana*, traditionally used in Southeast Asian culture. Meratrim has been proven to significantly reduce body weight, BMI, and waist circumference within 8 weeks when used in combination with a diet and exercise plan.

Meratrim appears to achieve this by modulating the accumulation of fat while simultaneously increasing fat burning. Toxicological studies on Meratrim have demonstrated a wide margin of safety.

Capsimax™ capsicum extract is a proprietary encapsulated form of premium, highly concentrated natural capsicum fruit extract manufactured from hot red peppers. Capsaicinoids are a group of compounds which cause the 'heat' found in hot peppers. In fact, over the past 30 years, studies including animal and human subjects support the potential of red hot capsicum and capsaicinoids as a safe, effective ingredient to aid in weight management. Capsicum and capsaicinoids help manage appetite, support healthy metabolism to burn calories, and help induce thermogenesis.

Zychrome™ is a unique, patent-pending chromium complex consisting of chromium, niacin and L-cysteine (chromium dinicocysteinate). Zychrome significantly modulates the levels of insulin and insulin resistance as well as the inflammatory cytokine TNF and protein carbonyl content, a marker of oxidative stress. Toxicological studies have demonstrated a wide margin of safety.

This product is obviously designed for the person who is overweight and wants to facilitate weight loss efforts. Athletes also may use this formula in their quest to reduce PBF (percentage of body fat).

I personally use this product on occasion when I'm doing intense workouts and want to reduce PBF.

SLEEP MAX

SLEEP MAX is designed to support natural sleep. It's a proprietary blend of *Magnolia officinalis* and *Ziziphus spinosa*, as well as a synergistic herbal blend, specifically designed to promote healthy sleep and support the body's normal nocturnal rhythms during stress.

For many individuals, the hectic pace of a Western lifestyle, lack of exercise and poor eating habits can lead to suboptimal health. Often, these same individuals do not receive enough sleep at night. The vast majority of health care providers now recommend that individuals receive at least 7-8 hours of sleep. This lack of sleep has been shown in studies to be a major cause of elevation of stress (cortisol) and appetite (ghrelin) hormones, which is thought to lead to a further progression of poor sleep and eating habits. These poor habits may be part of the factors that determine weight gain, cardiovascular fitness, mental alertness, immune health and other important indicators of optimal health and wellbeing.

SLEEP MAX (Seditol®) is designed to support healthy sleep patterns and help normalize stress hormones, thus leading to better sleep and relaxation patterns. The main ingredients of SLEEP MAX, Magnolia and Ziziphus, have been used in Traditional Chinese Medicine for hundreds of years and are well regarded for their roles in stress management.

In one clinical trial testing Seditol in adults, 87% of the participants agreed with the statements "Seditol helps you relax", "Seditol reduces fatigue due to lack of sleep" and "Seditol allows you to wake up feeling refreshed." In the same clinical trial, 83% of the participants agreed with the statement that "Seditol helps insure a sound night's sleep."

In a second clinical trial, over 87% of the participants agreed with the same aforementioned statements.

In addition to Seditol, chamomile, lemon balm and passion flower are included for the relaxing properties they can provide to assist the body's requirement for a restful night's sleep.

I personally never used SLEEP MAX, but the results my clients and some of my close friends get are amazing. Of course, they are also making efforts to live C.L.E.A.N and are taking the base supplements R3 ESSENTIALS and PURE OMEGA 3.

TESTO MAX

TESTO MAX is a *Hormone Specific Formulation™* of phytoandrogens, androgenogenic adaptogens, androgen agonists and androgen mimetics to help promote optimal testosterone function by maintaining the health of testosterone producing glands and by supporting the healthy functions of testosterone responsive tissues in both men and women.

TESTO MAX is a *Hormone Specific Formulation™* formulated by Dr. Joseph J Collins, created to support the optimal function of specific hormones through the use of hormone specific adaptogens, hormone specific agonists and hormone specific functional mimetics. This formulation may be used as part of a hormone health program with dietary and nutrient support. In addition, these formulations may be used by clinicians as adjuvants to support optimal hormone health in patients who have been prescribed bioidentical hormone therapies, including testosterone replacement therapy.

The primary functions of TESTO MAX are to support the natural production of testosterone and other androgens by gonadal tissue in both genders, and to support how tissues throughout the body respond to testosterone. This is accomplished by supporting the function of testosterone producing glands in both genders, and by supporting the function of testosterone tissues through the use of herbs that mimic the actions of testosterone.

The synergistic combination of specific herbs in TESTO MAX support important functions associated with optimal testosterone health in both genders:

• Promote production of testosterone by gonadal tissue.

• Promote production of other androgens by adrenal glands.

• Mimic specific functions of testosterone, thereby acting as testosterone functional agonists.

I personally use TESTO MAX 3 months on and 3 months off.

LESS STRESS

LESS STRESS is a synergistic combination of ten highly valued herbal extracts with adaptogenic properties designed to support healthy, balanced adrenal gland function.

These unique herbs were first used by the Russian Cosmonauts and elite citizens, and later successfully employed to enhance athletic performance. Many Olympic athletes enjoyed the benefits of these 'adaptogens'.

The plant adaptogens used in LESS STESS include Schisandra chinensis, Bacopa monnieri, Rhodiola rosea, Eleutherococcus senticosus, Magnolia officinalis, Rhemannia glutinosa, Bupleurum falcatum, Panax ginseng, Coleus forskohlii and Withania sominfera.

The plant adaptogens in LESS STESS effectively address all stages of both acute and chronic stress, support the body's ability to adapt to stressors and help avoid the damaging consequences from those stressors. Collectively, plant adaptogens can support symptoms of fatigue and enhance endurance as well as support normal mental and emotional wellbeing. Plant adaptogens also can increase the body's ability to resist and recover from stress while providing an overall feeling of balance and normalization.

While the primary benefit of plant adaptogens is the ability to restore healthy, balanced adrenal gland function, the effectiveness of these adaptogens is in large part also due to their ability to protect and promote the recovery of neurocognitive, neuromuscular, cardiovascular, glycemic, hepatic, thyroid, gonadal and immune system health.

I personally absolutely love this product, and take it when I feel my adrenals are exhausted (fatigued) in addition to catching up on some quality rest of course. I do recommend this product for people with lots of stress in their lives and urge them to learn how to take control over their emotions and feelings, and how to reorganize their lives to better manage the stresses.

L-ARGININE MAX

L-ARGININE MAX contains 700mg pure, crystalline L-arginine.

L-arginine is a versatile, conditionally essential amino acid. Amino acids have many functions in the body. They are the building blocks for all body proteins - structural proteins that build muscle, connective tissues, bones and other structures, and functional proteins in the form of thousands of metabolically active enzymes. Amino acids provide the body with the nitrogen that is essential for growth and maintenance of all tissues and structures. Proteins and amino acids also serve as a source of energy, providing about 4 calories per gram.

Aside from these general functions, individual amino acids also have specific functions in many aspects of human physiology and biochemistry. L-arginine is a conditionally essential dibasic amino acid. The body is usually capable of producing sufficient amounts of arginine, but in conditions of physical stress, e.g., trauma or illness, endogenous synthesis is often inadequate to meet the increased demands.

L-arginine can either be used for glucose synthesis or catabolized to produce energy via the tricarboxylic acid cycle. It is needed for tissue protein synthesis and ammonia detoxification via the urea acid cycle. L-arginine is required for the synthesis of creatine phosphate. Similar to adenosine triphosphate (ATP), creatine phosphate functions as a carrier of readily available energy for contractile work in muscles. Adequate reservoirs of creatine phosphate are necessary in muscle as an energy reserve for anaerobic activity.

L-arginine is also a precursor of polyamines, including putrescine, spermine and spermidine. Spermine and spermidine interact with DNA, act as physiological growth regulators of cell proliferation, and are involved in the stabilization of cell membranes and cell organelles.

L-arginine is a potent stimulator of insulin, glucagon, and growth hormone release, and functions as a representative signal to the endocrine system that dietary protein ingestion has taken place.

I personally don't use L-ARGININE MAX but I often prescribe it for friends or clients who suffer from neuropathies and muscular problems since L-arginine effectively promotes circulation and blocks pain.

BERBERINE PLUS

BERBERINE PLUS supplies high potency berberine combined with alpha lipoic acid and grape seed extract for blood sugar and cardio-vascular support. Grape seed extract is a well-known antioxidant with heart health benefits, and alpha lipoic acid helps to support proper insulin function.

Berberine is a naturally occurring alkaloid and a primary constituent of several plants including barberry, goldenseal, and phellodendron. Recent studies indicate that berberine is a helpful supplement for maintaining cardio-metabolic health and is considered effective and safe.

Berberine has been shown to regulate glucose and lipid metabolism, and support blood pressure and vaso-relaxatory effects.

Berberine's history of usage in Ayurvedic and Chinese medicine dating back approximately 3,000 years has shown to help maintain a healthy microbial balance. Polyphenols, part of a broad class of bioflavonoids, are commonly found in grape seeds. One type of polyphenols known as proanthocyanidins is highly regarded for their strong antioxidant properties, and for their functions in supporting the capillaries.

Proanthocyanidins appear to be especially effective in neutralizing highly reactive hydroxyl and singlet oxygen radicals. Both of these reactive oxygen species are involved in inflammatory processes.

Alpha lipoic acid is a nutritional coenzyme that is involved in the energy metabolism of proteins, carbohydrates and fats. It has physiological functions in blood glucose clearance, and is able to scavenge a number of free radicals. This important coenzyme appears to be necessary for the normal transport of blood glucose into the cell. This may be explained by its functions in the glucose-metabolizing enzymes, PDH and alpha-KGDH, but some researchers suspect a more direct role in cellular glucose uptake at the cell membrane.

NOTE:

The above mentioned supplements are some of the Health 4 Life Supplements. Please note that you don't need all of these supplements, and certain times or conditions call for certain supplements.

There are more supplements that I will recommend, for example Wasabia Japonica, Glutathione Plus, Milk Thistle Max and Turmeric Max during the liver detox phase of our detoxification program, or MSM and serrapeptase to combat inflammation and fibrin. Some of you may need specific supplements to resolve some lingering medical issues etc.

For more information (including the product label) of all Health 4 Life supplements, or to find out HOW to obtain other key supplements such as the Wasabia Japonica, please visit our website at www.Health4Life.info.

14.5 Key Points

We can all agree that we DO need high quality, natural supplements as an insurance policy to optimal health. Even organic, whole foods lose a significant amount of nutrients prior to consumption AND we are exposed to far more toxins today than ever before.

Supplements DO NOT REPLACE healthy foods and living C.L.E.A.N., they are exactly what's in their name: they SUPPLEMENT. Supplements assure a daily adequate amount of nutrients and facilitate regaining and restoring normal health.

Unfortunately, the vast majority of supplements have NO health benefits. To the contrary, many of them cause a negative nutrient balance. This is because few regulations exist, resulting in unsafe, useless products and false or misleading labeling.

To assure a high quality and safe supplement, one has to investigate the criteria that determine such a supplement. These criteria include: safety, absorption, potency, purity, identity, dosage, completeness, among others.

Single nutrients have no significant health benefits. All nutrients in our body work synergistically. Therefore, combination products or multi-nutrient supplements are recommended as a foundation.

Studies have indicated that only 1% of supplements comply with all these criteria. The Health 4 Life supplements and the liquid Vemma are part of these top rated products. Net proceeds of the Health 4 Life supplements go to one of my favorite charities: Children Incorporated.

Chapter 15 – Myths & Misconceptions

There are too many myths and misconceptions about health, foods, disease and drugs to explore in this chapter. However, we exposed many earlier in this book and I will continue to do so, on our website.

Below are some misconceptions that drive me crazy (luckily I'm getting much better at controlling my emotions LOL), mainly because conventional medicine, pharmaceutical companies, the FDA and manufacturers have PURPOSEFULLY misled the public for decades to gain profits while slowly killing us. These misconceptions are grained in our brains as truths while they all are nothing but habitual lies. We have come to accept them but it's time to overthrow these misconceptions, use some common sense and take control.

15.1 Cholesterol is NOT a deadly poison but a VITAL Substance

People continue to be confused about cholesterol. Cholesterol is NOT a deadly poison, but a vital substance. The fact is that our body makes and uses cholesterol. It's a natural, waxy substance produced by the liver and ingested through the foods we eat. Our body uses cholesterol for cell membrane function, hormone production, and for the conversion of vitamin D into a usable form.

It's the cholesterol-reducing drugs (including 'statin' drugs) that are the poison. Furthermore, recent studies show they even don't work. High cholesterol can indicate a health problem BUT also can be totally innocent by itself.

It's true that heart disease is the #1 killer in the United States (although I'm sure that it's drugs and ill advice from doctors along with lack of knowledge about health). Men over the age of 40 are particularly vulnerable for heart disease. But, the big pharmaceutical companies (and even your doctor because he or she doesn't realize) won't tell you that the majority of strokes and heart attacks have NOTHING to do with elevated cholesterol levels. Actually, recent reports from the American Heart Association indicate that more people with a low cholesterol die from a heart condition than people with high cholesterol levels, which is NOT a surprise.

The fact that the majority of all strokes and heart attacks have absolutely nothing to do with elevated cholesterol levels is a guarded secret. It's these statin drugs that are associated with major complications and side effects such as depletion of the body's essential energy molecule coenzyme Q10 (CoQ10), which can lead to congestive heart failure, extreme muscle weakness, neurological disorders and even death. Cholesterol is a vital substance and the drugs prescribed to lower cholesterol are simply dangerous.

What about cancer? All statin drugs have been associated with causing or promoting cancer in experimental animals. This is especially important since millions of Americans have been advised to take these drugs for the rest of their lives. The results of one study were especially frightening: statin drugs produced significant suppression of vital immune cells called helper T-cells. These cells play a major role in protecting us against cancer and fungal, bacterial and viral infections. The immune suppression was so powerful that authors of the paper even suggested that statins might be used to prevent organ rejection in transplant patients. The drugs tested in this study included Lipitor, Mevacor and Pravachol. Chronic immune suppression in these millions of people would mean that a tremendous number would be at high risk of developing cancer, and those already having cancer would see tremendous growth and spread of their cancers.

Statins do not seem to benefit postmenopausal women, or anyone without a history of cardiovascular disease. Yet, doctors are prescribing statins for anyone with elevated cholesterol levels, and also for all diabetics - no matter their cholesterol level.

My own mother, who still resides in my home country of Belgium, was put on Lipitor about 5 years ago. I wasn't aware of that, but she called and expressed pain and numbness in her legs. I tried to diagnose her over the phone and spent countless hours to figure it out...until I asked her: "Your doctor did not prescribe you cholesterol-lowering drugs, did she?" Well, she did. I advised my mother to discontinue the Lipitor immediately and within 3 days all her symptoms in her legs were gone. I also educated her on what to do naturally to treat the CAUSE of the high cholesterol (Live C.L.E.A.N), and more importantly on what to do to protect your heart. A Danish study found that those taking statin drugs long term were 4 to 14 times more likely to develop nerve degeneration leading to difficulty walking and painful extremities. Regardless, just read the side-effect profile of these statins on your drug label and you'll see.

Cholesterol is just a BIG HOAX!

An estimated 14 million Americans are taking these cholesterol-lowering drugs daily for their heart health while NOT knowing that they are just treating an unlikely cause for heart disease. The drugs are poisons and wreak havoc and toxemia in our body, while lowering cholesterol itself can be a dangerous proposal in itself since cholesterol is a vital substance.

Cholesterol-reducing drugs or statins are currently as common as aspirin, with commercials running non-stop on primetime TV. Drugs like Lipitor, Zocor, Pravachol, Crestor and Mevacor carry many serious health risks, including destruction of muscle, liver damage, increased risk of cancer, malformations at birth, and suppression of the immune system, just to name a few. Drug companies don't want you to remember that statins like Baycol had to be pulled from the market due to multiple deaths.

Let's face facts. If you or a loved one has been told you have elevated cholesterol or take cholesterol-lowering statins, invest 2 minutes out of your busy day and educate yourself, it will pay you a very healthy dividend.

My cholesterol is way above the established limits. I don't care at all because I know it's not important. Did your parents or grandparents take cholesterol-lowering drugs? Was there any talk about cholesterol a few decades ago? No. It's simply a big hoax. It's a manufactured idea by the pharmaceutical companies and medical world in a successful attempt to sell billions of dollars of these drugs. How did they come up with these ranges of 'good' and 'bad' cholesterol? Simple: they made sure that 90% of all people test above these 'man-made', unsubstanti-ated so called normal ranges so that their drugs can be prescribed. I got two words for all this: organized genocide.

My high cholesterol is partially genetics and is of no worry at all since I'm living C.L.E.A.N.

FACTS:

1. The whole **cholesterol industry is a BIG HOAX**. The 'supposed' dangers of dietary cholesterol have been strongly exaggerated and have made sure that most peo-ple would test 'positive' for high cholesterol levels so the drugs could be prescribed and sold to almost everyone. Yes, that's what happens when BIG money is involved.

2. **Statin drugs DON'T WORK anyway.** The mainstream media can no longer ignore the mounting evidence that these drugs are not a panacea. One study found that for every hundred people taking statins for three years, only one death will be prevented. Other studies hint that the number is far higher – that up to 250 people would have to take statins for at least three years to prevent a single death. A recent publication even shows that one such drug, Vytorin, simply does not even work for its intended purpose: the reduction of artery plaque. You read that cor-rectly – "does not work."

3. Having low cholesterol is not only bad for you, but can be

just as dangerous, if not more so, than having elevated cholesterol levels.

4. Cholesterol is only 'bad' if it becomes oxidized due to an insufficient amount of 'good' cholesterol or HDL which transports unused cholesterol back to the liver where it is recycled.

5. Lowering cholesterol will NOT improve your health or prevent heart disease. However, simple changes to your diet can protect your heart much better than expensive statin drugs.

6. Dietary cholesterol does NOT raise blood cholesterol and therefore does NOT cause hardening of your arteries (atherosclerosis). So please stop paying attention to these misleading products with labels like 'low cholesterol', they are trash. Instead, start focusing on eating your organic eggs again (they are one of the most nutritious food items available) and start living C.L.E.A.N.

7. Eggs (unlike milk) are a wholesome food. It is one of the most complete and versatile foods known to man. With all the media attention on cholesterol, consumers often lose sight of the fact that eggs are rich in nutrients and affordable contributors to a healthy diet. Not only do eggs contain the highest quality source of protein available, but they also contain almost every essential vitamin (A, E, K, and B-vitamins including B-12) and mineral we need (except vitamin C since chickens can produce vitamin C themselves). Eggs have a biological protein value (efficacy with which protein is used for growth) of 93.7%, compared to 76% for fish and 74% for beef.

Eggs also contain cholesterol but it is generally accepted that dietary cholesterol does not raise blood cholesterol levels. Eggs contain high levels of lecithin, a cholesterol-lowering agent, and an essential nutrient for every human cell. Lecithin is also a natural emulsifier (meaning that it helps liquefying fat inside the blood vessels and therefore preventing plaque build-up), and the primary source of choline, a precursor for acetylcholine (necessary for muscular contraction). Studies have shown that eating one to two eggs per day does NOT affect blood-cholesterol levels.

BUT, choose organic eggs! Organic eggs come from hens whose feed contains no pesticides, fungicides, herbicides or commercial fertilizers.

8. It's not eating eggs or foods with high dietary cholesterol that is the main problem. It's the BAD foods that stimulate cholesterol production. Consuming BAD foods (processed, synthetic foods, trans-fats etc.) forces the liver to produce more cholesterol. Why? Because the cell membrane has to increase its fluidity in order to absorb and break down these 'foreign' substances.

9. The production of cholesterol in our body actually increases when we consume less cholesterol. That's also why cholesterol-diets have very limited results.

10. Diet and exercise alone have limited results in lowering blood cholesterol. BUT one doesn't need to lower cholesterol. ONLY the ratio and balance between HDL ('good' cholesterol) and LDL ('bad' cholesterol) is important. Let's clarify: cholesterol is transported through the bloodstream by a lipoprotein. There are two main lipoproteins: low-density (LDL) and high-density lipoprotein (HDL). The LDL's take cholesterol from the liver throughout the body wherever it's needed as a vital substance, while the HDL are responsible for taking any unused cholesterol back to the liver for recycling. Only when there's a shortage of HDL's to take unused cholesterol back to the liver, LDL cholesterol remains in the tissues and becomes vulnerable to oxidation. Therefore, the key is a natural balance between HDL and LDL, not levels of cholesterol.

11. With a healthy lifestyle and optimal nutrients, optimal LDL – HDL ratios can be obtained and maintained. This is the ONLY way.

12. Many doctors have no or little knowledge about nutrition, vitamins and natural medicine and blindly and mistakenly follow the advice of drug companies...at the expense of your health.

So *if you want to protect your heart,* you need to focus on eating heart-healthy foods and consume or supplement with specific nutrients. Avoid saturated fats and consume more oat bran, avocados, fresh garlic, and phytostyerol-rich foods such as olive oil, nuts, flax and other seeds, and beans. Supplement with fish oils or krill and powerful antioxidants including CoQ10.

For some of us, high cholesterol levels may indicate poor health. However, chasing man-made symptoms on lab reports won't improve your health, to the contrary. Even if you wanted to lower your cholesterol, drugs are the worst choice. Simply improving your diet and adding high doses of pure omega 3 will do the job, much better and without an extensive list of adverse reactions and health impairing impact.

Take control. Throw those drugs in the garbage (don't flush them or you will end-up drinking them later) and start the Action Plan in this book if you are serious about regaining your health.

IMPORTANT NOTE

Many drugs such as those for cholesterol, digestive problems (heart burn or acid reflux), pain, inflammation etc. should be discarded immediately to reduce the toxic load in your body. However, if you have been taking drugs for your heart condition, seizures, type I diabetes and other more serious so called diseases for a long time, I suggest to gradually reduce the dose of these drugs with the cooperation of your physician who can monitor your progress until you can safely omit these drugs. I know that your physician will most likely discourage you from this plan but that's because he or she is more concerned with legal ramifications than with your health, and frankly doesn't know anything about health in the first place. You are in control of your health, not your physician. You should let your physician know that and ask for his or her cooperation in reaching your goals by safely monitoring your progress.

A good example is Coumadin (blood thinner) that is prescribed like candy. This rat poison is so dangerous that it even scares me and I don't take it. I'm not going to bore you with the course of action of this drug in the body, the short-term adverse reactions and the apparently unknown long-term ramifications. But you easily could google them.

Getting off this drug has to be done gradually and with the cooperation of your cardiologist to avoid sudden dangers, but it has to be done. A healthy lifestyle automatically results in thinner, healthier blood and additionally there are many natural alternatives available to thin your blood as opposed to rat poison, including fibrolytic and anti-inflammatory enzymes such as serrapeptase.

15.2 Milk & Dairy Products

Let's put the **MILK** argument at rest forever. But first I would like to applaud the amazing marketing success of the American Dairy Board in portraying milk as a good, nutritious drink... congrats! People today still believe that they need to consume large, daily quantities of milk to achieve good health.

In general, most animals are exclusively breast-fed until they have tripled their birth weight, which in human infants occurs around the age of one year. In NO mammalian species, except for the human (and domestic cat) is milk consumption continued after the weaning period. Why? Because there's no need for milk! Furthermore, the milk of most mammals varies considerably in its composition...the milk from cows, goats, elephants, camels, and wolves have remarkable differences. Each was designed to provide optimum nutrition for the young of their respective species. So, last time I checked we were not calves. Drinking the milk of another species is yet another strange perversion... just think about it.

That's also why cow's milk is the number one allergic food in our country. It has been well documented as a cause of diarrhea, cramps, bloating, gas, GI-bleeding, iron-deficiency, anemia, skin rashes, arteriosclerosis, and acne. It's also the primary cause of recurrent ear infections in children. Ear specialists frequently insert tubes into the ear drums of these children...many times unnecessary, since just stopping the consumption of milk would solve the problem in over 50% of the cases.

Milk consumption is also linked to Type 1 diabetes (Insulin dependent), rheumatoid arthritis, infertility and leukemia.

And that's only the truth when you consume raw milk. What if, like most people, one consumes processed and pasteurized milk? The problem gets worse! I'm not going to bore you with the entire milk processing procedure, but I can tell you that during these processes all precious enzymes are destroyed and the milk is transformed into allergens and carcinogens. The FDA also approved the use of BGH (Bovine Growth Hormone) which now is responsible for the fact that more than 50% of the milk is heavily contaminated with antibiotics. Let's put our hands together for the FDA again and applaud their sincere efforts to protect public health (choking would be better than applauding).

Any farmer also knows that if you feed pasteurized milk to a baby calf it will die in 6 weeks due to malnutrition. Mother's breast milk is high is phosphorus, a brain food, while cow's milk is high in calcium, food for the bones. One needs to understand that human babies develop their brain first while the baby calf develops its bones first. That's also why cow's milk contains 300 times more casein, which furnishes the necessary amino acids to build bones and support body weight, than mother's milk. A cow develops twice its weight in 7 weeks while a human baby develops twice its weight in 7 months. Can you see now why it's totally absurd to feed a human infant cow's milk?

The above are not opinions, but merely straight-forward facts as is the following fact of human biology. Our body produces an enzyme 'lactase' to break down lactose which is contained in mother's milk. However, our body stops producing this enzyme around the age of 1. This simply means that Mother Nature doesn't want us to drink any more human milk after we reach the age of 1. After the age of 1, drinking milk results in all kinds of problems as outlined earlier because there's no enzyme available to break down lactose. Ever heard of lactose intolerance? In short, there's is no single reason to consume milk after the age of 1; water is what we should drink.

Oh, I almost forget...what about calcium? Isn't milk a good source of calcium? Well, raw milk is a fairly good source of calcium, but most milk contains the wrong type of calcium (which then leaches calcium from our bones to process that wrong type of calcium, resulting yet again in a negative calcium balance).

Guess why cows' milk contains calcium? Because cows eat grass and leafy greens. Again, humans do NOT need milk, and as far as calcium goes....eat more leafy, green vegetables which are a far better source of calcium then any milk. Plus, these vegetables have many other health benefits such as alkalizing your body and providing essential nutrients.

Next time you reach for the milk or think about buying milk, I truly hope you reconsider. It's not nutritious, it's poisonous! Take responsibility and STOP giving your kids and loved-ones milk, or any dairy product for that matter. Should you stop having cornflakes and cereals for breakfast then? Well, breakfast is overrated, but if you must have some useless cornflakes use some almond milk (Silk brand). Almond milk is just the juice of almonds; they call it milk because it's white. Almond milk also tastes sweeter so you won't need to add any sugar (and you will get used to it in a week).

Other dairy products such as cheese and yogurt should be banned from your diet also, or its consumption at least minimized and then gradually omitted. Cheese and yogurt are fermented milk products which simply means that they are rotten milk... from another species. WOW!

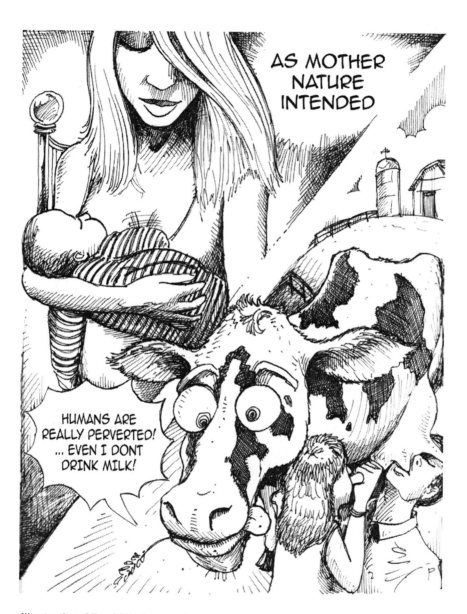

Illustration 27 – Milk Perversion

15.3 Soda & Diet Soda - The Killers For Real?

A True Killer, No excuses, ONLY FACTS! Yes, I know you are addicted to soda (no matter which one it is) and therefore you try to find 'excuses' to keep swallowing gallons of this toxic waste or liquid toxic candy down your throat. If you drink this waste, do yourself the BIGGEST favor EVER, Stop RIGHT NOW! Even if it's the ONLY THING you ever do to improve your health, this one will make a HUGE difference.

Here are the FACTS:

Both soda & diet soda are VERY **ACIDIC** (pH: 2.5 - 3.5), corroding the teeth by eroding its enamel. Phosphoric acid, present in carbonated drinks is violently poisonous and de-oxidizes the blood. In detergent manufacturing industries, phosphoric acid is used to produce water softener. In the human body, it removes calcium from bones causing osteoporosis (porous bones). Besides causing tooth decay and osteoporosis, soda and soft drinks cause indigestion, kidney stones, skin problems, malnutrition, and much more (toxemia will do).

In most carbonated beverages, **caffeine** is deliberately added to make it addictive. Caffeine in carbonated drinks is more readily absorbed than any other drink (like coffee, chocolate etc.). Caffeine disturbs sleep by stimulating the nervous system. It also makes premenstrual syndrome worse, causes dehydration and induces the stomach to produce acids, aggravating hyperacidity. Since caffeine disturbs sleep, the body is more likely to produce C - reactive protein, which plays an important role in heart disease.

Soft drinks are mainly composed of filtered H2O, artificial additives and **refined sugar**. Thus, they lack nutritional value and only add up calories through their refined sugar. Therefore, sodas (including the diet products) make you gain weight and are a contributing factor to the rise of obesity (also amongst our children). The high amount of sugar consumed through soft drinks (an average of 12 teaspoons or 40 grams/can) leads to the development of bacteria that attack the teeth thus aggravating dental problems.

Even though there is no 'real' sugar in diet soda, the artificial low-calorie sweeteners such as **aspartame** make you feel hungrier and increase the craving for food. The release of insulin is still stimulated and the so called 'diet' soda has NO EFFECT whatsoever on your sugar metabolism. Also, people who drink the diet soda wrongly assume that they ingest less sugar, and usually feel that they are 'allowed' more other goodies.

Diet soda is EVEN WORSE than regular soda because it contains ASPARTAME & Benzene!

The official story is that aspartame was discovered in 1966 by a scientist developing an ulcer drug (not a 'food additive'). Supposedly he discovered, upon carelessly licking his fingers that it tasted sweet. The chemicals industry was blessed with a successor to saccharine, the coal-tar derivative that foundered eight years later under the pressure of cancer concerns.

Aspartame found early opposition in consumer attorney James Turner, author of "The Chemical Feast" and a former Nader's Raider. At his own expense, Turner fought approval for ten years, basing his argument on aspartame's potential side effects, particularly on children. His concern was shared by Dr. John Olney, Professor of neuropathology and psychiatry at the Washington School of Medicine in St. Louis. Dr. Olney found that aspartame, combined with MSG seasoning, increased the odds of brain damage in children.

Other studies have found that children are especially vulnerable to its toxic effects, a measure of the relation between consumption and body weight. The FDA approved this sweetener in 1981, and it's found in hundreds of foods, including iced tea, chocolate milk, milk shakes, chocolate pudding, pie, jello, ice cream etc. The FDA is ever mindful to refer to aspartame, widely known as NutraSweet, as a 'food additive' and not a 'drug'. A 'drug' on the label of a Diet Coke might discourage the consumer. And because aspartame is classified a food additive, adverse reactions are not reported to a federal agency, nor is continued safety monitoring required by law. NutraSweet is a non-nutritive sweetener. The brand name is a misnomer. Try Non-NutraSweet. Once again we applaud the FDA.

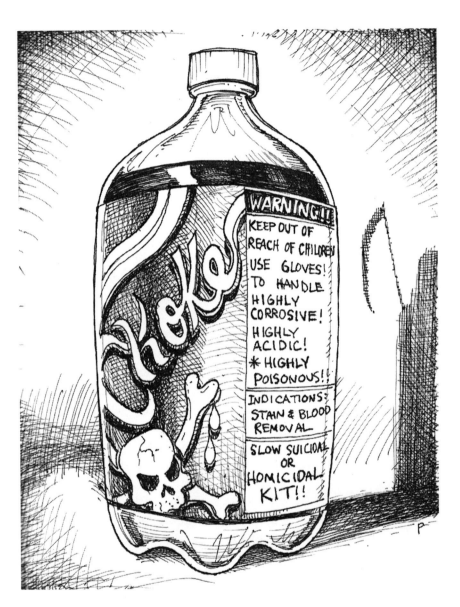

Illustration 28 – Choke

Food additives seldom cause brain lesions, headaches, mood altera-tions, skin polyps, blindness, brain tumors, insomnia and depression, or erode intelligence and short-term memory. Aspartame, according to some of the most capable scientists in the country, does. In 1991 the National Institutes of Health, a branch of the Department of Health and Human Services, published a bibliography, "Adverse Effects of Aspartame", listing more than **167 reasons** to avoid aspartame.

Aspartame is an rDNA derivative, a combination of two amino acids. The Pentagon once listed it in an inventory of prospective biochemi-cal warfare weapons submitted to Congress. But instead of poisoning enemy populations, the 'food additive' is currently marketed as a sweet-ening agent in some 1200 food products.

I could easily go on and on, but I guess I made my point.

Benzene is a known carcinogen, a common industrial chemical, and one of the primary causes of leukemia in the U.S. Benzene carries FDA's 'carcinogenic to humans' status (formerly 'Class A'). What is most shocking is that the FDA knew of this public threat for over a decade before it informed the public. Benzoates (carbon based crystal com-pounds) are preservatives added to acidic packaged food to prevent the growth of mold, yeast, and some bacteria. Benzoates can be found in such products as pickles, certain Asian condiments, and sodas.

Many soft drinks and sodas contain a form of vitamin C (for flavor). What the FDA knew as early as 1990 is that Vitamin C ('ascorbic acid' to food scientists) can break benzoates down into, yes, you guessed it: benzene.

Enough said about sodas and soft drinks. To sum it up: SODA & SOFT DRINKS are probably the WORST FOOD on planet earth. They are HIGHLY ACIDIC, contain extremely high amounts of sugar or – even worse – artificial sweeteners (listed as biological warfare weapons) that are TOTALLY TOXIC to living cells and GUARANTEE severe damage to all living tissue. And let's top it all by adding some carcinogens to assure this elixir of DEATH really works. Allowing your kids soda is defi-nitely committing homicide, period.

TIP: replace your sugar with Stevia or raw honey. But pay attention because most honey is just syrup (which is nothing more than glucose). Try some REAL honey from your local market place.

15.4 Soy & GMO

We've all heard it before: "Soy is the healthy plant protein, the alternative to evil killed animal flesh". What's interesting about this is that common belief and expert opinion state that soy has a myriad of health benefits. Truth is that soy is merely a poison, the end.

Well how can this be? "The person at the health food store assured me that soy was so critical to life and has the power to cleanse me of my food sins, deliver me from my evil appetite for delicious steak, and set my place at the right hand of Gaya". What's even MORE astounding, is that the pervasive nature of this bold face lie is so ubiquitous in our society that a cornucopia of people from highly educated professionals to the uneducated blind-following masses just go along with these lies, goose stepping to the voice of some soy-god telling them that this junk is 'healthy'.

Look, here is a quick synopsis. SOY contains naturally occurring and built-in insecticides called 'isoflavones'. Remarkably, although these Isoflavones have been designed by nature to KILL predatory bugs using a neurological disruptor akin to Raid, they are actually advertised as beneficial to people. Ask yourself: in what universe could Raid be health promoting to any living being?

Isoflavones are a 'phytoestrogen', an estrogen like substance that can have analogous effects on your body in a similar manner as 'home grown' estrogen. So what are the ramifications of an excess of estrogen then? Excess estrogen or estrogen dominance stimulates the production of fibrin, which impairs blood flow throughout the body and reduces mechanical function of tissues and organs. Too much estrogen in the body is also implicated in the development of the majority of cancers known to men. In addition to preventing pregnancy and promoting infertility, frigidness, and ED (Erectile Dysfunction), excessive estrogen contributes to irritability, mood swings, fat accumulation, breast disease and uterine fibroid formation.

As if all that wasn't enough, estrogen affects one's 'manhood?' If you are a male and you knew drinking beer would kill testicular tissue and eventually contribute to turning you into someone 'less than a man' with extra breast tissue (funny how those big beer drinkers could use a bra, right?), would you still drink beer? If your answer is "yes," you wasted lots of time reading this book. Go to the bar and swallow down some beers, buy a nice bra, or go to Starbucks and pound down those 'Venti Soy Latte's'.

Studies indicate that isoflavones (Genistein and Daidzein) permanently reduce testicular function and lower Androgen (man) Hormone production, like Lutenizing Hormone (LH), a hormone that signals your testicles to 'work'. As the result of decreased androgens, estrogen dominance skyrockets, leading to baldness, fat belly, prostatitis and cancer in men. Baby boys and young males fed soy formulas and soy products (by good intentioned but ignorant moms just following the 'conventional wisdom') produce more female hormones and display more female characteristics.

Isoflavones have been shown to decrease thyroid hormone production. A compromised thyroid gland results in excessive fatigue, inability to recover from even moderate activity and accumulation of fat. Female children consuming the estrogens in soy formulas and their derivatives often hit puberty prematurely. We have been seen this trend in the last few decades, not only as a result of soy products, but the presence of hormones in a multitude of food products.

It gets worse... pregnant women ingesting soy products have the potential of affecting sexual differentiation of their offspring. Yet, day after day, we see a 'health conscious' pregnant woman jamming down a 'Tall Double Soy Latte' at Starbucks. So pervasive is this Soy epidemic that it has reached almost ubiquitous levels in our culture. In exactly the same way we were erroneously led to believe cigarette smoking had no deleterious fetal impact, current peer reviewed literature indicate that soy can lead to aberrations of the reproductive tract, alterations in brain development, and children born with undifferentiated male and female sexual organs. There goes our species... down the drain!

The list goes on and on. Isoflavones impede 'GOOD' cholesterol (HDL) and allow 'BAD' cholesterol (LDL) to proliferate. Soy contains an additional chemical called Phytin, which leeches essential minerals out of the body wreaking havoc on our system. Soy contains Trypsin inhibitors that block a vital anti-cancer enzyme and an anti-fibrosis enzyme (explaining the heightened risk for fibrotic conditions and all kinds of cancers). Soy is connected with a high rate of Vascular Dementia (Alzheimer's disease) and a host of other diseases. It all makes sense. Soy increases the levels of toxemia AND toxemia is the one and only cause of ALL so called disease. When it comes to soy, just say "NO."

We've all heard a barrage of reasons as to why we should avoid non-organic foods, fruit, veggies, meat etc. The research supporting these assertions is not insignificant. However, the main reason we consume non-organic foods: bugs. They're gross. Bugs kill the plant, eat the plant, shit on the plant, have sex, deposit eggs in the plant... everybody knows it, it's gross. So 'Better Living Through Chemistry' became a part of our lives and mainstream science promised to rid our lives of such pesky problems like bugs in our food.

But consuming non-organic foods is far worse. These foods (fruits and veggies) have been deluged in mostly petrochemical based pesticides. These chemicals act as additional estrogen in the body. In fact, MOST (if not all) organophosphate agra chemicals, from bug spray to fertilizers, are extremely estrogenic. Remember that many cancers, fibrosis based diseases, infertility, miscarriage, etc, may be driven by estrogen.

Non-organic meat is FILLED with Hormones and antibiotics. Which hormone you ask? Well, estrogen of course, estrogen is given to animals to fatten them up. Wait a minute, if we give estrogen to animals to make them fat, how do you think that translates to the end user? Ever heard of 'you are what you eat?'

What about the Hybridized GMO foods WE eat? What about the animals fed GMO foods and how we eat those animals? GMO foods have no seeds, no ability to reproduce.

These Hybridized foods are overly LARGE as compared to their organic cousins. Now look down the side walk of America at all the FAT and overweight people waddling around eating non-organic, GMO, Hybridized food and tell me there is no connection.

Finally, remember that these animals are also pumped full with antibiotics to fight the diseases inherent to our farming, feeding, and slaughtering techniques. The over -and improper use of these chemicals has been implicated not only in creating resistant strains of super bugs that attack us, but more importantly in providing us with a daily amount of dangerous toxins.

It should be easy: Say NO to SOY and NO to GMO.

But it doesn't seem to be easy. In November of 2012, California's Proposition 37 was presented to the voters requiring that all food products be labeled if they have been genetically modified. Monsanto apparently funneled hundreds of millions of dollars into California to defeat the measure. They were successful in defeating Proposition 37. It is beyond my comprehension why people would vote down a proposition disclosing what's in their food products. Never underestimate the actions of ill-informed American voters I guess.

15.5 Vaccines

Vaccines for measles, mumps, rubella (MMR), polio, influenza (common cold), swine flu (lmao) and meningococcal vaccines, as well as vaccines containing pertussis, diphtheria, and tetanus are all another huge threat to our health.

When you get sick, your body creates special proteins called antibodies to fight the infection. The next time you are exposed to that same virus or bacteria, those antibodies keep you from getting sick again.

The premise of vaccines is that they do the same thing without making you ill. "Vaccines induce the protective immunity that is a consequence of natural infection, without having to pay the price of [becoming sick with] a natural infection," says Paul Offit, chief of the division of infectious diseases and the director of the Vaccine Education Center at the Children's Hospital of Philadelphia. Oh my dear Paul, you may have to review that statement of nonsense. "Without paying the price of becoming sick with a natural infection", meaning without symptoms or without the natural course of action the body undertakes to fight pathogens and return back to normal or optimal health. This approach not only makes the organism (yes, that is you) weaker and ineffective, but loads that organism (that's you again) with a toxic load.

Like so much of Medicine, the root cause of so called diseases like Parkinson's, Alzheimer's, Autism etc., have been misunderstood. However, in this 21st century, because of advancements in technology like F-MRI in the above examples, many degenerative changes in the brains of these patients can be observed like never before. I don't want to belabor you with the details of how protein cross linking is implicated in a de-facto short circuiting of nervous system transmission or how aluminum shards in DNA strands disrupt bodily function. Suffice it to say that the egregious overabundance of exogenous (from OUTSIDE the body) toxins, like those found in vaccines contribute not only to a decrease in neurotransmitters, but also a shrinking of the brain as the result of a decrease in its fat content (as an oversimplification, it is helpful to imagine the brain is comprised of mostly cholesterol).

But these conditions and considerations are the end results of an abnormal terrain in the body and not its direct cause. Low grade inflammation, constant, ongoing and lingering, both in the body and in the brain (brain inflammation: encephalitis) is what is implicated as the root cause of these and other conditions.

In Parkinson's patients, a particular component of the brain becomes inflamed and as a result, begins to decay. If left unchecked it will eventually become necrotic. As this degradation occurs, over time, the patient will lose more and more ability to function. It's a horrible, insidious thing because the part of the brain being destroyed is credited with Dopamine production amongst other functions. Dopamine 'connects' the brain to the body, which explains the symptom complex in Parkinson's.

Then we have Chronic Fatigue, another so called disease, but fatigue is nothing more than a symptom. Do you know what they call a 'quarter pounder with cheese' in Europe? They call it a 'Royal' with cheese. Do you know what they call Chronic Fatigue in Europe? They name it 'Myalgic Encephilitis', in other words: swelling of the brain (inflammation). Chronic Fatigue patients have a brain swelling that triggers the symptoms and manifestations of the so called disease.

Now wait a minute, Chronic Fatigue has a gazillion things in common with other disease states like Mononucleosis (Epstein Barr Virus) or Post-Polio Syndrome, commonly diagnosed in patients who were inoculated with the live Sabin polio inoculation. Mononucleosis, Polio and Post-Polio all have a brain inflammation associated with the condition and all have inoculation in common. You do the math.

But wait, let's not forget Autism. Autism has been linked to brain inflammation and also to mercury poisoning. Each inoculation contains 5 times the OSHA standard for toxic levels of mercury. Five times the toxic levels multiplied by the number of inoculations administered and there you have it: mercury in your baby or child's brain. Does anybody still think MERCURY isn't deleterious and can negatively impact development? It may or may not be the cause of Autism, but it certainly adds greatly to toxemia and any so called disease.

What about you Mr. & Mrs. Grown up? Do you get annual flu shots like you're told on morning talk shows or by a brainwashed doctor? That flu shot has analogous mercury preservative for you, so don't feel left out. LOL.

As if that wasn't bad enough, there is strong evidence suggesting that the inflammation that leads to the disease states stems from the viruses in the vaccines themselves. "Oh, but they're weakened (attenuated) versions of a live virus and so they are not harmful" would be a dump reply from a manufacturer or doctor.

Every virus 'family' we've ever acquired either via exposure or inoculation, is viable and hosted/housed in our body in a state that could be best thought of as suspended animation. You may or may not be aware that the Chicken Pox virus we were exposed to as kids can manifest as Shingles as adults or Hepatic Neuralgia (permanent nerve pain caused by the Herpes virus later in life). Many of the viruses we were inoculated with as children in the good faith effort to keep us healthy have come home to roost. How does that happen you may ask? The body simply neutralizes the toxin as long as possible, preserving life. At an older age, when health is further compromised by unhealthful living, other emergencies become more important and the dormant virus is released.

We can just conclude that these unnecessarily inoculations or vaccines simple contribute to toxemia. But worse is that these excess, strong poisons are administered in high, frequent doses to our young ones. Can you imagine how that 'perfect' creation of a baby or child has to react and neutralize these toxins to preserve life? How we poison them? It's clearly homicide and genocide. It's criminal to interfere and poison a human being in perfect health.

How do we protect against these epidemics and diseases like polio, small pox and chicken pox then? LOL. Answer: BE HEALTHY. Only the weak suffer and the weak just get weaker by the arrogant, wrong, and fraudulent interventions of today's medicine. Our body has the answer to pathogens, nature has the answer to pathogens, and human quacks are arrogant enough to think they also have the answer with these vaccines and pharmaceutical poisons. It's sad, but true.

Final note: epidemics only rise when pathogens invade an entire population. This can only happen when that population is weak and sick, or malnourished. In this case, to preserve life, poisons such as vaccines may save lives of course... in the short term. But you can see that the cause is not addressed and merely a band aid has been provided.

When traveling to underdeveloped countries, with lack of hygienic conditions such as unclean water and food, vaccines also could save a life in case the traveling individual exhibits impaired health at the time of exposure.

In general, vaccines are unnecessary poisons and shouldn't be injected just because the schools and doctors want everyone to do so without rationale. In a perfect world, we can eliminate these vaccines but as we know, in economically deprived, Third World, underdeveloped countries, these diseases run rampant. Also, in a highly mobilized world where any location in the world is just an airplane ride away, these diseases will always be a threat to the weak among us.

15.6 Allergies

In western medicine terminology, many so called diseases end in "itis" or "osis." While "itis" indicates inflammation, "osis" indicates fibrosis (hardening), scar tissue and adhesions. We learned that chronic inflammation leads to hardening of the tissues, in other words: "itis" becomes "otis" in an effort to preserve life. Our body's inability to manage the mediators of inflammatory levels, prostaglandins and cytokines for instance, often lead to a hyperactive immune system that manifests as, among other things, 'allergies'.

An allergy, (overly) simply stated, may be thought of as an overreaction by our immune system to almost any stimulant it perceives to be a threat. As an example, particular types of food, dust mites, weeds and/or pollen can trigger an allergic event. For people without allergies, these stimuli are harmless. But when someone develops an allergy, their immune system 'sees' these stimulants as hostile foreign invaders. In an effort to drive these invaders out, the immune system mobilizes all its resources: the INFLAMMATORY RESPONSE is initiated. Elimination efforts such as sneezing, tearing, vomiting, sweating and pooping may be called into battle.

In fact, it's not too much of a stretch to suggest that practically every presentation of an allergy begins its journey with inflammation COMBINED with exposure to certain mediators, like an unusually occurring protein, in the body. These unusual proteins interact with the immune system and generate antibodies and, are subsequently flagged by the body as allergens that are now the target of the immune system response.

Examination of these allergens suggests that they have a common denominator: they bind to something in our body called heparin. Heparin is released from cells in conjunction with histamine and may be released into the intestines to block pathogens from binding to the intestine surface. Heparin is anti-inflammatory in nature and contributes to minimizing the inflammatory response of the intestines, to food for example.

Abnormal inflammation may reduce heparin production and utilization. Inflammation that reduces heparin production thereby increases immune response to FOOD, food antigens and other antigens (think outside stimulus like weeds, pollen, dander). This cascade of events may result in de facto hyper immune system response leading to the presentation of allergy symptoms. NORMALLY, inflammation is self-limiting.

Unfortunately, numerous toxins we become exposed to over time lead to a shift from local inflammation that usually protects us, to *systemic* inflammation that gives rise to inflammatory mediators in the blood stream and can lead to coughing, sneezing, achy stuffy head etc.

Allergy medicines and anti-histamines of all kind yet again just deal with the symptoms, which are nothing but the effort of the body to deal with the toxins. Inhibiting these efforts by inhibiting the symptoms only worsens the inflammation and causes hardening or thickening of the mucosa later on. Yet again, the cause is not taken away and the symptom complex worsens. So can a simple allergy turn in to a severe pneumonia or bronchitis, and eventually respiratory failure or cancer. One just needs to take away the cause (toxins) and AVOID the progenitors of inflammation that lead to all that mess!

Implementing the ACTION PLAN in this book will rid you of many toxins, most likely many of them responsible for your allergies. If you want to find out what toxins are triggering your specific allergies, you may opt to do an LRA test.

The following test is optional but may be of great benefit in the short-term. A LRA test reveals the food items we should eliminate from our diet.

LRA-Test

One of the major advancements in medicine in recent years has been our expanded understanding of the immune system and its far broader and more important role in general health and wellness. Initially, it was thought that our immune system was only involved in defending our bodies against threatening agents such as bacteria, viruses, and environmental 'invaders'. Medical science has recently come to recognize that the immune system has defense as well as repair capabilities. This repair component plays an important role in restoring tissue and organs from damage that a disease state may have caused. Recent studies have shown that when lymphocytes (white blood cells) are mobilized to fight off invaders, the vital repair process suffers. As a result, organs and tissue weaken over time and the body's ability to fight off future assaults is reduced. The effect of immune system dysfunction can be chronic inflammatory and auto-immune diseases that always defy treatment (the only cure is to take away the cause).

The most common assaults that pose the greatest burden to our immune system on a daily basis are digestive remnants and environmental antigens. An antigen (from antibody-generating) is a substance that prompts the generation of antibodies and can cause an immune response. By identifying these antigens and eliminating them from our exposure, the immune burden can be lifted or eliminated, allowing both the defense and repair systems to return to optimal function. The result is improved, sustainable overall health.

By living C.L.E.A.N. this result will be obtained automatically, but it doesn't hurt to find out exactly what substances are causing a heightened immune response in your body.

How is the LRA by ELISA/ACT testing different from a RAST test?

RAST (IgE) only detects immediate allergic reactions to approximately 100 dietary or environmental substances. This test is useful to assess hives, wheezing, or shock that may appear minutes after being exposed to a reacting food or chemical.

The LRA by ELISA/ACT is a comprehensive, reliable test able to identify the causes of delayed allergy/hypersensitivity reactions. These can occur from hours to weeks after exposure. Most people do not realize they are reacting to these substances since the onset of symptoms does not occur quickly. For example, people may develop achiness hours to days after a food or chemical exposure.

This test measures sensitivities up to 450 items including foods, additives, preservatives, environmental chemicals and toxic minerals, molds, danders, hairs and feathers, medications, therapeutic herbs, and food colorings.

How does it work then?

A blood sample is taken and at the lab these different items are introduced one by one to your blood. The test basically measures the antigens produced against each of these items. If the body produces a high number of antigens against a certain item, it means that your body is 'sensitive' to that item...the body doesn't like that item (for whatever reason) and is constantly fighting it. This causes your defense system to be in a constant 'war' which burdens the repair system and eventually the immune system....resulting in so called disease.

Once we know what items our body is sensitive to, we need to eliminate those items from our diet or avoid exposure to them. The defense system can take a break, the repair system starts working better, and the immune system regains optimal function.

Note: This test is also VERY beneficial as part of a weight loss program, since an impaired immune system and therefore a body-out-of-balance limits effectiveness of diet, exercise and supplementation. Eliminating the items your body is sensitive too will indirectly speed up (read: bring back to normal) your metabolism, which was sluggish and part of your weight problem.

The downside is that this LRA-test is expensive. For more information visit our website.

Let me share with you one more pearl of insight. The majority of so called allergies are actually toxicities and all too often the substance you are 'allergic' or 'toxic' to is NOT the one recorded in your medical chart.

For example, if you are injected with 2% artichoke extract (a natural lipolytic and diuretic) or 2% lidocaine and you develop a so called allergic reaction (read: toxic reaction since the body is trying to expel the toxin), your medical record (for your lifetime) will indicate you are allergic to lidocaine (in the latter case). Now, think about this please. What is the change that you are actually 'allergic' to lidocaine when lidocaine only makes up 2% of the solution? Indeed, the likelihood is only 2%. It's far more likely you are 'allergic' to any of the poisonous junk that makes up the other 98%, including preservatives, proteins, colorings, fillers, etc.

Exposure to toxins and ingestion of a host of processed foods often contribute to inflammation, which can occur in the adrenal glands secreting hormones and therefore destabilizing insulin and blood sugar levels. Elevated levels of insulin may cause your body to hold on to and inappropriately deposit fat, rather than allowing it to be employed by the Krebs cycle for energy. In this manner, food allergies may contribute to weight gain, and subsequently, that adipose tissue or extra fat further promotes inflammation, exacerbating the problems of allergies. This is yet another example of a never ending, vicious cycle of suffering, caused by toxemia.

Many environmental allergies that we suffer from may actually be considered secondary immune system manifestations being driven by primary allergic responses to foods (among other things).

Since it seems apparent that all modern so called diseases have a significant inflammatory component, and since conventional diets are bereft with inflammatory mediators, we recommend avoiding synthetic, nearly unidentifiable processed foods from your diet.

For many people, the elimination of the potentiators and progenitors of chronic inflammation, and therefore eliminating a basic food allergy, obtains results in 3-7 days. Often times an increase in energy, enhanced clarity, improved digestion and a reduction of all kinds of symptoms is felt and seen.

Chapter 16 – Dr. Mike's Health Freedom Wellness Model

Many of us assume that just starting to eat healthier, taking some supplements and exercising a little bit more will turn things around. Unfortunately, this is NOT how it works. Agreed, it's better to do something than doing nothing at all, but let me explain.

Your body is like a tree or plant, and when the tree or plant is diseased and needs nurturing, we can do something about it. We can make sure the tree gets plenty of sunlight, water the leaves, and trim them. It may all help. However, what we really need to do first is to nurture the root. We need to provide the root with the appropriate nutrients and an adequate water supply. If we nurture the root, the root will nurture the whole plant or tree.

Our body functions in the same way. We need to establish a health foundation. If we establish this basic health foundation and balance the body, it will flourish. Biochemical reactions will function optimally, bodily systems and organs will work effectively and efficiently, the immune system will fight invaders and health is promoted.

Doesn't it make sense to balance the body and provide a foundation for health prior to trying to combat a so called disease? I thought so.

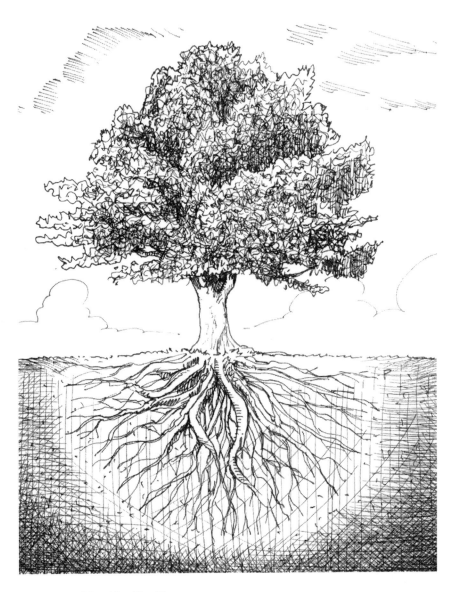

Illustration 29 – Healthy Tree

Another analogy we used in the beginning of this book is the one of the wounded soldier. Instead of giving this soldier powerful weapons to defeat the enemy, wouldn't it make more sense to first heal that wounded soldier and only then sent him or her back on the battlefield with those powerful weapons? Of course.

As such we need to RESTORE our health prior to RESOLVING any medical problems or so called diseases.

16.1 R3 - Restore, Resolve, Rejuvenate

R3 is my HEALTH FREEDOM WELLNESS MODEL. First we need to RESTORE or regain our health. We need to get back to 'NORMAL'. What I mean with 'normal' is a body, mind and soul in balance. How do we balance our body, mind and soul? By respecting the laws of human life and living C.L.E.A.N. We need to reestablish a balance in our body and put it in the RIGHT CONDITIONS to REGAIN and OBTAIN optimal HEALTH.

Once the body is back in balance and 'normal' health is restored, our body has now the ability to heal itself and RESOLVE any current health issues: from chronic pain, fibromyalgia, fatigue, high blood pressure, high cholesterol, insomnia, low libido, depression to more severe conditions including heart conditions, diabetes, degenerative disease, Alzheimer and cancers, you name it.

We already know the root or cause of all these symptoms and so called diseases (toxemia) and we also know the one and only solution: take the cause away. We even know HOW to take the cause away: by living C.L.E.A.N. However, in the RESOLVE phase of the R3 wellness model, we will facilitate and accelerate the abolishment of symptoms by introducing specific nutrients, supplements, behavior modification techniques etc.

I can already share with you that when you put phase 1 (RESTORE) into practice, the majority of your symptoms will disappear and eventually they all will be gone (the body heals when placed in the RIGHT conditions). The RESOLVE phase is merely a phase of facilitation as specific nutrients and conditions are introduced based on the specific symptom profiles.

One more task awaits us after we RESTORE 'normal' health and RESOLVE our current 'medical' problems: REJUVENATE ourselves.

We need to OPTIMIZE health and PREVENT disease. We need to assure LONGEVITY. We need to continue to provide our body with the necessary nutrients but simultaneously supplement with CUSTOMIZED nutrients and continue to improve our habits of C.L.E.A.N. living. Stephen R. Covey explains this in his 7th habit: SHARPEN THE SAW.

As we age, our body needs even more essential nutrients as tissues start to naturally wear down more and more, and repair is crucial. We need to neutralize more free radicals with more potent ANTIOXIDANTS so that we defeat oxidation and prevent so-called disease.

Also, as aging continues we need to replace more and more essential nutrients, and continue to monitor pH and metabolism. We need to anticipate depletion of nutrients and proactively replace them; we need to check hormone imbalance and replace (not substitute) them with bio-identical hormones, and we need to continue to modify our plan of action as our age, environment, activity level, and health changes. We also need to continue to learn how to respond to emotional and traumatic experiences we encounter in life, and understand how these experiences (if not coped with properly) significantly affect our health in a negative and harmful manner.

The Health 4 Life Action Plan outlined in the next chapter will provide you with the steps and actions to take in your quest to successfully RESTORE your health.

This is the BIG PLAN: Restore, Resolve, Rejuvenate. But, let's start with the most important step: RESTORE. We have to provide our mind and body with the basic foundation to regain, obtain and maintain optimal health.

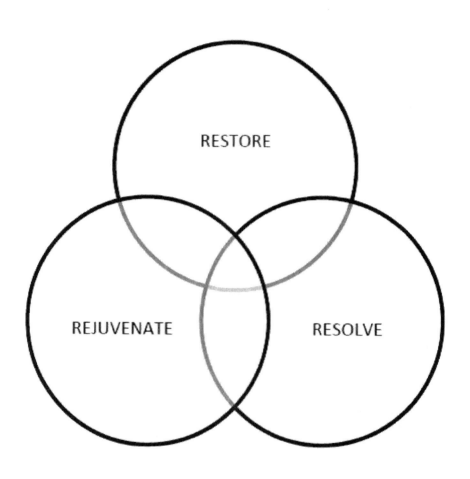

Illustration 30 – R3 Wellness Model

RESTORE:

This is the MOST IMPORTANT phase by far. Nothing will change without the proper implementation of this RESTORE phase.

The RESTORE phase is 90% of the Health 4 Life Action Plan. It's about learning HOW to live C.L.E.A.N.:

Control your emotions and feelings.
Listen to the warning signs of your body, avoid overstimulation and overindulgences.
Enough Rest, Sleep and Sunshine.
Active Lifestyle.
Natural and Clean food, water and air.

RESOLVE:

Trying to RESOLVE your current medical issues or problems without RESTORING health is like trying to catch fish in the air. It just won't happen. By implementing the RESTORE phase, your mind and body are regaining BALANCE, and your body will be able to HEAL ITSESLF when placed in the RIGHT CONDITIONS.

During the RESOLVE phase, we merely facilitate the resolution of lingering symptoms and speed-up the healing process by introducing more specific nutrients based on the symptoms or so called diseases that present themselves.

Look up your medical condition or problems online and search for natural remedies. Do some diligent research and also consult with a local naturopathic doctor or a doctor with knowledge in natural medi-cine. Find out what NATURAL nutrients are recommended to RESOLVE your 'medical' condition.

Again, make sure that you consume organic, whole foods and that the nutrients or supplements are purchased from a reputable company and that these supplements are able to be absorbed by your body.

EXAMPLE 1: RHEUMATOID ARTHRITIS

If you suffer from rheumatoid arthritis or another condition that causes pain or symptoms due to inflammation (injuries, arthritis, colitis and anything else ending with –itis), we need to provide our body with some highly effective, all natural anti-inflammatory supplements or foods. The following nutrients can assist your body in managing and even abolishing chronic inflammation:

1. Liquid Vemma (decrease in C-reactive protein).

2. MSM supplement (unless you are 'allergic' to sulfur).

3. Since our pancreas drastically reduces the production of fibrolytic and proteolytic enzymes after the age of 27 (yeah, I know...how did they come up with this number... who knows), we need to ingest high quality fibrolytic and proteolytic enzymes. Serrapeptase would be an excellent enzyme to reduce inflammation and fibrogenesis.

4. Fish oils (pure omega 3 only), fresh pineapple (bromelain), ginger and many other alkaline foods also have strong anti-inflammatory properties.

The next step would be to identify 'other' problems that come with the disease, and repeat the process above. In this example of Rheumatoid Arthritis we not only deal with the pain caused by inflammation, but we also have to deal with damaged cartilage and tissues surrounding the inflamed joints. We need to find out which nutrients could assist in rebuilding the cartilage and tissues. In this case, it may be sulfur (such as in onions and garlic), glucosamine, chondroitin, and others.

Besides placing emphasis on nutrients that help reduce and abolish existing symptoms, make sure you also limit nutrients that may aggravate your symptoms. For example, milk, red meat and table salt in the case of Rheumatoid Arthritis.

I know, you will need to do some research...but guess what? It's easy to collect lots of data online in a minimum amount of time. Once you educated yourself, you may (or may not) consult with a knowledgeable person on the subject. Once you know what nutrients you need, make sure you get the RIGHT ones (read: the ones that 'really' work). But be aware about the information you find online: lots of that information is bogus and skewed, trying to sell you something.

When in doubt, please contact us anytime. But ALWAYS REMEMBER that without restoring your health (including alkalizing your body and consuming wholefoods), the measures presented in the RESOLVE phase are virtually obsolete.

EXAMPLE 2: FIBROMYALGIA

This so called disease is not only misunderstood (just like any other so called disease because there simply is no disease) but has been treated by conventional medicine in such a profoundly wrong way that it could drive me to drink (water that is LOL). I say 'so called' because there are no diseases, only symptoms. However, I do recognize the REAL pain and problems these patients suffer.

I could write an entire book about this so called fibromyalgia (or myofascial pain syndrome) but it would be a waste of time since all so called disease is cured by simply resolving toxemia, including this fibromyalgia. In other words, the answer is in this book as is for any symptom or so called disease.

But let's simply dissect the word 'fibromyalgia'. Myalgia means muscle pain and fibro indicates fibrin. Fibromyalgia then means that the person suffers from muscle pain caused by the production of excess fibrin in the body.

Fibrin is like scar tissue and when in excess it forms a network within, in this case, the muscles and tissues. This fibrin network impairs circulation in the muscles and tissues, resulting in what we call hypoxic pain (pain due to a lack of oxygen). Poor circulation brings poor oxygenation.

Conventional medicine has a ridiculous chart with 18 palpation points. If more than 12 of these 18 points are tender upon palpation, the diagnosis is made. I guess we are back in kindergarten! We are dealing with a systemic issue and if the issue is real, all points will be tender.

The cause is – of course – toxemia. However, what situation or condition causes the bucket to overflow, resulting in more toxins being produced versus eliminated? There are two main causes when it comes to our fibromyalgia syndrome (which is nothing more than a symptom complex):

1. Estrogen dominance: excess estrogen relative to progesterone. A simple blood test can indicate whether one is estrogen dominant or not. The solution is simple also: a natural (or bio-identical) progesterone crème. Explanation: excess estrogen stimulates the production of fibrin.

2. Excess cortisol: cortisol is vital to life but when in excess stimulates the production of fibrin. Cortisol is also called our stress hormone.

Now, if you think about this, it all makes sense. Most people with so called fibromyalgia are women. These women are usually pre-menopausal, post-menopausal or in their menopause and their hormones are out of balance (estrogen dominance) AND/OR extra STRESS came into their lives.

The onset of this 'fibromyalgia' often correlates with a time indicating an increase in stress. This stress may be a divorce, a car accident, a loss in the family, job change, unemployment, etc. This extra stress causes an increase in cortisol and subsequently an increase in fibrin.

So, what's the ONLY solution to fibromyalgia? RESTORE health by living C.L.E.A.N. and stopping toxemia. Hormones will be balanced and stress levels under control.

As part of the RESOLVE phase, we can recommend fibrolytic enzymes such as the previously mentioned serrapeptase (cocoon of the silk worm) to 'eat away' the fibrin in the muscles and tissues, L-arginine (to

413

increase circulation and reduce pain), and maybe even some magnesium citrate (to relax the muscles).

Without the RESTORE phase, even this common sense approach will be limited in its results, but with the RESTORE phase, fast and lasting results are achieved ... EVERY SINGLE TIME.

As part of the RESTORE phase we will have to achieve hormonal balance (in case of estrogen dominance) and/or we will have to reduce stress and learn HOW to control our emotions and feelings in order to avoid the excess production of cortisol. If your husband causes all your stress, maybe counseling or a divorce is necessary. If your job is stressing you out, you may need a career change. If you lost a dear family member and several years later you are still in grief, you may need some professional help etc.

Masking symptoms without addressing the cause NEVER gives lasting results. In the case of fibromyalgia, many doctors prescribe anti-depressants ... really? Because they themselves are oblivious as to the nature of this so called fibromyalgia, their patient must be imagining all of this or is exaggerating. The reason these patients become depressed is because conventional medicine doesn't have a solution.

Men, even though not reported in conventional statistics, suffer as much from this symptom complex as women do, as any other symptom complex. Men indeed don't suffer from menopause, yet they do suffer from andropause and encounter similar stresses of life.

REJUVENATE:

WHEN you successfully resolved your medical problems and issues, and regained your health, it's time to REJUVENATE. You are back to 'normal'. But we don't want to be just 'normal', we want to be OPTIMAL.

We need to boost energy, boost immune, prevent disease, and continue to be proactive in dealing with the challenges of aging. We need to build up an energy reserve that can be tapped into during emergency situations.

We need to continue to maintain our 'body in balance' by continuing to follow our RESTORE plan and living C.L.E.A.N. We need to continue to work on our MENTAL aspects (positive thinking and HELPING OTHERS) and fine tune the skills that control our emotions and feelings in our search for true happiness.

We need to continuously and relentlessly 'sharpen the saw' by improving on every aspect of C.L.E.A.N. living.

16.2 Key Points

The Health Freedom Wellness model is unique in that it advocates to RESTORE health prior to try and RESOLVE a 'medical' problem.

R3 stands for: RESTORE – RESOLVE – REJUVENATE. The R3 model, unlike any wellness model, shows you HOW to remove the cause of all disease and REGAIN, OBTAIN and MAINTAIN OPTIMAL HEALTH.

The RESTORE phase is by far the most important phase since it rebuilds the foundation for optimal health and simultaneously teaches one HOW to remove the cause of all disease: toxemia.

The RESOLVE phase is a symptom-targeted phase in which we will use conditions or nutrients to facilitate and accelerate the resolution of symptoms. This phase is ineffective without the RESTORE phase for the obvious reasons.

The REJUVENATE phase is the phase in which we can build up vitality and energy reserves and work on prevention. It's also the phase in which we continue to improve upon the RESTORE phase and all aspects of living C.L.E.A.N. It's the SKY IS THE LIMIT phase when it comes to health and happiness.

CHAPTER 17 – GRAND CONCLUSION

This chapter gives the reader a quick review of the most important concepts of this book and summarizes the most important conditions in our quest to regain, maintain and sustain optimal health.

17.1 THE WRONG CONDITIONS

Most of us have been living in violation of the laws of human life and as a consequence have suffered so called diseases as an inevitable consequence. Just remember that health, not disease, is the natural or normal condition of all organisms.

Sickness and suffering are consequences of breaking the laws of nature and human life; they cannot be escaped. Almost the whole practice of medicine is an effort to enable us to escape the inevitable and necessary results of our transgressions of the laws of human life. We attempt to drug and dose away the effects of violated law but unfortunately that never works.

Every so called disease is a plea for desistance (opposite of assistance). Pain is not a plea for pain killers but for rest and desistance. Discomfort does not call for sedatives or tonics but for desistance. Loss of appetite is not a call for tonics and digestive aids but is simply a sign that our shop (stomach and digestive system) is closed for repair and no food should be taken. Nausea and vomiting are not a plea for anti-emetics and digestives but for abstinence of food. Pain in the stomach following a meal does not call for Malox or Pepsin or Nexium but rather for abstinence of food. Nature continues to cry out for you to cease abusing your stomach so the natural forces of repair and recuperation can do their job, etc.

To conceal a symptom or condition by sand-bagging your senses is utter nonsense and certainly harmful. Every measure directed at the removal of symptoms and not at the removal of the one and only cause is simply evil.

A great analogy was used in 'Human Life – Its Philosophy and Laws' by Herbert M. Shelton. In repairing a house the carpenter uses the same materials, tools and methods that were employed in its construction. No man attempts to repair a house built of lumber with brick and mortar. He employs a hammer and other tools for working with wood (and not a trowel and other tools for working with brick and mortar). Carpenters are employed to repair wooden structures and masons to repair stone structures. Any other methods and materials of repair would not be tolerated by an intelligent home owner.

The process of repair in houses is the same as the process of construction. This is also true for any other structures, machines etc. We do not even consider that it would be otherwise. However, we seem to use far less intelligence when dealing with our human body. We substitute food for poisonous drugs, rest for stimulation, cleanliness for antiseptics and sterility, sunlight for electric lights and pure water for coffee, sodas, alcohol and bottled mineral water. No man expects his house to be repaired instantly but he does want instantaneous cures.

Health comes through healthy living and there are no substitutes.

Few people realize how much time and money they spend trying to cover up evidences of their ill health instead of improving their health. For example, if they are constipated they blame the constipation for their ill health instead of blaming the impairment of their health for the constipation.

Another example is that one of a foul breath or an unclean mouth. The unclean mouth is not the cause of disease; it's an effect, a symptom. You don't improve your health by scrubbing your teeth, rinsing your mouth, and gargling your throat. These actions remedy nothing. Good health is the best mouth wash, the best tooth brush, and the best deodorant.

One has to just listen to the warning signs of the body and make the RIGHT choices. Man's normal instincts are a reliable guide in the matter of feeding and fasting, but under current conditions few men reach maturity with normal instincts and sound warning signs. Man has become a master of perversions by ignoring his natural warning signs and making the wrong choices.

The materials used in health are therefore the same materials that should be used in disease.

Isn't it about time that the millions of people suffering today should know the grand truth that health, not disease, is their birth-right... a birth-right they continually sell for a bunch of indulgences?

Isn't it about time that you realize WHAT the remedy is for any so called disease? The discovery of the cause is the discovery of the remedy. The cause is always the same: TOXEMIA. Therefore the remedy is always the same: REMOVE TOXEMIA.

The old school physician, the drugs, and the therapeutic methods are ALL FRAUDS attempting to mask symptoms out of plain ignorance or for monetary gain. These frauds that INTERFERE with our body contribute to toxemia and are hazardous to our health. There is no argument. It's time to make a shift and finally choose the road to optimal health. YOU, and only you, are in TOTAL CONTROL and you need to take it.

WAKE UP and stop being brainwashed by your so called doctors, pharmaceutical companies, alternative medicine practitioners and therapists of all kind AND start taking away the CAUSE of all your ailments.

It should be obvious and known that any benefit to health must come through the ordinary physiological acts. Medicines and therapeutics possess no power to antagonize or neutralize the cause of so called disease or to assist the organism in its work. They simply cannot add power to the organism, but only stimulate the physiological functions to a certain extent, robbing the body of vital energy.

Current medical practice is based on chasing symptoms, and 'curing one disease while producing another', and inducing a drug disease to 'cure' a primary disease. Think about the following: we don't give medications to the healthy because then they will get sick, so why is it that we give medications to the sick? In both the sick and the healthy, medications add to toxemia.

To throw an immense quantity of medicine into a diseased body, and accidentally kill or cure, as the event may happen to be, requires but little science and skill.

Drugs and medicine merely suppress symptoms, and the effects of suppression are:

1. Prolonged course and severity of the so called disease,

2. Cause complications and more symptoms,

3. Cause a build-up of toxins in our system and contribute to toxemia, causing many other so called diseases,

4. Kill the patient.

Dr. Trall stated: If the medical man with good intentions administers one of these drug poisons, or a hundred of them, and the patient dies then the patient dies because the medicine can't save him. But if a malefactor with murderous disposition gives the same medicine to a fellow-being, and the fellow-being dies, he dies because the poison killed him. Does the motive of the one who administers the drug alter its relation to vitality?"

I often get the argument that people do get better when taking drugs or after some kind of treatment. This merit of 'cure' is that of coincidence in time, nothing more. Nature always strives for perfection and health and gradually overcomes those conditions that are in conflict with that aim. These conditions that are in conflict with that aim can be both spontaneously or artificially induced. It's just a delusion of the patient and the physician that their prescription would have some potency that affects the desired result. Without interference, the problem would have resolved better and faster.

Medications and therapeutic measures only add to the problem, and if by some coincidence the patient gets better it must have been the drug or therapy. This happens over and over again (in their fraudulent clinical trials based on hypothesis and principles that are fundamentally wrong) so the drugs must work because the results are consistent. What's really happening is that the body not only overcomes the so called disease but also overcomes the conditions in conflict with the healing process (medication and therapeutics). That's how strong our body is. But it will NEVER be cured unless placed in the RIGHT CONDITIONS.

Remember that our organism is a self-curative thing and that it is capable of putting up a winning fight against great odds. It's not the chemotherapy or radiation that 'cured' the cancer, it's the power of the organism that not only survived the cancer but also survived the radiation or chemotherapy. Again, if the patient dies, the chemotherapy didn't work and if the patient survives the chemotherapy did work... really? This is laughable. Without the chemotherapy the patient would have a far bigger change to survive.

17.2 THE RIGHT CONDITIONS

We learned that living matter ALWAYS strives for perfect health and that what we call disease is nothing more than a beneficial process that does NOT need any interference of any kind. So called disease and its symptoms are healing actions of our body in an attempt to restore optimal health.

Only our body, so complex our human brain is incapable of understanding, has the ability to cure itself. Ignorance and short-sightedness have done much mischief in the treatment of human illness. Only nature is the true physician. The restorative power is inherent to the organism.

There is only ONE cause of so called disease: TOXEMIA. Therefore, there is ONLY ONE solution to all so called disease: REMOVE the CAUSES of toxemia. HOW?

1. We must STOP all practices and habits that cause toxemia and consequently prevent proper elimination and recuperation.

2. We must STOP the absorption of ALL internal and external poisons. Internal poisons are the result of normal metabolism and are effectively eliminated by a healthy body, but when health is impaired toxins built up. External poisons DO NOT need to be added to these internal poisons. External poisons include all man-made, unnatural foods and drinks, drugs, unnecessary vaccines, serums etc.

3. We must SUPPLY ourselves the RIGHT CONDITIONS for optimal health. A MODE OF LIVING, not a plan of treatment is the road to optimal health. The RIGHT CONDITIONS include natural wholefoods, fasting, pure water, fresh air, natural sunlight, rest and sleep, activities (exercise), mental poise (in control of emotions and feelings), physical comfort (shelter, not too cold or too hot), and HYGIENE.

With hygiene I do not mean the use of soaps, shampoos, mouth washes, antiseptics etc. These are totally unnecessary and most often harmful. When taking a shower or cleaning the body, or when the throat and mouth demand cleansing, or when other body parts require cleansing (eyes, nose, ears, vagina, wounds etc.) use plain, pure water. If true cleansing is indicated, you may dilute lemon juice or pineapple juice. Keeping the body clean also includes limiting the wear of clothes.

With hygiene I both refer to physical cleanness and mental cleanness. Mental cleanness refers to keeping the mind clean from perversions and negative thoughts, and being able to control emotions and feelings.

4. We must continue to ACCUMULATE VITAL ENERGY. This should be done by avoiding all influences that waste vital energy (see 1), and by supplying our body and mind with adequate rest, sleep and relaxation in order to allow for optimal repair and recuperation.

5. We must be patient because removing toxemia and restoring optimal health takes TIME. Cure is an evolution in reverse and does not happen instantaneously. A common mistake is to regard so called disease as cured and health restored when the symptoms have ceased, In reality, the person is now in just the same condition he or she was just prior to the appearance of those symptoms, and the way back to optimal health is still far. The process of repair is slow and gradual and therefore the return to firm and vigorous health requires several weeks, months, or even years... based on favorable or unfavorable influences and circumstances, and habits of life.

6. We must ACCEPT the HIGHEST POSSIBLE STANDARD (optimal health and nothing less). All we have to do is supply the favorable or RIGHT CONDITIONS so that our body can do its job. Besides protection from trauma and provision of shelter, we just need to LIVE C.L.E.A.N.:

CONTROL EMOTIONS AND FEELINGS
LISTEN TO THE WARNING SIGNS OF OUR BODY – AVOID
OVERSTIMULATION AND OVERINDULGENCES
ENOUGH REST, SLEEP AND SUNSHINE
ACTIVE LIFESTYLE
NATURAL AND CLEAN AIR, WATER AND FOOD

Furthermore, we must not become one-sided in our manner of living. One cannot be healthy by exercising alone, or through a healthy diet alone, or with plenty of rest and sleep alone. Life must be lived as a whole and don't even think YOU are exception to the laws of life.

These conditions will allow the body to restore itself and regain optimal health. Our bodies have enough vitality to live and survive (for a while) under the wrong conditions, imagine what it can do under the right conditions...

Acute Disease

The approach to any ACUTE so called disease and its symptoms: DO NOT TREAT.

The body simply requires:

1. Physical, mental and physiological rest,

2. Abstinence from all food,

3. Pure water when thirsty,

4. Fresh, clean air,

5. Hygiene.

Do not use pain killers or other treatments to relief pain: pain killers are an unmitigated evil and produce more pain eventually than they ever can relieve. Pain is merely a symptom and therefore beneficial and protective. If not suppressed, pain serves as a great diagnostic guide. My advice: grin it and bear it.

Nothing would be better for a sick person than a high fever. The higher the fever is, the faster the recovery. Do not suppress the fever in any way, shape or form: no medicine to stop or reduce the fever, no cold baths. The misconception that 2 to 6 degrees of fever destroys the tissues in the body is nonsense, and a fever of 104 is certainly not the burning process some would have us believe it to be.

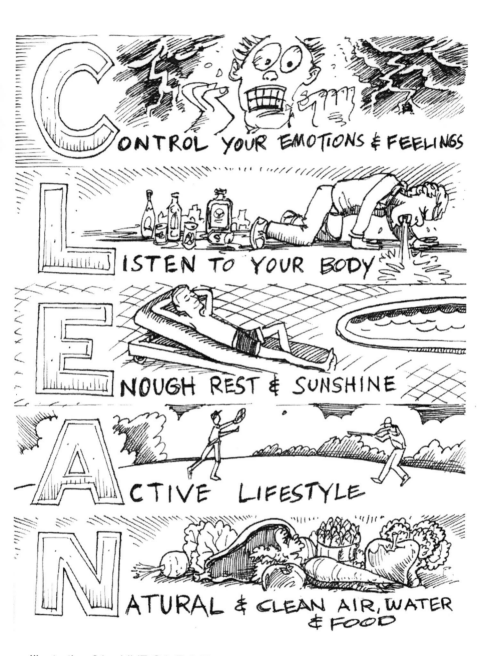

Illustration 31 – LIVE C.L.E.A.N

Even delirium and convulsions are just symptoms (RIGHT ACTIONS) and should NOT be suppressed. They never kill, however their causes may kill as well as their interventions. Collapse only occurs as a result of interventions so the treatment is simply removing those interventions.

Once the sick patient has recovered and feels better, rest and sleep are essential. The body has just emerged from a major fight and is weak from expending a lot of vital energy. The patient is in NO condition to return to normal activities until he or she is fully recuperated. Recuperation can be fast under the RIGHT CONDITIONS: C.L.E.A.N. (don't allow negative emotions, don't get excited, don't overstimulate your mind, gradually introduce light activities, eat clean and wholesome foods, drink pure water, breathe fresh air and get plenty of sunlight).

This works for any so-called acute disease...all the time! This is a very simple approach and it doesn't even seem possible that it would work. But if you read and understood this book, you now understand why it is possible; you can see it's the only logical way to treat the person with acute symptoms.

Chronic Disease

As with acute symptoms, all so called chronic disease must be cured by correcting the causes. Therefore all cure is self-cure. The physician is guided by only a limited number of subordinate facts, which, being isolated from their true connection, are untrustworthy. Only you (the sufferer) know all the facts and only your body tells you what's going on.

In order to overcome chronic so called diseases, the mind of the sufferer and the minds of his or her relatives and friends first need to be freed of the perverted views and erroneous theories of disease being fostered by the medical profession (this book may help). Even the very expression 'cure' as used today is misleading and wrong. We established clearly that all cure is self-cure and that cure cannot be established by outside therapies, skills, or medications. It is on the fallacy of curing disease that doctors are drugging the world to death.

The most difficult part for the chronic sufferer will be to overcome his or her own ignorance and prejudices (hopefully that has been successfully done by reading this book) and counteract the traditions and habits of society, the feelings and opinions of relatives and friends and the misguided opinions of the physicians. You must either get your loved-ones on your side and have them support you, or you must get a good club and empty the house. Often one's worst enemies are of his own household and his worst foes are his best friends.

Man is capable of possessing a higher degree of health and vitality than any other animal on the planet, yet he possesses far less. It's man alone that thinks he requires to be in shops for repairs and therefore supports doctors, nurses, hospitals, pharmacies etc. unlike any other animal (except those animals he has enslaved).

The effort to beat the laws of nature, to cheat cause out of its effect, by the use of remedies or medicines is so childishly absurd and so inherently impossible that man should long ago have realized his folly in persistently attempting such a thing.

The medical profession even admits they cannot cure chronic disease, and that's because they are chasing pathologies instead of studying the cause of all disease.

So what is chronic disease and how do we treat it?

If the body fails its acute reaction against any pathogen, it will accommodate itself to the condition and carry on the battle vigorously and over a longer period of time. This is what we call chronic disease. The failure of the body to overcome the acute crisis is usually due to the suppressive methods used by the physician.

The chronic sufferer, not aware of the cause of his so called disease, continues his WRONG HABITS. Toxemia increases and the body becomes weaker and weaker until death puts an end to the suffering.

Just remember that there are NO INCURABLE DISEASES, although there are incurable cases. By this I mean that all cases are curable if the causes are corrected in time BUT if progressed too far they may be incurable. Degeneration may reach a point where regeneration is impossible, often accelerated by medical intervention.

So if you are sincere in correcting your chronic so called disease and regain your health, take action and implement our Health 4 Life Action Plan. Make up your mind to abandon all your bad habits, bad food choices, stimulants, overstimulation and overindulgences once and for all... not one at the time, not by some ridiculous transition program but abruptly. Get it over with: go through the pain and the withdrawals, the discomfort and the depression. You will recover faster and with much more certainty.

Tapering off methods don't work. It's in vain to attempt gradual methods to abandon bad habits. So called stimulants such as coffee, alcohol, tobacco, weed, sugar etc. keep alive the craving for their use. Those who attempt to 'taper off' usually end up in failure and free themselves (by returning to their bad habits). The morbid desire for these sub-stances is kept alive by the least indulgence in them. There is simply no safety for the user until the morbid irritability of the nervous system has been overcome and normal sensibility is restored.

The approach is the same: LIVE C.L.E.A.N. But below you will find some more advice specifically for chronic sufferers.

REST: a chronic sufferer needs MORE rest and sleep. A prolonged period in bed (3 to 6 weeks) would speed up recovery in many cases. Remember that the mind should be at ease too! Go to bed early and sleep as long as you can. Insomnia is often caused by drugs (also sleeping drugs) and worry or other emotions. Never TRY to fall asleep, the trying in itself will keep you awake. You need to learn to repose the mind and relax before going to bed. This may take practice and time. Do not resort to sleep aids and if you are taking them, flush them now.

BE AWARE that you will experience some CRISES. Symptoms may appear to grow worse and your doctor and loved-ones will keep insist-ing that this is wrong, but be assured that it is not. Do not expect to move forward in a steady, uniform course without hurdles and crises. You may encounter worse symptoms and extreme fatigue, after all your body is correcting the disease and eliminating toxins. If you encounter an acute crisis, it's handled like all other acute crises. Welcome them and rejoice in the improved health that follows them.

In order to recover successfully and faster, keep the following recommendations in mind regarding your diet:

1. Improve your diet and eat less. Fasting is not necessary but a 3 to 10 day fast will speed up repair, elimination and recovery.

2. The diseased organ or part should be made the standard of the ability of the entire system. For example, if one has a diseased liver or lung but a vigorous stomach, then the quality and quantity of the food should be regulated NOT by the ability of the stomach but by the ability of the diseased organ (liver or lung in this case). Practically, it means to eat ONLY clean, natural, alkaline foods in the right combinations AND follow the back to basics rules (eat only when hungry, no breakfast etc.).

3. If doing a fast, I suggest preceding the fast with a few days of only fruits and vegetables to increase peristalsis and provide proper nutrients for cleansing. The fast itself will cause more or less distress and discomfort based on the eating habits prior to the fast (life-long eating habits).

4. Make sure you review the instructions in reference to breaking a fast (chapter 8).

What if permanent damage has been done?

In liver cirrhosis (hardening of the liver), kidney failure, deforming rheumatoid arthritis, cancer, overgrowth of connective tissue etc. only little can be done. The damage is too severe and degeneration has exceeded regeneration capabilities. Cure will depend on the amount of functioning tissue left in the affected organ or part of the body.

The degeneration has been going on for decades and the body has pre-served life for all that time, putting out countless fires and accommodating, encapsulating, storing, and purging as many toxins as it could. We ignored all the signs and kept feeding our body with toxins. For these people, repair is not likely to happen BUT QUALITY OF LIFE can be drastically improved by committing to the action plan in this book and living C.L.E.A.N. At least the disease process will be stopped at this point and there will be no further progression of the disease or damage to the cells and tissues. One can still live in a fair degree of health and comfort WHEN living C.L.E.A.N.

If enough vital tissue and cells are available in the diseased organ or part of the body, the body will use it powers to establish physiological compensation to correct the condition.

Let this be a lesson and a WARNING SIGN for the ones among us that feel well, look well, eat well and live an active lifestyle. The mere fact that you are not currently sick doesn't mean your mode of living is not harming you.

The REAL LESSON is that ALL so called diseases are PREVENTABLE and it's much better to restore and prevent than try to resolve.

FINAL NOTE:

One must recognize also that our Health 4 Life Action Plan works for every human being. The human constitution is ONE; there are no constitutional differences in the human race which would prevent adopting one general regimen. The Health 4 Life Action Plan is healthful to all.

Heredity and genetics require some attention also. Whether you have a good organism at birth depends partially upon heredity and partially upon the nutrition received from the mother. What that organism will become after birth and whether it will reach its highest potential or fall short of its inherent possibilities ONLY depends on HOW that organism LIVES.

It's all too common that people blame their sickness and ailments on their genetics... if the parents are obese it explains why the kids are obese and leaves the kids an excuse to be lazy and indulge on whatever. The truth is that both parents and kids LIVE WRONG and that's the cause of their sickness or obesity. Even if one would be predisposed at birth (genetics or poor nutrition from the mother), one can still work for the betterment of these things for the future and reach their full potential.

CHAPTER 18 – HEALTH 4 LIFE ACTION PLAN

Access to success is attitude, and regaining optimal health is accomplished by applying the knowledge you gained in this book and being proactive. Follow the Action Plan and stick with it, no matter what.

Without a plan to succeed and without setting firm goals, you actually plan to fail by default.

You are a creature of habits and without stepping out of your comfort zone, nothing will change. Only you can make changes to your life and relieve yourself from your own restrictions. But this takes courage, conviction, and some risk taking. It also takes perseverance to succeed and to overcome all obstacles on your way to success.

It's about being focused on the end-result and refraining yourself from complaining in order to prevail.

It's about doing NOW what others won't do so that you can have LATER what others never will have: health and happiness. It's an investment now to reap the benefits later. Don't worry about the past, don't worry about the future, but rather live in the present. Enjoy today, face today enthusiastically, and focus on the important things in life. We often get carried away with the small stuff in life and forget to work on our dreams. Your daily to-do list should contain activities to reach your life goals and dreams, not just day-to-day activities focused on putting out fires. Life is not a treasure hunt, life itself is the treasure.

Stephen R. Covey talks about the Time Management Matrix. This matrix divides your time in 4 quadrants in which you should organize and execute based on priorities. Quadrant 1 activities are urgent and important (crises, pressing problems, deadlines), quadrant 2 are activities that are not urgent but important (taking care of yourself, relationship building, recognizing new opportunities, planning, recreation), quadrant 3 are urgent but not important activities (some calls, some meetings, some pressing matters, popular activities, interruptions), and quadrant 4 are not urgent and not important activities (trivia, time wasters, pleasant activities, some work, some calls). We need to learn to limit quadrant 3 and 4 activities, and prevent (through planning) many quadrant 1 activities so we can allow significant time for the most important quadrant 2 activities. For a more detailed understanding, please study habit 3 – Put First Things First in Stephen R. Covey's bestseller 'The Seven Habits of Highly Effective People', or employ any time management tool that allows you to work and focus on your dreams and the important things in life.

Taking this road to optimal health alone is though. It would be wiser to take on this task with others: family and loved-ones, friends, or like-minded people. Find support with us and with others implementing this Health 4 Life Action Plan.

Once you are on the road to optimal health, you need to help others by guiding them, exciting them, fostering self-confidence in them, and energizing them. Show them the way, HELP them, GIVE to them freely, pay-it-forward. It's part of your own action plan anyway.

Step by Step Action Plan

The Health 4 Life Action Plan is also available for download or print on our website. Our Health 4 Life Interactive App allows you to keep track and stay the course in your quest for optimal health, all in a fun and motivating environment.

The plan below is set-up in a check-box format. Every time you successfully implement an ACTION, you may check off that box. This format allows you to change the order of actions you implement as to accommodate your individual needs. Remember that postponing the harder actions by skipping them will not be beneficial; it only puts more pressure on you at the end. If you can, just follow the plan step by step.

RESTORE

Let's get started. You must complete (1) goal setting, and (2) start NOW in this order. The following phases (3), (4), (5), (6) and (7) address all the recommendations to be implemented and achieve your ultimate goal: LIVING C.L.E.A.N. It's not necessary to complete one entire phase and then move to the next one. I suggest that when you start (3) CLEAN air, water and food, you start completing some sections of all other phases and work simultaneously on them until all your boxes are checked.

It's possible to complete the entire Health 4 Life Action Plan is 15-30 days. Of course, that doesn't mean you regained optimal health at that point... it means you have set up everything correctly and are making all the changes and modifications necessary to regain that optimal health.

Initial health benefits can be felt and observed within the first 10 days and will continue to show as you get through the plan and succeed the implementation of my 5 rules of C.L.E.A.N. living.

1. Goal Setting

☐ Write a short 2-5 page essay on WHAT really caught your attention reading this book. Explain what health and disease REALLY is and WHY it's easy to regain optimal health without the interference of current medical therapeutics. Finish with a brief statement on where you think your health is lacking and give yourself a health score (%) knowing that 100% is perfect health and 0% is dead.

☐ Write down THE MAIN 3 REASONS WHY you want to change your health. Explain and elaborate. Tape a copy on your bathroom mirror and read it every morning.

☐ Write down ALL previous attempts you may have made to

improve your health or lose weight. Write down WHY you think each of these attempts failed.

☐ Write down WHAT you will DO DIFFERENT to succeed this time.

☐ Write down your personal strengths and weaknesses in regards to (1) self-esteem, (2) self-confidence, (3) ability to change old habits.

☐ WHAT are the obstacles and FEARS you expect during this life changing journey? HOW are you going to overcome them?

☐ Are your fears stronger than your desire to succeed? Explain. If your fears are stronger, you won't succeed. How will you cultivate your desire? Are the main 3 reasons why you want to change your health fueling your desire to succeed?

☐ What (other) important but unpleasant tasks in life have you been postponing? Why?

☐ Are you currently doing what you like to do in life? Explain.

☐ WHAT do you really imagine for your future?

☐ Make a list of the people around you that are positive and supportive of you, and who may want to be interested in regaining optimal health also.

☐ Make a list of people that look up to you and whom you can empower (at home, at work, in your community).

☐ Use a time management technology (I personally use Stephen R. Covey's Time Management Matrix) and start using it. Make sure you establish enough time daily to work on this Health 4 Life Action Plan.

2. Start NOW

☐ Go back to (1) Goal Setting and FINISH the entire goal setting section. You MUST write it all down. You may continue to adjust and fine-tune your answers, but you need your initial draft finished TODAY. Tape a copy of the 3 MAIN REASONS WHY you WANT to change your health on your bathroom mirror... not tomorrow, but RIGHT NOW.

☐ Make a budget and start saving to purchase the following: commercial blender (I use Vitamix), water purification system, live plants (don't put them in your bedroom), pH-strips, supplements, books (unless you borrow them from the library), and maybe new cooking utensils. As you will start getting healthier and implement this action plan, you will start saving money on foods. So besides a small initial investment, you will be able to redirect your spending (the savings on food will allow you to purchase your supplements etc.).

☐ Visit our website at www.health4life.info and get familiar with the site. Become a member and enjoy the daily informational and motivational information and videos, attend the calls and webinars, and take advantage of our high-tech apps and interactive member forums. Get involved and share your experiences and your successes.

☐ Download (for free) your RECORD KEEPING forms online, and keep track daily.

☐ Purchase a binder to organize all your forms, lists and records. If you are computer savvy, save paper and keep track online.

☐ Effective immediately:

☐ No more milk (use coconut or almond milk if you wish).

☐ Drink water (you may use lemon or lime) and OMIT coffee, alcohol and sodas.

☐ Omit desserts.

3. CLEAN Air, Water & Food

There is no time limit on when to implement the recommendations listed below, however my suggested deadline for this phase (3) is 10-14 days. For each of the recommendations below, set yourself an implementation deadline within these 10-14 days. Get to work and JUST DO IT!

☐ Read Chapter 6 again and make a check-off list of ALL the things you must do to improve air quality. Keep adding to the list as you think of new or better ways (and share them with us online). Implement at least 3 items on the list immediately (e.g. open windows and have air circulating in the house or office, turn off the A/C, eat or sit outside, replace the air filters, remove toxic household products etc.).

☐ Take 20 minutes (with your family and/or friends if you can) and practice diaphragmatic breathing. Incorporate this breathing protocol 3 times daily and whenever fatigued.

☐ Purchase a water purification system ASAP.

☐ Make a list of all the things you must do to improve the quality of your water. Keep adding to the list as you think of new or better ways (and share them with us online). Implement at least 3 items on the list immediately (e.g. alkalize drinking water, install purification system, limit the use of soaps and shampoo etc.).

☐ Make a list of all the things you must do to conserve water. Keep adding to the list as you think of new or better ways (and share them with us online). Implement at least 3 items on the list immediately (e.g. close tap while brushing teeth, limit your shower time, re-use water for plants, etc.).

☐ Read chapter 5 again, feeding versus feasting. Make a list (and add to it during the next few days) indicating WHAT situations or emotions trigger your appetite and WHEN they occur.

☐ Read chapter 12 again, behavior modification. Make a list (and add to it during the next few days) indicating your 'bad' habits AND the strategy you will employ to convert those 'bad' habits into good ones. Implement the items from your previous list (appetite triggers).

☐ Make a EATING schedule on paper based on the 'BACK TO BASICS' section of chapter 5.

☐ Review the 'ALKALINE MODEL' section of chapter 5 and follow the implementation instructions (including measuring your pH, shopping for alkaline forming foods, avoiding acid forming foods etc.). Download and print the ALKALINE – ACID FORMING FOODS LIST from our website (for free).

☐ Now review the 'FOOD COMBINING' section of chapter 5, and download and print the food combining chart from our website (for free). Use magnets to post both the food combining charts and alkaline – acid forming foods list on your refrigerator.

☐ Review the 'ORGANIC FOODS' and 'CLEAN FOODS' section of chapter 5, and replace some cooking utensils if indicated.

☐ Using the alkaline – acid forming foods list and the food combining chart, put together your meals for next week. Ideally you only need 1 main meal per day. Breakfast and lunch can be omitted, or replaced with a simple piece of fruit, salad, homemade veggie juice or pea protein shake.

☐ Organize your meals in advance and make a weekly shopping list (I usually shop during the weekend for the entire week, but I run into the store for fresh fruits and veggies more often, or visit the farmers market).

☐ Review chapter 13, the truth about supplements, and purchase your essentials. I personally take the Vemma and Pure Omega 3, but you may purchase other high quality products of course. Just be aware that the majority of supplements don't work and harm your health.

☐ If you want to get a head start and are determined to boost your health, I recommend to ONLY juice during these 10-14 days while getting organized and making your lists. Load up on all kinds of vegetables (the more variety the better, and buy some you never bought before) and fruits (80% veggies and 20% fruits is a good guideline). Just juice them and drink them. There is no limit as to how much, so you don't need to feel hungry. Take your supplements with the juice. The first 3-5 days will be very hard (you will crave food), but after the first week things will get easier as you start feeling the initial health benefits.

☐ Continue to update and modify your lists, and continue to educate yourself on CLEAN AIR, WATER and FOODS.

☐ Keep track of new, healthy, clean foods you implement in your regimen, and record the unhealthy, man-made foods and drinks you successfully omit (dairy, coffee, soda, alcohol, meat, pastries, hydrogenated oils, salt, condiments, refined sugar, enriched flours, fermented products etc.).

4. Enough Rest, Sleep & Sunshine

☐ Read chapter 8. For 3 – 5 days, record sleeping and rest habits (time of day, length, quality, reasons for disturbed or incomplete sleep).

☐ Write a 1 page essay on whether or not you think you get

enough rest and sleep, and explain WHY. HOW can you make practical changes to assure enough rest and sleep if needed?

☐ Make a list of the improvements you can make to assure a better QUALITY of sleep (eg. time when you go to bed, activities prior to going to bed, overstimulation such as noise and light, emotions such as worrying etc.).

☐ Copy or download my 30 day DETOXIFICATION program and review it. Take out a calendar and set a date within the next 90 days in which you will START this program. The earlier you fast and detox, the better. Schedule accordingly and keep in mind that some phases of this program may have to be during a weekend based on your working schedule etc. Also make sure you purchase the necessary foods and supplements prior.

☐ Review chapter 7 and make a complete list of practical things you can do to get more exposure to sunlight (not heat). These may include: lighter or limited clothing as much as possible (especially inside the house and your back-yard), T-shirts versus long sleeved shirts and shorts versus pants, schedule more outdoor activities (and limit clothing), going outdoors for lunch or dinner, open doors and windows and allow sunlight to enter, open the sunroof, remove sunglasses and hats, etc.

5. Active Lifestyle

☐ Review chapter 10 and write a short essay on your current lifestyle in reference to exercise and activity. Remember that it's not necessary to engage in sports or organized exercise classes in order to achieve an optimal activity level.

☐ Write down a list of activities you would love to do and/or learn. You can think about activities you can do by yourself, or activities you can do with your family and/or friends.

Outdoor activities would be the best choice of course (air and sunlight). Implement 2 new activities within the next 2 weeks. Activities could be as simple as taking a walk during lunch (since you may opt not to have lunch anymore or consume a light salad only... after that walk), riding the bike to work or to the store, playing ball with the kids or the dog, joining your first yoga class (you should encourage your yoga instructor to offer outdoor classes), learning a new dance, taking the family on a hike or nature trail, or planning a canoe trip etc.

6. Listen to your Body

Listening to our body requires a conscious effort for most of us. We need to start learning to do it. Our biological clock is most likely messed up as well as our sense of hunger and thirst.

☐ During the next entire week, record all the things your body is telling you and record what your USUAL response would be and what your ACTUAL response should be.

Some examples:

☐ My stomach feels full but I'm going to eat that delicious dessert anyway.

☐ My friend offers me a drink while I'm not really thirsty.

☐ There are donuts in the lunch room at work so I may as well eat one.

☐ I'm tired but I want to watch the end of this football game.

☐ I'm exhausted but I'm going to the gym anyway because I need to lose weight.

☐ I eat breakfast because my doctor says it's the most important meal of the day.

- My boss stresses me out and I'm in fear of getting fired all the time.

- Every time I worry about something, I get diarrhea and feel dizzy.

- I feel lonely and eat for comfort.

- I have back pain but I need to clean my house regardless.

- I have a headache so I'll lie down in the couch and watch a movie.

- I'm constipated and I'm going to eat a pulled pork (acidic meat) sandwich (white bread or enriched flour).

- I'm tired so I'll drink a red bull or coffee (both depressants).

- I'm running a fever so I'll take some ibuprofen or Tylenol.

- I'm sick so I'll take some medicine and eat to stay strong.

- Etc.

 Review Chapter 5 and write down WHAT we should drink, WHEN we should drink, and HOW MUCH we should drink. Do you currently exhibit signs of dehydration? Explain. What are you going to do about it?

 Make a list of all the things and/or items that may cause overstimulation in your life (eg. electronics, phones, TV, radio, computer, games, noise, sound, light, emotions etc.). Be specific and write down HOW you can limit or eliminate each one of them? Take action!

 Make a list of all overindulgences you are guilty of in your life (eg. excess food, drinks, partying, sex, masturbation, exercise, work, drugs, medicine etc.). Be specific and write down HOW you can practically limit or eliminate them. Take action!

7. Control your Emotions

☐ Read chapter 9 again.

☐ Make a list of all the things that stress you out. Write down HOW you are going to eliminate these stressors.

☐ Start your 'JOE' (Journal of Emotions) and go through the 5 steps to complete your list.

☐ Take ownership of your emotions and write down in your JOE in what situations you blame others for your emotions.

☐ Write down at least 4 options you have to CONTROL your emotions. Now choose one option for each emotion or feeling you have listed in your JOE.

☐ Each day, pick one emotion and consciously control that emotion the next time it pops up. Record your failures and successes. Practice all emotions until you can control all situations.

☐ Write a 1-2 page essay. Are you a reactive or proactive person? List at least 5 things you can do to become a more proactive person.

☐ Write a 1-2 page essay. Describe what a self-fulfilled prophecy is. Are you optimistic or pessimistic? Do you have a positive 'YES' attitude or a negative (I complain a lot) attitude? List at least 5 actions you can implement to change your attitude.

☐ List all false core beliefs you may have. Write down WHY each one of them is false. Work on eliminating these false core beliefs through rationalization.

☐ List all thoughts and ideas that stimulate negative emotions in your life. How will you control or overcome them?

☐ Make a list of things you can DO to HELP others. Make sure you do something on this list on a daily basis.

☐ Read a motivational book and listen to motivational audio regularly (minimum once a month). This can be Anthony Robbins, Steven R. Covey, Napoleon Hill, Jeffrey Gitomer, and hundreds of other inspiring men and women.

☐ Consider relaxation, meditation, yoga, tai chi, or any other form of activity that may reduce your stress, help control your emotions, and repose the mind.

☐ Consider BHRT if you suspect hormonal imbalances.

RESOLVE

This second phase of my R3 Wellness model should only be initiated after ALL recommendations of the RESTORE phase are successfully implemented.

Based on your current medical so called diseases and symptoms, you should facilitate the resolution of these.

☐ Look up what foods and nutrients can help with your symptoms and so-called diseases. Record them. Now look up which whole foods contain these nutrients and add them to your diet in abundance. Supplements may be beneficial but be aware that most of them simply don't work.

REJUVENATE

This third phase of my R3 wellness model is meant to build-up the vital energy reserves and 'sharpen the saw' (habit 7 in Stephen R. Covey's book). Sharpen the saw means that we continue to assess and evaluate our C.L.E.A.N. living efforts and continue to improve upon them.

- ☐ Continue to implement regular fasting and detoxification.

- ☐ Read the book again and mark the sections, items, or rec-ommendations you are not implementing fully yet or at all. Make a plan on HOW to implement them successfully.

- ☐ Make a list of the recommendations in the action plan that you have difficulty with. WHY do you think this particular part is difficult for you to implement? WHAT can you do differently to assure successful implementation?

- ☐ Continue to check new information and new recommen-dations on our website. Which recommendations could benefit you? HOW and WHEN will you implement them?

- ☐ Become a certified HEALTH 4 LIFE Consultant (no prior education required) and show others the ONLY path to optimal health.

- ☐ Consider becoming a HEALTH FREEDOM INSTRUCTOR (contact us for more information).

END NOTE

We must view life as a struggle between self-control and self-indulgence. We must realize that self-control leads to strength, health and happiness and that self-indulgence leads to sickness and misery.

There is absolutely NO NEED for any action or habit that impairs life and produces weakness and so called disease. But people are enslaved by their habits and focused on the pleasures of the moment. People lack self-control and are unable to free themselves. SELF-CONTROL is our greatest need and SELF-DISCIPLINE is our only saving force.

I hear it over and over again: "I would rather live as I do now and only live to be 70 years than live as you have outlined in your action plan and live a 100 years". Don't you see that this is the despairing cry of a SLAVE? These people (yes, this may be you too) are hopelessly enslaved by their bad habits and thoroughly perverted in both mind and body. Their mind and body are dominated by their habits and they are most likely beyond redemption. They will declare that they derive more satisfaction from their cigarette or cigar, or drink, or fast food than from anything else in life.

Their cry is "We live but once, let us enjoy life while we are here". I do believe also in enjoying life... REAL LIFE though! I mean life in the highest and fullest sense, not life in the gutter as these slaves are referring to. They should rephrase their cry: "We live but once, let us make it short and fun".

These slaves desire to be saved IN THEIR SINS, not FROM them.

The 'satisfaction' they derive from their overindulgences and stimulants (read: depressants) is poor satisfaction compared to the higher joys of real health based on wholesome living.

TAKE ACTION NOW AND CHOOSE HEALTH FREEDOM
YOU WILL ABSOLUTELY LOVE THE BENEFITS

TO LEARN AND NOT TO DO IS REALLY NOT TO LEARN

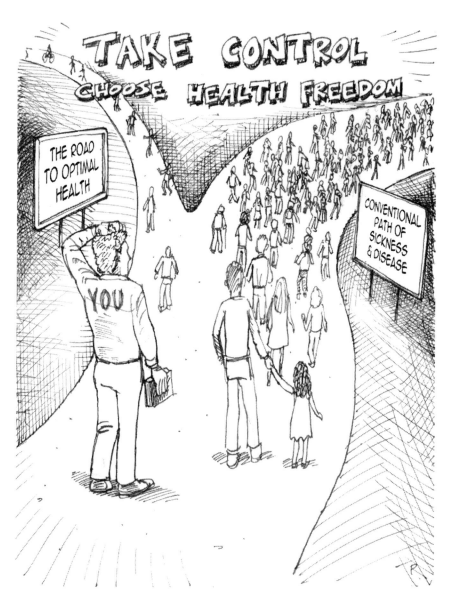

Illustration 32 – Choose Health Freedom

REFERENCES

My references: everyone and everything that entered my senses since the day I was born.

Short explanation:

Frankly, I don't know or recall all my references. I have just been typing away and used some info and insight from books, articles, online texts etc. The main references are listed in my book. I give credit to the people and books that personally influenced me and prompted me to write this book.

In my modest opinion, references are unnecessary. If I reference a book, then you would have to look at the references of that book, and yet look again at the references of that one and so on. Bottom line is that we all are born with zero knowledge and that today our knowledge is a result from our environment, the input of our parents and other people, teachers, instructors, books, articles, media, TV, radio, online articles etc. Who are we to claim copyright? I don't. Copy away and share this information with as many people as you want.

If I used some of your information and I didn't mention you in my book or references, or you think it's YOUR information, which it can't be since your knowledge at birth was also zero and the words you use are already in the dictionary, I'll thank you sincerely for your contribution. You helped establishing this work which may help thousands of people around the globe regain control of their health.

Yours in Optimal Health,
Dr. Mike.

TABLE OF ILLUSTRATIONS

Illustration concepts and ideas by Dr. Mike Van Thielen

Illustrations created by Artist PEREGO.

CPSIA information can be obtained at www.ICGtesting.com
Printed in the USA
LVOW07s0421030914

402069LV00004B/6/P